Y0-COU-830

RESEARCH IN HUMAN CAPITAL AND DEVELOPMENT

Volume 7 • 1993

HEALTH CARE IN THE CHANGING ECONOMIC AND SOCIAL ENVIRONMENT

RESEARCH IN HUMAN CAPITAL AND DEVELOPMENT

HEALTH CARE IN THE CHANGING ECONOMIC AND SOCIAL ENVIRONMENT

Series Editor: ALAN SORKIN
Department of Economics
University of Maryland

Volume Editors: P.C. HUANG
Department of Biochemistry
Johns Hopkins University School of Hygiene and Public Health

RUEY S. LIN
College of Medicine
National Taiwan University

L.P. CHOW
Department of Population Dynamics
Johns Hopkins University School of Hygiene and Public Health

VOLUME 7 • 1993

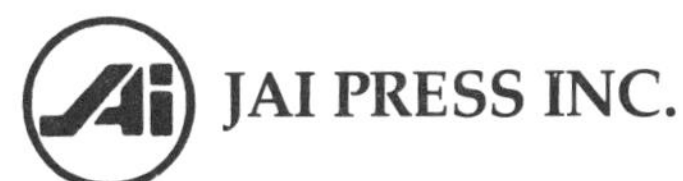

Greenwich, Connecticut *London, England*

55 Old Post Road, No. 2
Greenwich, Connecticut 06836

JAI PRESS LTD.
The Courtyard
28 High Street
Hampton Hill, Middlesex TW12 1PD
England

ISBN: 1-55938-132-9

Manufactured in the United States of America

CONTENTS

PART IV. THE ECONOMICS OF HEALTH CARE

LIST OF CONTRIBUTORS

Gerald F. Anderson	Johns Hopkins University School of Hygeine and Public Health
M. Harvey Brenner	Johns Hopkins University School of Hygeine and Public Health
Ming-Cheng Chang	Taiwan Provincial Institute of Family Planning Taichung, Taiwan
Po-Ya Chung	Bureau of Health Taipei, Taiwan
Ted Chen	Tulane University Medical Center New Orleans, Louisianna
Ching-Yeh Chiang	Taiwan Provincial Institute of Family Planning Taichung, Taiwan
Bernard Choi	Faculty of Medicine University of Toronto
L.P. Chow	Department of Population Dynamics Johns Hopkins University School of Hygeine and Public Health
Jacqueline K. Corn	Department of Environmental Sciences Johns Hopkins University School of Hygeine and Public Health
Morton Corn	Department of Environmental Sciences Johns Hopkins University School of Hygeine and Public Health

Karen Davis — Johns Hopkins University
School of Hygeine and Public Health

Lorraine Davis — Department of School and Community Health
University of Oregon

Jan Garrard — Health Department
Victoria, Australia

Ryumon Honda — Department of Hygiene
Kanazawa Medical University

P.C. Huang — Department of Biochemistry
Johns Hopkins University
School of Hygeine and Public Health

Kao-Chia Hsieh — Department of Sociology
National Chengchi University
Mucha, Taipei, Taiwan

Eriko Ikai — Department of Hygiene
Kanazawa Medical University

Masao Ishizaka — Department of Hygiene
Kanazawa Medical University

Teruhiko Kido — Department of Hygiene
Kanazawa Medical University

Ching-Mei Lee — Department of Health Education
National Taiwan Normal University

Phillip Lee — Institute of Health Policy Studies
University of California
San Francisco

Jersey Liang — School of Public Health and Institute of Gerontology
University of Michigan

Hui-sheng Lin — Taiwan Provincial Institute of Family Planning
Taichung, Taiwan

Ruey S. Lin	Institute of Public Health College of Medicine National Taiwan University
Tracey McDonald	Department of Nursing The University of Wollongong
Gilbert S. Omenn	School of Hygiene and Community Medicine University of Washington
Michael Rabinowitz	Harvard Medical School and Marine Biological Laboratory
Monica Slattery	Monash University Victoria, Australia
Alan Sorkin	Department of Economics University of Maryland
Wei-Tsuen Soong	College of Medicine National Taiwan University
Ikiko Tsuritani	Department of Hygiene Kanazawa Medical University
Gilles P. Theriault	School of Occupational Health McGill University
Jung-der Wang	School of Public Health National Taiwan University
Kenneth E. Warner	University of Michigan School of Public Health
Alvin Winder	School of Public Health University of Massachusetts
Shwu-chong Wu	College of Medicine National Taiwan University
Yuichi Yamada	Department of Hygiene Kanazawa Medical University
Seung-Hum Yu	Yonsei University College of Medicine

ACKNOWLEDGMENT

From 1978 until 1991, Dr. Ismail Sirageldin was the Series Editor for *Research in Human Capital and Development*. Under his expert guidance, six volumes appeared focusing on a wide variety of substantive themes including health and development, population and development, the economics of education, economic and social aspects of migration, and the labor force participation of women in developing societies. One supplementary volume, focusing on Manpower Planning in the Oil Countries of the Mideast, is still a highly relevant work for this vitally important region of the world.

While several of the papers provided a synthesis of the appropriate literature, the bulk of contributions represented original work. Many of the papers provided important advances of a methodological and empirical nature.

Dr. Sirageldin did an outstanding job as series editor. His high standards regarding the quality of the chapters prevented the uneven level of papers that are so common in volumes composed of contributed works. His incisive comments helped numerous authors to greatly improve on earlier drafts. In addition, the volumes prepared under his editorship always had an appropriate blend of contributions from new Ph.D.s and senior scholars.

It was my pleasure to assist Dr. Sirageldin with several of the previous volumes. I hope that the experiences obtained from working with him will help me in my new role as series editor.

Alan Sorkin
Series Editor

PREFACE

Strategies for the delivery of health care to the public differ around the world, with each nation's approach reflecting its unique economic and political setting. Yet all communities share the same goal and expectations in health care, that is to sustain and prolong life with dignity—adding life to years. Indeed, for the past millennium a prolonged life expectancy has been regarded as the ultimate aim of living in many a civilized society. The outcome of it is a steady increase in the age of survivorship over the past decades since the dawn of modern clinical and preventive medicine.

The increase in longevity is attributable to a substantially reduced infant mortality, a drop in death rate in the middle age and healthier old age. Meanwhile, better care during pregnancy, more precise prenatal diagnosis and counseling, and universally effective vaccination have helped the decline in the rate of death among newborns and children. More pertinent medical advice and intervention through surgical, therapeutic and pharmacological procedures make many forms of diseases, whether hereditary or infectious, amendable to prevention and cure. Better nutrition and exercises have also brought about better overall fitness, hence a longer life span in the more priviledged, developed countries

While the general health of the populace is continuously being maintained and in some case improved, health care reform is perhaps the most prominent social-political issue today in both developed as well as developing countries. What exacerbates the problem is the spiraling increase in costs, as a result of a combination of factors. Continued rise in malpractice premium, litigation awards, and fraudulent claims have elevated the demand for medical payments. Shifts in the composition of the population, such as in age or in socioeconomic status, have increased the societal burden for health care. New technologies are often costly at their initial stage of application, albeit more sensitive and accurate then the conventional methods in diagnosis or treatment. The cost for health care has reached such a point that many find it unaffordable. The United States, for all its richness, is currently being besieged by a large number of uninsured (about 38 million), in spite of various cost containment programs, numerous health plans, and a diversity of tax credit proposals that were designed to deal with this warning of calamity. The question is thus not whether but how to reform and to implement.

The state of health in many countries are being further challenged by an ever-increasing burden of environmental and/or occupational stresses, and subsequently an expected increase in demand for a broader provision of services beyond the care of debilitating diseases. An agenda to relate current medical practice through emerging new technologies to ensure appropriate, cost effective and quality health would seem to be urgently needed. It would also be appropriate to have the focus on health shifted from the intervention of illness by traditional medicine to maintain wellness with preventive measures. Instead of dealing with health crisis when it has occurred, it may be more sensible to fashion the pattern of life style which underlie and undermine our health.

We find it timely to have some of these health care issues addressed in a collected volume, so that health professionals, physicians, insurers, legislators, economists, biomedical scientist, and the public alike can examine the problems and evaluate approaches that exist or are applicable.

This volume thus consists of four interrelated parts. Part I addresses the impact of socio-demographic changes in our living environment on the perception of its populace, which in turn affects the health care of individuals. Taiwan is given as a prime example in which culture, tradition, family, economic security, and societal attitude interplay, and the sense of value and purposefulness of life very much dominates one's state of mental health. These parameters will determine to a large extent whether a comprehensive health care plan to be carried out in two years can be effectively executed in a society which traverses a successful economic transition from developing to being recognized as developed (Chang, pp. 3-27). As one consequence of economic development is intensive industrialization which brings about a shortage of endogenous labor and influx of migrant workers, the ability of migrants to adapt to a new environment is an interesting factor which can well determine whether his or her health would be jeopardized (Hsieh, pp. 29-51). Demographic changes in the composition of population, whether caused by migration, birth and death, can therefore dramatically alter the nature of health care needs and the means necessary to deal with it. In this regard, we consider it relevant to include papers on the problems of shifts in the proportion of the aged among populations. Lifestyle of the elderly can change abruptly upon retirement or when incapacitated by sickness, hence worsening the aging process (Liang, Wu, & Chiang, pp. 53-68; Chang & Lin, pp. 69-91). The problem of long term care of the elderly is often unique (McDonald).

The significance of life style on health is addressed in Part II of this volume. Evidence is presented to show that social attitude affects the propensity of substance abuse, as in smoking (Lee & Davis, pp. 115-134). The positive effect of an anti-smoking campaign (Warner, pp. 135-148), and the measurements of its cost versus benefit are analyzed (Choi, pp. 135-148). While the space limitation of this volume does not permit a more comprehensive coverage of addiction and diseases such as AIDS due to societal attitude and lifestyle, we have included a paper on the ill effect of alcohol on hypertension by Ishizaki, Yamada, Kido, Honda, Tsuritani & Ikai (pp. 177-187) and a case history from Australia on the issue of drug abuse by Slattery & Garrard (pp. 189-207). In these cases, potential use of a pedagogical approach is evident.

We included one paper on efforts through education to improve mental health as measured by behavior changes responsive to stress by Chen & Winder (pp. 209-221). Such an approach echoes the finding that drug use in the USA has experienced a continuous decline in the past five years among the teenagers. The decline is explained by the speculation that these youths have grown up watching anti-drug messages in the media, in their classrooms and in their homes, and are therefore better informed. If this can be substantiated, the strategy of using media to inform would be one way for effectively combating a health problem at its very root.

The general topic of health and changing environment is addressed in Part III. We call to question whether the rapid deterioration of the environment we live in, in developing as well as developed countries, poses threats to our health, and what has transpired with the experience so gained in attempting to cleanse the sources of pollution or hazards in the work place. It is clear that our work environment is being bombarded with insults heretofore unknown until the discovery of laser, microwave, computer chips, heavy metal alloys, automobiles, noise, not to mention repetitive motion and competitive enterprising, and so forth, within this past century. Do these conditions cause stress? Would stress lead to substance, such as alcohol abuse and deterioration of mental and general health as discussed in Part II?

As we become aware of our surroundings, we realize that factories and offices are not the only places which present themselves as stressful environments to health. Homes and classrooms have also been shown to be contaminated, innocently or inadvertently, by undesirable compounds such as the unwanted radon and excess carbon monoxides. At home the effect of damage is often endemic and delayed in its onset with age, women are particularly vulnerable.

Its impact may be antecedent to the understanding of environmental effect on the health of infants and the young. In schools, the presence of lead, from old paints, is a case in point (Rabinowitz, Wang, & Soong, pp. 253-272) for which the United States is to embark on a one billion dollar multi-agency clean up program to eliminate this health nuisance.

In view of the fact that epidemiological method is one of the most powerful tools in deducing disease etiology, we call attention to a special paper on its application (Theriault, pp. 239-251). We would like to recognize new avenues which may be useful in tackling our environmental problems (Omenn, pp. 273-283).

The last part of this volume, Part IV, is devoted to the economics of health care. Whereupon individuals may opt for the extent of care to be provided based on available resources, a close examination of the expenditure at the national level rings serious alarm. The cost of health care is growing at an unsustainable rate in many countries. The United States alone spent 666.2 billion dollars on health care in 1990, a 10.5 percent over the 1989 level, more than twice the 5.1 percent growth rate of the gross national product. This is the third consecutive year that health spending increased at double digit rates, yet about 4 percent of the population remain without health insurance. By comparison Canada spends 39 percent less, and Germany and Japan spend half per capita on health care than United States but every one is covered with high quality health care. Why? Is the U.S. system worthy of the cost? What can be done to make it more economical and quintessential?

In this volume, we contrast the evolving practices in a well developed country, United States (Davis, pp. 287-306; Sorkin, pp. 307-327), and one that is being planned for in Korea, a newly developed country (Yu, pp. 359-368), which like Taiwan (Chang, Part I, pp. 3-27) is being chosen for her miraculous success in economic development. Special consideration for physician's compensation (Lee, pp. 329-345), and technology assessment (Anderson, pp. 347-357) are also included.

While the care of health is an economic issue, economic development of a society affects health. We conclude with a thesis that stable economic growth is the fundamental source of improvement in health and longevity (Brenner, pp. 369-391).

Clearly, the intricate permutations for choice between various socioeconomic paradigms, whether a classical market place theory, a new managed care practice, tax credit incentives, or the time honored public financing initiatives, would have to be weighed against social, economic, legal/political and technical determinants in the much heated debuts in the months to come. As change in health care strategy is the only certainty in our predicament, past experience and future innovations can coexist. With this conviction, we dedicate this volume to the cause of public health, which must transcend national boundaries, with faith and anticipation.

We thank Profesor Alan Sorkin, editor of *Research in Human Capital and Development* for suggesting the publication of this volume, and to the authors for their valuable contributions. The basic doctrine and findings expounded in several papers were presented earlier in a symposium on "Health, Environment and Social Change; Emerging Health Problems in Rapid Socioeconomic Development" held in Taipei, July 2-5, 1990, and are revised for this volume.

P.C. Huang
Ruey S. Lin
L.P. Chow
Volume Editors

PART I

SOCIO-DEMOGRAPHIC CHANGES AND HEALTH

SOCIAL AND ECONOMIC DEVELOPMENT IN TAIWAN:
HEALTH POLICY IMPLICATIONS

Po-Ya Chang

I. INTRODUCTION

The Republic of China on Taiwan (hereafter referred to as Taiwan) has achieved an economic miracle. The economic success and prosperity have induced profound social and environmental changes. Consequently various health, environmental and social problems have emerged or are emerging. The "demographic and epidemiologic transitions" have altered the disease pattern and, therefore, the health needs of the people. In spite of the impressive economic success, parallel improvement in the quality of life of people has not occurred; contrarily, there have been signs indicating deterioration of social and physical environment.

In line with the theme of this volume "Health Care in the Changing Economic and Social Environment," it should be of interest to examine the interactions among socio-economic development, environmental changes and the health of people, and to review the health policy implications of these changes. The

Research in Human Capital and Development, Volume 7, pages 3-27.

ISBN: 1-55938-132-9

experience of Taiwan should provide valuable lessons for other countries in the region and the world, which have been actively following the path of Taiwan in pursuing economic development.

II. ECONOMIC DEVELOPMENT AND SOCIAL AND ENVIRONMENTAL CHANGES IN TAIWAN

The achievement of Taiwan in economic development during the past four decades is frequently cited as a success story of the developing world. Taiwan's per capita GNP which was no more than $100 in 1952, increased to nearly $8,000 in 1990: a 80-fold increase within less than four decades.

Taiwan's economic growth has been achieved largely through industrialization and international trade. For example, agriculture, which used to be the staple industry in Taiwan, has now been replaced by manufacturing. The contribution of the agricultural sector to the total domestic products declined from 35.9 percent in 1952 to 7.6 percent in 1984 and 4.3 percent in 1990. Contrarily, the contribution from manufacturing and other secondary industries increased from 18.0 percent in 1952 to 39.2 percent in 1984 and 43.2 percent in 1990 (Council for Economic Planning and Development, 1990). Tables 1 and 2 show some of the indicators of economic and social development in Taiwan.

Industrialization, and its inevitable consequence of population urbanization, has caused significant changes in the natural and working environment of the people. In spite of efforts made by the government to prevent environmental deterioration, only limited progress has been made. The quality of air and water surrounding larger cities in Taiwan in fact has deteriorated (Council for Economic Planning and Development, 1990).

III. DEMOGRAPHIC CHANGES

The demographic changes that have occurred in Taiwan, caused partly by the deliberate policy to reduce fertility and partly by the natural consequences of modernization and development, will continue to occur in the future and will have the most profound impact on the health of the population, and therefore on the health policy of Taiwan for the next century and beyond.

The total population in Taiwan was approximately 6 million in 1941, doubling to 12 million in 1964 when the island-wide family planning program was started. In 1990 the total population in Taiwan was 20 million, with a density of 1,429 persons per square mile of land area. It is projected to increase to 24 million in year 2030 according to a medium fertility assumption (Council for Economic Planning and Development, 1988).

Table 1. Economic Development in Taiwan Area, ROC (1986 value)

Year	Mid-Year Population		Per Capita GNP		Per Capita Income		Per Capita Expenditure		Consumer Price Index (1986=100)	Growth rate %
	1000	Index (1952=100)	NT$	Index (1952=100)	NT$	Index (1952=100)	NT$	Index (1952=100)		
1956	9,234	15.5	22,537	18.8	21,623	17.8	14,842	11.9	—	5.50
1966	13,021	59.9	37,412	97.2	35,466	93.2	22,767	71.7	25.1	8.97
1976	16,329	103.1	77,406	307.9	71,572	289.9	41,909	216.2	55.4	13.70
1986	19,357	139.4	151,148	696.1	137,992	651.8	70,593	432.5	100.0	12.57
1987	19,564	142.0	167,301	781.7	154,838	743.6	77,702	486.2	100.5	11.87
1988	19,788	144.4	178,376	840.1	164,229	794.8	86,883	555.4	101.8	7.84
1989	20,006	147.4	189,367	898.0	174,407	850.2	97,053	632.1	106.3	7.33
1990	20,233	150.5	197,404	940.4	181,319	885.9	104,443	687.9	110.7	5.24

Notes: Real number of the year/real number of base year (1952) 100 — 100.
Exchange rate in 1990: One US $ = 27 New Taiwan Dollars (NT$)

Source: National Income of Taiwan, ROC, Directorate-General of Budget, Accounting and Statistics E.T. (Figures for 1990 are estimates).

Table 2. Indicators of Social Development

Year	*TV sets per 1000 population*	*Number of Newspaper magazines per 1000 population*	*Percentage of Households having airconditioners*	*Automobile per 1000 population*	*Correspondance posted per capita/year*	*Telephone per 1000 population*
1975	169.1	89	6.5	82.3	49.5	4.84
1984	222.4	178.4	60.2	208.0	64.5	20.89
1990	275.2	201.2	158.9	283.1	84.0	30.87

Source: Council for Economic Planning and Development, Republic of China, 1991.

The crude birth rate declined from the peak of 50 in 1951 to 17.6 in 1990. The crude death rate also declined sharply from 18.2 in 1951 to 5.1 in 1990. The total fertility rate in 1990 was 1.7, having declined from 5.1 in 1964 when family planning program was started.

Because of this sharp decline in fertility, Taiwan's population has been rapidly aging and will accelerate its aging process in the future. As shown in Table 3, the proportion of population under 15 years of age had declined from 45.5 percent of the total in 1964 to 27.2 in 1990 and is projected to decline further to 14.6 percent in 2030. Contrarily, the proportion of people 65 years old and older increased from 2.5 percent in 1964 to 6.1 percent in 1990 and will increase to 19.8 percent in 2030 (Council for Economic Planning and Development, 1988). After 40 years, one in every five persons in Taiwan will be "elderly"—65 years old or older. Since older people consume a disproportionate amount of medical care resources, the impact of aging population on the nations' health policy and medical care system is obvious.

Low or negative population growth and sharp rise in old age dependency in the future have created considerable concern about the long-term economic outlook among some political and social leaders. However, a recent article by Easterlin, a well-known economic demographer, indicated that there is little empirical evidence that declining population growth has slowed the rate of economic growth. Increased old age dependency will be more than offset by reduced needs to support younger dependents (Easterlin, 1991).

Urbanization of population, increasing movement of people within and outside of Taiwan, breaking down of traditional extended family structure and increasing proportion of nuclear families, changing social institution of marriage and social mores regarding sexual behaviors, as well as changing characteristics of the population such as education, employment and sex ratios, will have substantial and sustained impacts on the health of people, therefore greatly impacting on the future health policy.

The demographic transition, however, also has its bright side. As can be seen from Table 3, the dependency ratios of Taiwan's population decreased

Table 3. Age Composition of Population in Taiwan by Broad Age Groups: 1964-2030

Year	*Total population Million*	*Proportion of population* 0-14	15-64	65+	*Dependency Ratio*
1964	12.28	45.5	52.0	2.5	92.3
1988	19.79	28.2	66.2	5.6	51.1
1990	20.25	27.2	66.7	6.1	49.9
2030*	24.02	14.6	65.6	19.8	52.4

Note: * Projections of the Population of the Taiwan Area, Republic of China, 1988-2030, Council for Economic Planning and Development, Executive Yuan, Taiwan, R.O.C. (medium assumption)

from 92.3 in 1964 to 51.1 in 1988 and 49.4 in 1990. The ratio is expected to increase only slightly to 52.4 in 2030. Taiwan will continue to enjoy relatively low dependency burden for the next 30-40 years, during which period efforts can be made to improve the quality of the life of people.

Technological changes, improvement in medical technology in particular, have largely been a blessing, keeping some people alive who otherwise would not have survived; however, it has also has had its negative side. Aside from increasing iatrogenic risk, modern medical technology complicates the already complicated health care system. Most modern technologies are expensive, adding to the already strained medical care cost and, at times, with only marginal or no appreciable benefit.

Social and economic development has caused political changes and reform —democratization of the political system. People of diverse and frequently conflicting interests are demanding health and social services of higher quality with greater access. More vocal groups with political clout are demanding a greater than justifiable share of attention and resources, resulting in an unbalanced, ineffective, and inequitable allocation of increasingly competitive health resources, thus sowing the seed of social disharmony.

IV. HEALTH STATUS OF POPULATION IN TAIWAN

Economic development has had both positive and negative impacts on the health of people in Taiwan. People have generally become better educated. They will have better knowledge about health and generally will have more desirable personal hygiene practice. Basic sanitary facilities, including safe water supply, adequate sewer system, and better housing can be procured with money. People are better nourished, as indicated in the increase in average daily caloric intake and intake of protein.

There are now more hospitals with better equipment. More medical personnel are available to serve people. More people are now able to afford more and earlier health care (Table 4).

Table 4. Practicing Physicians, Hospital Beds and Nutritional Intake

Year	*Number of Practicing physicians**	*Number of Hospital beds***	*Total calorie intake (Keal)****	*Protein intake(gm)****
1956	6.3	3.4	2262	53.9
1976	7.0	19.9	2771	75.9
1986	9.2	41.8	2969	85.1
1990	10.4	43.1	3017	89.5

Notes: * per 10,000 population (including practitioners of traditionall medicine)
** per 10,000 population.
*** per person per day.

The negative aspects of economic development include its impact on the natural and social environment because of its accompanying urbanization and industrialization. There are greater risks of air and water pollution. Overcrowding of people in urban centers intensifies the stress and strain of daily life and increases crimes, suicides and mental health problems. The chance for cross infection also increases. More automobiles mean more traffic accidents and more air pollution. Indulgence in unhealthy behaviors increased: smoking, drinking, substance abuse, and "illicit" sexual practice. "Diseases of the affluent" such as diabetes, obesity, and hypertension have also increased. Epidemiologic transition, coupled with demographic transition, has greatly increased the prevalence of various chronic and degenerating diseases. In spite of these negative impacts of economic development, the health status of people in Taiwan, in general, has significantly improved.

Mortality rates have declined significantly among all age groups. Improvement is especially significant in infant mortality, which has declined from 44.7 in 1952 to 6.0 in 1990. Similarly, maternal mortality has declined sharply from 1.97 to 0.09 in the same period (Department of Health, 1991) (both per 1,000 live births).

The expectancy of life at birth was 71.1 years for male and 76.5 years for female in 1989, lengthened from 53.1 years and 57.3 years for male and female, respectively, in 1956 (Figure 1).

The causes of death have shifted from the pattern of a developing country to that of a developed country with various chronic diseases ranking at the top of the leading causes of death. This process of change is generally known as the "epidemiologic transition" (Figure 2).

Fortunately, Taiwan is relatively small area-wise with good communication and transportation systems. Income distribution in Taiwan is relatively even. A concern of "epidemiologic polarization" has not happened.

Some age-old health problems remain. Although several major communicable diseases, such as plague, small pox, rabies, and malaria have been eradicated, control of some other communicable diseases has not been

Year of age

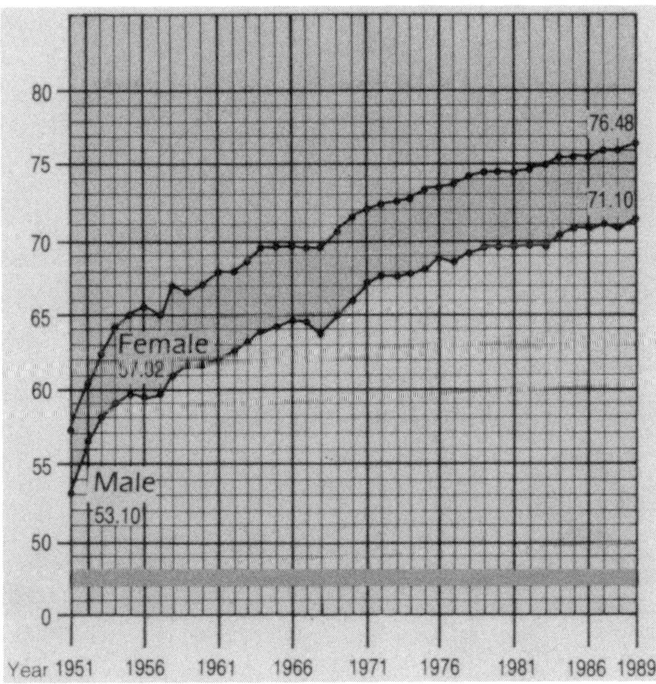

Figure 1. Life Expectancy in Taiwan Area, ROC, 1951-1989

as successful. For example, various vaccine preventable childhood diseases, such as measles, poliomyelitis, Japanese B encephalitis, and diphtheria-pertussistetanus (DPT) still exist. Outbreaks of Dengue fever occurred from time to time in the past. Mortality from tuberculosis, although significantly lower, remains higher than desirable. Hepatitis A and B are major public health concerns. Sexually transmitted diseases, including the much feared AIDS, will have the potential for increase. Parasitic infections, especially ascaris, hook worm and pin worm, are still prevalent among children in rural areas (Department of Health, 1991). Pneumonia, bronchitis and influenza continue to be health threats, especially for the very young and very old.

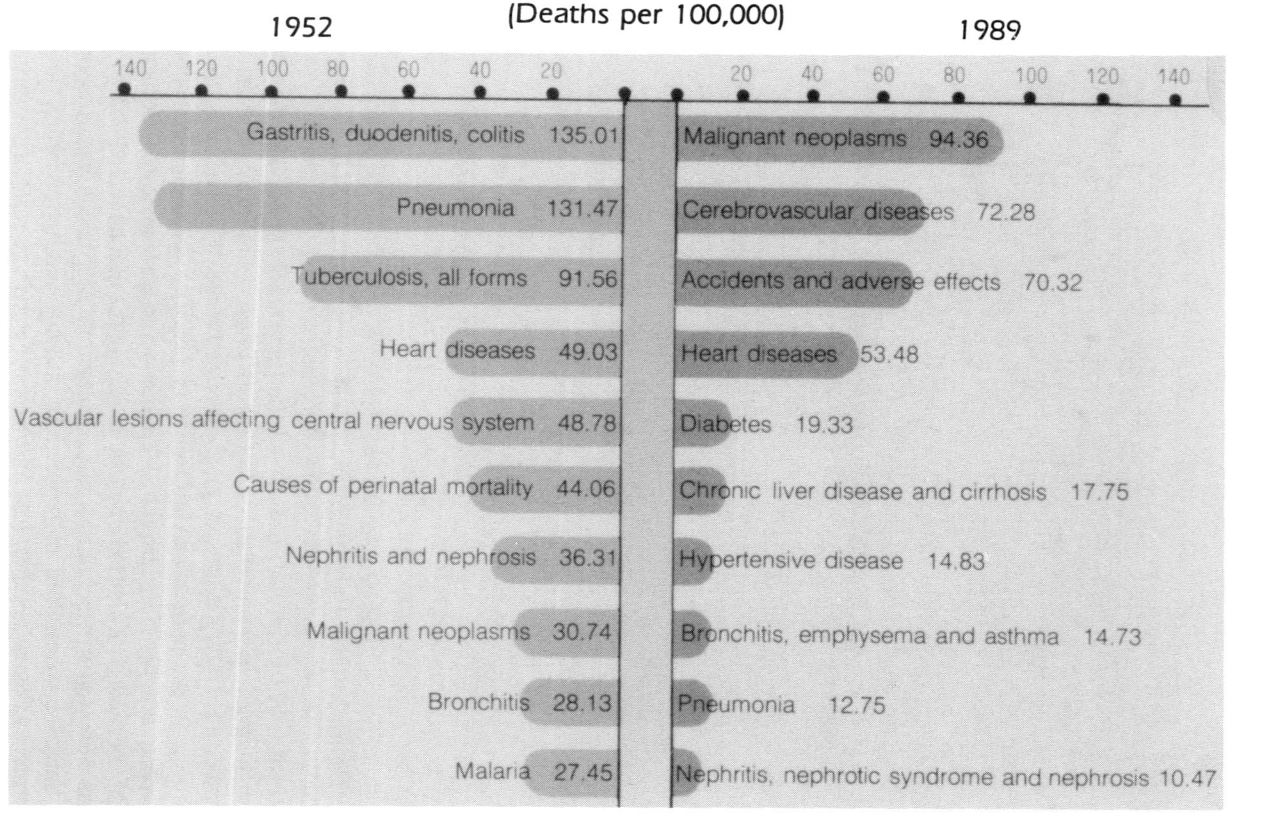

Figure 2. Changes in Ten Leading Causes of Death, Taiwan Area, 1952 and 1989

Table 5. Deterioration of Social Environment

Year	Crimes per 10000 population	Automobile accidents per 10000 population	Fires per 10000 population
1980	28.1	6.5	1.5
1984	27.6	3.8	4.5
1990	45.4	3.1	3.8

Source: The Ministry of Interior, Executive Yuan.

The sharp increase in the number of crimes and fires, as shown in Table 5, suggest the potential risk of "deteriorating" social environment.

V. SOCIO-ECONOMIC DETERMINANTS OF HEALTH

For better understanding of the interactions among economic development, social and environmental changes, and health, ascertaining the socio-economic determinants of health or of diseases is essential. Strategies can then be designed to counter these determinants to reduce the risks.

Health had long been considered a "medical problem," and therefore within the exclusive "prerogative" of medical professionals. According to this medical mode (Dever, 1984) the responsibility of the health care system is to treat the disease when it occurs, as in the figure below.

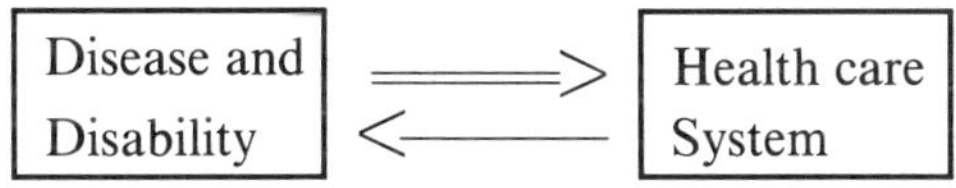

Evans and Staddat considered this simplest feedback model analogous to a heating system controlled by a thermostat. When the health of individuals or a population deteriorates to a pre-determined level, the system responds by activating the remedial care services mechanism. The level of such response is determined by the "access" to care which a particular society has provided for its members. In a poor community such "access" will be more difficult, and people either will not seek care or will not be treated (Evans & Stoddart, 1990).

Because of this "reactive" nature of the health care system, it has frequently been dubbed "sickness care system." In most countries, both industrialized or otherwise, most health resources are directed to this "health care system." Health care policy has dominated the nation's health policy.

Under the above simple framework of health policy, the major concern at the present time in most of the economically developed countries, especially in the United States, is the ever increasing health care cost, which is frequently referred to as the "health care cost crisis." Various new ideas for containment of health care cost have been advanced and tested in the United States, including prospective payment, DRG, HMO, PPO, IPA and "managed care" (Dougherty, 1988). More recently, the concept of "rationing" health care has been advanced and is being tested in a few states, such as Oregon, in the United States (Aaron, 1991). With the impending implementation of a universal health insurance program in 1994, the health care cost spiral is also a real concern for Taiwan, when she continues to pursue the course for economic development and expand her "health care system."

The "four health field" framework proposed that the determinants of health status be categorized under four headings: Life style, Environment, Human biology, and the System of health care organization (Lalonde, 1974).

This model implies that control and manipulation of three other factors—life style, environment and human biology—may in fact contribute more to the improvement of human health than further expansion of the health care system. This health field concept was a call for a broader and more active social policy for the improvement of health, going beyond the provision of health care services.

However, the implicit assumption of the model is that life style and, to a lesser extent, living environments are "chosen" by the individuals concerned and that people are largely responsible for their own health status. The health field model, therefore, tends to lead to "victim blaming" (Allukien, 1990).

The health field model, however, has created among health administrators and scientists an awareness of the need for the study of socioeconomic determinants of diseases and to undertake risk analysis, investigating the social, environmental, psychological, behavioral and biological determinants of health and illness.

The strategy for intervention has widened accordingly. Taking cancer as an example, the responsibility of the health care system used to be to treat cancer when it is diagnosed. Under the health field concepts, there are more alternatives in the interventions: one may choose to modify his/her life style, such as abandoning smoking. Or one may improve the natural or working environment to reduce the risk of exposure to cancer-causing agents. Alternatively, one may choose to invest in research on cancer in the hope of discovering a better way of treating cancer. One may improve the resistance of the host by improving or modifying his/her diet and nutrition (Jamison & Mosley, 1990).

A controversy with respect to this health field model is the fact that the life style seems to have the largest measurable effect on health, which is also portrayed as under the control of individuals. This has led to the "politically innocuous, inexpensive, highly visible, but relatively ineffective health communication and education campaign." It has also been unintentionally used to "justify" inaction of the government. For example, the Health

Objectives Years 2000: United States, have been criticized by some health scientists as a "justification for the lack of action by the Federal government" (Allukien, 1990).

More recently it has been realized that not all "life styles" or human behaviors are voluntarily "chosen." For example, it is known that smoking behavior is strongly related to socioeconomic status, indicating that smoking is a form of social conditioning. Arguing that individuals are responsible for their own health, or blaming the victims for their ill-health is neither justifiable nor helpful.

In the extended model of Evans and Stoddart, human behaviors are considered in response to social, physical and genetic environmental changes, not entirely the individuals' voluntary "choice." Their model implies that most public policies concerning the interest and obligation of individual citizens are, in fact, all related to "health policy" because they will affect the health of individuals and the health status of the population (Evans & Stoddart, 1990).

An over-expansion of the health care system may, in fact, adversely affect the health of the population. With a finite amount of resources, optimum allocation of resources for all health-enhancing programs and activities is essential.

VI. THE FUTURE OF PUBLIC HEALTH IN TAIWAN

Further economic development will cause more social and environmental changes, affecting the socio-economic determinants of health and risk factors of diseases. The future health problems and health status of the population also depend on the aging process of the population and the advance in medical sciences and technology.

The health of people in Taiwan is most likely to continue to improve but at decelerating rates. Life expectancy will be prolonged but also at a slower pace. The gap in life expectancy between male and female will narrow when females gradually lose some of their advantages, such as lower risk of work related morbidity and mortality; social and behavioral factors which traditionally favored females, such as smoking and drinking; and stress and strain, which have been more severe for males. As more women are employed, doomsayers had predicted that they would collapse under the stress of "role overload" as they juggle work, children, and homemaking.

It should be possible to eradicate several childhood communicable diseases which are vaccine preventable: poliomyelitis, measles and DPT. The prevalence of tuberculosis, hepatitis and parasitic infections will be gradually reduced. However, the mortality rates of various chronic diseases, such as cancer and cardio and cerebro-vascular diseases are likely to increase, as will death from external causes: accidents, suicide, and homicide. Deterioration of the natural and working environment will become major health concerns unless intensified and concerted efforts are made in time.

Senile dementia, espcecially Alzheimer's disease, will surely increase sharply along with the aging of the population. By year 2030, it is estimated that there may be more than 400,000 Alzheimer victims in Taiwan if the prevalence rate of the United States prevails in Taiwan). The disease is not only devastating for the victims but also for the family members and care givers, causing a tremendous burden on society.

From the programmatic viewpoint, the concern of the nation's health care system may be more of morbidity than mortality. An argument is whether morbidity compression or morbidity extension theory is going to materialize.

Fries, in 1980, advanced the theory of morbidity compression (Fries, 1989; Fries et al., 1989). Improved health status of population through various preventive measures, according to the theory, will not eliminate but will delay the onset of diseases. Morbidity will thus be "compressed" to a shorter period of later life.

However, a contradictory view expressed by the extension theory is that modern medicine will let the sick and infirm survive longer without significant change in the age of onset of illness (Olshansky, 1991). This will increase the disease prevalence and the disease burden of a population.

Between 1970 and 1980 the life expectancy at age 65 in the United States was prolonged by 1.2 years for male and 1.6 years for female. However, a large proportion of the prolongation was with some disability; disability-free life had been lengthened only by the same 0.2 year for male and female (Crimmins et al., 1989).

Are people in Taiwan going to live longer but be sicker? Are various public health programs simply "adding years to people's life" without "adding life to people's years?" While making efforts to prolong longevity, it must be a goal of future public health programs to improve the quantity of life to extend "active life expectancy."

VII. NEED FOR HEALTH POLICY RESEARCH AND DEVELOPMENT

Confronted with the challenge of ever increasing complexity of the "environment" of modern society, the persistence of various infectious diseases, the possible increase in the burden of chronic-degenerating diseases and the conflicting demands of multiple constituencies, and yet faced with the increasingly competitive resources for health care, there is a real need for health administrators in the industrializing countries to research and develop appropriate health policy to guide their future course of action. Such health policy must be developed and in place well ahead of the problem. Social and environmental changes may occur within a relatively short period of time.

However, most chronic diseases have long lead time. It will be too late to take any effective action when the problem is already in sight.

Consensus must be reached in regard to the ultimate goal of the health program: it must be for the "production of the maximum amount of health" not the "consumption of more health care resources." This consensus may not be particularly difficult to reach in theory. In practice, the health administrators in the rapidly developing economy will be hard-pressed to resist the political and social pressure to divert more money to expand the health care system, neglecting other more effective health-enhancing activities.

Problem Identification and Need Assessment

Use of various conventional measures, known as the health indicator method, is the most common approach for problem identification and need assessment. Infant mortality rate, maternal mortality rate, mortality rates specific for age, sex and causes, and expectancy of life at birth and at specified age are all useful indicators frequently employed. The standard mortality ratio (SMR) is another simple yet useful health indicator, especially for the prediction of future problems and setting the program's priority and goal (Brownlee, 1922).

Table 6 shows the mortality ratios of Taiwan standardized to the age specific mortality rates of 15 leading causes of death in the U.S. in 1988. Attention will be drawn immediately to the unusually high SMR of 309.7 for cerebrovascular disease (stroke) in Taiwan, followed by nephritis and nephrosis (SMR–260.9), accident and adverse effects (SMR = 202.9) and chronic liver diseases (SMR = 204.0). These high SMRs indicate the need for epidemiologic studies to disclose the reasons for the higher mortality rates from these causes in Taiwan and to find effective intervention strategies. The higher SMRs point out the direction for future public health program efforts. Higher SMRs also suggest the possibility of lowering the mortality rates from these causes if effective programs are implemented.

Lower SMRs of Taiwan are both good and bad news for the health administrators. The good news is that Taiwan is ahead of the U.S. and that the future program effort is to maintain these "achievements." The bad news, however, is that there is a possibility for the mortality from these causes in Taiwan to increase to the level observed in the United States if the process of socioeconomic development in Taiwan continues. How to contain these rates from increasing will be the challenge for the public health program.

Survey approach is also frequently used for identifying health problems and community's health need. However, the conventional interview survey using structured questionnaires have been criticized for being superficial with questionable reliability. Margaret Mead, the renowned anthropologist, disdained the use of "statistics for problems that required complex situational

Table 6. Standardized Mortality Ratios of Taiwan: Fifteen Leading Causes of Death, Standardized unto The U.S. Population: 1988

Cause of death	°*Number of death expected in Taiwan if US 1988 ASMR prevail*	*Number of death observed in Taiwan 1988*	*Standardized Mortality Ratio US = 100*
1. Diseases of heart	27,309	14,847	54.4
2. Malignant neplasms	22,172	18,233	82.2
3. Cerebrovascular diseases	4,865	15,067	309.7
4. Accident and Adverse effect	6,766	13,730	202.9
5. Chronic obstructive pulmonary diseases	3,241	3,457	106.7
6. Peneumonia and influenza	2,325	2,648	113.4
7. Diabetes mellitus	2,322	3,883	167.2
8. Suicide & self-inflicted injuries	2,164	1,790	82.7
9. Chronic liver diseases and cirrhosis	1,731	3,532	204.0
10. Nephlitis and Nephrosis	791	2,064	260.9
11. Atherosclerosis	549	182	33.2
12. Homicide & Legal Intervention	1,800	493	27.4
13. Septicemia	931	1,123	120.6
14. Perinatal conditions	1,422	424	29.8
15. Human Immundodeficiency Diseases (HIV)	1,253	0	—
All causes	174,532	101,055	57.9

Notes: * Applying the age specific mortality rates of the disease of interest in the US in 1988 to the population of Taiwan in 1988.

and emotional statements of contexts" and likened her own role to that of "an insightful diagnostician" (Peggy, 1979; Stycos, 1981). She and other social science researchers frequently use some "qualitative survey techniques" known as the "consensus reaching approach," including such techniques as community forum, key informant interview, participant observation, nominal group process, focus group research, and Delphi technique. Application of these "qualitative" research techniques will add depth to the understanding of nonsuperficial aspects of human emotion, motivation and felt-need (Kidder, 1981).

Estimating Disease-burden of Population

Estimating the burden of various diseases on population will greatly facilitate priority determination in health policy formulation and development. Year of Life Lost (YLL), Potential Year of Life Lost (PYLL) or Year of Productive Life Lost (YPLL) are the indicators frequently used by health economists for quantifying the disease-burden (Romeder & McWhinnie, 1977; Reynolds &

Gaspari, 1985). More recently the importance of quality of life has been realized and consequently the Quality Adjusted Year of Life Lost (QAYLL) or Healthy Year of Life Lost (HYLL) concept and indicators have been introduced (Ghana Health Assesment Project Team, 1981; Barnum, 1987).

Over the past two years the World Bank has undertaken, with a number of collaborators, a Health Sector Priority Review (HSPR) utilizing the HYLL (lost) as the measure. The World Bank is encouraging various developing countries to undertake country-specific review and analysis to estimate the disease-burden of the country for health policy formulation and priority determination (Measham, 1991). Taiwan is among the few countries in the developing world where vital and health statistical systems are well developed. A plan is to undertake such HSPR in collaboration with The Johns Hopkins University to facilitate health policy development, and also to demonstrate to other countries as well as various international health organizations the feasibility and usefulness of such review.

Evaluating Alternative Intervention Strategies

Controversies exist and debates ensue in regard to the "best" intervention strategies for the "production of health." The debates frequently polarize around issues such as prevention versus curative approach, research versus action program, selective versus comprehensive approach, vertical versus integrated program, and use of high technology versus appropriate technology in health care (Jamison & Mosley, 1990).

Prevention Versus Curative Approach

An age-old adage says, "An ounce of prevention is better than a pound of cure." It is "fashionable" for politicians to preach the virtue of prevention. However, not all preventive measures are more cost-effective than the curative or case-management approach.

There is little question about the effectiveness of immunizations against various vaccine preventable childhood diseases. The health benefit of behavioral changes, such as smoking, is well established if people are willing to modify their unhealthy behaviors. However, there is cost as well as risk in inducing behavioral change. Even such simple behavior as exercise, which appears to be cost-free, is not "free" (Russell, 1986).

The cost-effectiveness of some other preventive measures, especially screening, depend on many factors, including the prevalence of the disease, diagnostic cut-off point, sensitivity and specificity of screening, compliance of people with screening and treatment, and the cost of screening itself. Costs will include the opportunity cost of lost time as well as the cost for side effects (e.g., injuries) and their treatment. The psychological "cost" of being labelled "sick" and the "cost" of the false sense of security of false negative of a screening test must also be considered (Jamison & Mosley, 1990).

In general, if the prevalence of the disease is high, the method of screening is highly sensitive and specific, the consequence of untreated disease is serious, and if the method of treatment is effective, a screening program will produce large benefit. Mammography for screening of breast cancer and papanicoulas test screening for cervical cancer, targeted to high risk women, are examples. Contrarily, labelling a "healthy" but somewhat hypertensive man as "sick" and treating him with medication may not produce the desired benefit.

Cost-effectiveness analysis of alternative intervention strategies has revealed a number of neglected and emerging health problems which deserve higher priority. Curative care for tuberculosis and acute respiratory infection (ARI) appear to be extremely cost-effective, according to Mosley and his associates. Even a relatively expensive curative approach, such as the management of angina or insulin dependent diabetes, can be moderately cost effective because of the relative ease with which the interventions can be targeted (Jamison & Mosley, 1990).

Contrarily, provision of ORT in low mortality environments is estimated to be about 20 times less cost-effective than tuberculosis control using passive case-finding and short course of chemotherapy, based on the analysis by Mosley and his colleagues.

Research Versus Action Program

Research generates new knowledge to guide action and help develop new "tools" to solve the problems. The discovery and development of antibiotics, vaccines, new diagnostic modalities, and new clinical procedures are but some examples. Epidemiologic research identifying cigarette smoking as a major risk factor has enabled the health administrators to design an effective strategy for the prevention of lung cancer.

People generally respect scientific undertakings and therefore usually support investment in research. A heavy investment made by the United States to establish the National Institutes of Health (NIH) is a distinctive example. NIH is considered the "gem" of the nation and has contributed greatly to improving the health and well being of people all over the world.

In the developing countries, the question is not only the money; more important are the people who can make good use of the money to produce the anticipated research results. Moreover, strategic considerations and priority determinations are needed if the money for research is to be well-spent.

Research does not only mean the highly sophisticated biomedical research at the molecular level such as the recombinant DNA technology. Although they undoubtedly are important, other types of research should not be overlooked, especially for the developing countries. They are the research which will enhance the quality of life of people. The related disciplines may be jointly called the Life Enhancement Sciences (LES), which include basic research to identify the etiology of diseases; epidemiologic and social sciences research to identify the risk factors and socio-economic determinants of health and illness; research to determine the risk factors associated with ill-health; clinical research to discover better ways of diagnosing and treating patients and alleviating their suffering; rehabilitation research to disclose methods and procedures of facilitating the regaining and recovery of impaired functions, including biomedical engineering research to better design robots and various prostheses to assist the elderly and disabled. In addition, there must be health services research to test and determine effective and efficient ways of organizing and delivering health care services; and above all, health policy research to identify the nation's health problems, estimate the burden of various diseases, set their priority for intervention, design appropriate intervention strategies, ensure optimum allocation of resources, and monitor, control and evaluate the effectiveness and efficiency of various health research and services program.

In the developing countries, since the disease-burden is heavy and research infrastructure is poorly developed, the highest priority must be given to building up research capacity for Essential National Health Research (ENHR) by strengthening the existing research institutions and research manapower development, then gradually expanding the capability to move into various "research-frontiers" (Commission of Health Research for Development, 1990).

From the programmatic viewpoint, research should not end in "research." The results must be utilized to improve the health of people and enhance the quality of their lives. Unfortunately too many research results are unknown to the health administrators and therefore are seldom utilized to help health policy formulation or service improvement.

In regard to other issues, such as selective versus comprehensive approach, vertical versus integrated approach, and high technology versus appropriate technology and so on, they can be argued both ways, perhaps depending on the local conditions, organizational infrastructure, and individual perception.

Four Basic Approaches for Social and Behavioral Change

The health administrators must remember that there are four basic approaches which may be used to induce social and behavioral changes to promote health: educational, economic, legislative, and technological. All of them should be employed as appropriate in dealing with the health problems of modern society.

Health educational activities should not be the monopoly of the departments of health. Various private sectors can and are making significant contribution, usually motivated by their own self-interest. Many voluntary organizations are "marketing" health messages to promote their causes. The Cancer Society,

Heart and Lung Association, Red Cross and Planned Parenthood Association are but some examples. Their advocacies are referred to as "social marketing."

For-profit commercial and industrial firms, by promoting their products, are disseminating health messages to advocate for behavioral changes.

Food industries are advertising low calorie and cholesterol-free products. McDonald's has recently added a new product line of lean hamburger. Even the tobacco companies, being accused of "promoting death," have been advertising low tar cigarettes, thereby enhancing the awareness of people of the health hazard of cigarette smoking.

Health education program should adopt the marketing technique which is being successfully used by the business sector. The technique includes market research to identify problems, analyze consumers, review organizational strength and weakness, ascertain influence channels, and segmentation of the market. Strategy fully utilizing the market mix of 5-Ps—products, price, place, promotion and people—are then designed and developed to actively promote the products by appealing to the "want" of people (Kotler, 1982).

Economic development has "produced" more sophisticated and better informed customers. In response, business and industry, despite or because of their profit motive, have become increasingly conscious of their social responsibility to maintain a cleaner environment and better health of the public. Use of biodegradable material for wrapping by the fast-food industry in the United States is an example. Many supermarkets are recycling shopping bags and beverage containers.

Economic incentives and disincentives have been widely and effectively used by the government and private sector to encourage or discourage certain behaviors. The government has the power of taxation and by levying higher sales taxes it is possible to discourage smoking or drinking. Insurance companies usually charge higher premiums for smokers because their life expectancy is shorter and the risk of fire hazard is higher than for nonsmokers. Higher insurance premiums for drivers after traffic violations make automobile drivers more careful in driving. Although still controversial, some U.S. firms are providing both positive and negative economic incentives to modify the behavior and lifestyle of their employees.

The government has the power and authority to regulate human behavior for health benefit. The enactment of seat belt laws in most states in the United States is an example. Legislation and regulation governing the environment, work place, restaurants, food and drug industries are other examples. Setting safety standards for automobiles and speed limits on highways are still others.

Human behaviors can be modified also by technologic improvement. A simple example is the design of the automobile seat belt. For example, many new models of automobiles now have an automatic seat belt buckling system. When the driver and passenger are seated and the doors closed, the seat belts automatically come in front of them. Compliance with the seat belt law will be nearly complete with such a device.

The development of 28 pills per cycle of oral contraceptive, 21 with hormones and 7 placebo, is another example indicating that a simple technologic innovation can promote compliance of women in regularly taking the pills. If a "perfect" contraceptive is developed, the solution of the world's population problem will be greatly facilitated.

Priority Determination

Priority of health problems has been determined qualitatively. The scoring system based on five criteria developed by Brackett and his associates of the World Health Organization has been used in the past. These five criteria are: extent, seriousness, preventability, local concern and time trend of the problem (Brackett, 1984). The "most important" health problem perceived by the community may not always be the best target for intervention either because an effective intervention method is still lacking or the cost of intervention is exorbitant. The combined scores obtained from the scoring system will give health policymakers some objectivity in guiding decision-making.

The use of cost-effectiveness analysis of various intervention strategies, following the estimation of socio-economic burden of diseases on population, have enabled health administrators to determine priority on quantitative terms. Use of the Basic Priority Rating (BPR) model, as advocated by Vilnus and Dandoy, is another possibility (Vilnus & Dandoy, 1990).

However, health policy decisions can seldom be made entirely on "cold" quantitative or economic terms. Frequently political considerations are needed and non-quantitative priority-setting with human elements is essential. Use of PEARL system will facilitate the process of priority-setting. The first consideration is the political feasibility (P) followed by economic consideration (E). Acceptability (A) by the community and the people is of course important. Resources (R) for the solution of the problems must be available, and the actions to be undertaken for the solution of the problems must be legal (L). Decisions can be made more objectively by using such management technique as the Force Field Analysis.

Implementation and Management

"Management" had been jargon used mostly by business people. Since physicians do not consider their practice as a kind of "business," most health professionals had only a marginal interest in management. However, this is no longer true. Increasing use among medical practitioners of such business jargon as "clients," "customers," "products," "product lines," "reimbursement," and "marketing," and so forth, attest to the increasing "commercialization of the health industry" and the need for effective managers (Vilnus & Dandoy, 1990). Several universities in the United States have started to offer courses for training "physician administrators" whose responsibilities will include social marketing their "products" (Kotler, 1982).

In order to effectively deal with the intricate environment, health administrators in the rapidly developing economy must improve their management capability for planning, decision-making, organizing, directing and controlling their organizations and programs. They will need conceptualizing and human relations skills in addition to the technical skills which they presumably already have. They need not only the quantitative skills to analyze the problem but the human relations skills to organize, motivate, direct and lead their people for them to willingly strive to achieve the common goal.

An effective manager is usually an innovator who is willing to take risks for testing new ideas and new approaches.

Monitoring and Evaluation

Development of health policy will be facilitated by establishing an effective health information system to routinely collect health statistics and information to monitor the program's performance and evaluate its effectiveness and impact. The health information system should attempt to regularly collect and analyze socio-economic and demographic statistics, vital statistics, health services statistics and health resources statistics (National Center for Health Statistics, 1989). In addition, surveillance systems to constantly monitor the outbreak of communicable diseases, occupational diseases and injuries, environmental quality and changing risk factors, and congenital birth defects are also needed.

Sampling survey to periodically ascertain the changing environment, and changing health problems, health status, health needs and risk factors of population, their demand and utilization of health care facilities and services should be conducted as appropriate and feasible. Monitoring the changing health status of population is especially essential when the universal health insurance program is started in Taiwan in 1994.

The "sentinel health events," as described by Rutstein and his colleagues, is a useful method to guide the formulation of health policy and to monitor the performance of health program and the quality of health care (Rustein et al., 1976). A list of conditions which are termed "sentinel health events" including unnecessary disease, unnecessary disability and unnecessary and untimely death is developed. These events are considered preventable or manageable and their occurrence indicates that something is wrong with the health care system and changes or improvements are needed. For example, occurrence of infant death or maternal death may be considered warning signals. The occurrence of various vaccine preventive childhood diseases may be other "sentinel health events."

International Collaboration

While pursuing the goal for economic prosperity, one should not overlook the suffering of those less fortunate poeple in other less developed countries. It should be an obligation as well as a privilege for the more developed countries to allocate a part of the accumulated wealth to help improve the quality of life of those people. Health is the most appropriate and desirable subject for such international collaboration and assistance because of its humanitarian nature.

International collaboration in health research should be highly promising and extremely rewarding. Health problems of significance can be addressed more effectively and efficiently through collaborative efforts of scientists in the region and around the world. Recently, the Commision on Health Research for Development (CHRD), an independent international initiative formed in 1987 with the objective of improving the health of people in the third world countries, recommended that in addition to undertaking Essential National Health Research (ENHR) to facilitate solution of health problems of national interest, efforts should be joined together with the research for world-wide attacks on the highest-priority health problems (Commission on Health Research for Development, 1990).

No country can be a responsible member of the international community if she closes her eyes and ignores the needs of the people in the developing world. Taking lessons from the experience of various developed countries, such collaborative efforts should attempt to design an alternative development strategy which preserves the ecology, environment and social fabrics of the local communities, and respects the sensitivity, pride and culture of the local people.

VIII. CONCLUSION

The economic success of the "four little dragons," including Taiwan, must have inspired the leaders of many developing countries to vigorously pursue the same goal toward economic prosperity. In fact, many of these countries, including several on the Pacific rim, are not far behind Taiwan in their development.

The achievements are indeed something to be proud of. However, with hindsight and the viewpoint of health administrators, there were problems which could have been prevented, avoided, or at least contained to minimize their adverse impact on the health of people on the island. The objective of this article is to review the past in order to learn lessons for planning a better future. The need to monitor and analyze the socio-economic determinants of health in line with the rapidly changing physical and social environment is emphasized. Development of a sound health policy by evaluating the disease-burden, setting priorities, and evaluating the cost-effectiveness of alternative intervention strategies is recommended. Administering public health programs without such health policy to guide the operation is similar to navigating troubled water without a compass.

There seem to be at least five major misconceptions about health policy. First, the "get-rich-first" mentality among the economic planners and political decision-makers. They all agree that good health is a goal worth pursuing but promise that "we will do more for health when we become richer." This is a priority set in reverse order. A country cannot be rich if her people are sick or otherwise disabled and discontented.

A good health policy, therefore, corresponds to a good economic development policy and vice versa because both share a common aspiration for better quality of life and a common goal of enhancing the well being of people. "We cannot create a city surrounded by heavily polluted air and severely contaminated water and call it 'development'" as said by the former president of the World Bank.

The second is to consider that when a country becomes wealthier, health problems will be easier to solve because more resources are available. In fact, the reverse will be closer to the reality. When a country becomes more propserous economically, the accompanying social, environmental and behavioral changes will make the health related problems more complex. More sophisticated "clients" with a diversity of conflicting interests will each demand attention and resources, making the job for health administrator increasingly demanding. Policy research to facilitate the design and development of sound health policies and program strategies will become imperative.

The third is to equate health care policy with health policy. The responsibility and functions of the health department (or ministry) are not just to provide health care; it should be the "production of health." Expansion of the health care system may actually reduce health, not enhance it.

The fourth is to consider health problems as "medical problems" and attempt to impose "medical solutions." In fact, many health problems are social problems in a broad sense. Identification and modification of socioeconomic and environmental determinants of health and diseases may be more effective. The government health department will have at least four policy options to choose intervention strategies from: educational, economic, legislative and technological approaches. To be effective, all or some of these options should be employed as appropriate in promoting health.

The last but not the least important is to regard the promotion of health as the concern only of the government health department and to overlook the potential contribution of private sector enterprises. In fact, various private businesses and industries can and are making substantial contribution, and their potentials should be harnessed to supplement the public program efforts. A good administrator is the one who is capable of motivating and coordinating the efforts of others to help achieve his/her own goals.

Expenditure for health was once considered a "consumption." Subsequently economic justification of good health in terms of enhanced productivity was realized and such terms as "investment in health" was used. Health was then considered as a mean for economic prosperity. A World Health Day slogan of "Health is Wealth" was then considered mere rhetoric, but has become more realistically appreciated.

The concept for health has recently changed further. Health is now considered the end in its own right, not a mean to economic development. As said by Dr. T. W. Schultz, a Nobel Laureate, "...the wealth of nations (has) come to be predominantly the acquired abilities of people—their education, experience, skills, and health" (Schultz, 1981). In this regard, it is less meaningful to measure the country's development by such indicators as GNP or per capita income. Rather, the nation's wealth and strengths should be measured by such variables as education, skills, health, and above all the quality of life of the people.

The future health policy-makers and health administrators in the changing society and environment must have the dual qualifications of being administrators and scholars. They must not only be effective managers but also dynamic leaders.

Managers and leaders differ in that managers preside over processes by which the organization functions, such as allocating resources prudently and making the best possible use of people. Leaders must think in terms of renewal. Leaders must think longer term, not just worry about day-to-day business or monthly reports. They must attempt to reach and influence constituents beyond their jurisdictions, such as legislators and political leaders. They must have the political skills to cope with the conflicting requirements of multiple constituencies (Gardner, 1989).

The leaders must not only be concerned about the organization they head; they must grasp its relationship to the larger system and reality. Above all, the leaders emphasize vision, values and motivation. The countries undergoing rapid economic development and social changes will require such dynamic leadership in effectively dealing with the ever increasing complexity of epidemiologic reality.

ACKNOWLEDGMENTS

This paper was prepared for the "1990 International Symposium on Health, Environment and Social Change: Emerging Health Problems in Rapid Socio-Economic Development," held in Taipei, Taiwan, Republic of China, July 2-5, 1990. The author is deeply grateful to Dr. L. P. Chow, Professor, Department of Population Dynamics, The Johns Hopkins University School of Hygiene and Public Health, for his assistance in editing the manuscript of this paper. Dr. Chow and Dr. W. Henry Mosley, Chairman of the said department, jointly made several valuable comments and suggestions which are incorporated into the chapter. Thanks are due also to Mrs. Ruth Skarda of the said department for wordprocessing the chapter.

REFERENCES

Aaron, J. (1991). *Serious and unstable conditions: Financing America's health care.* Washington, DC: Brookings Institution.

Allukien, M. (1990). Healthy people 2000 and our domestic gulf crisis: President's column. *Nation's Health.*

Barnum, H. (1987). Evaluating healthy days of life gained for health projects. *Social Science in Medicine*, 24(10): 833-841.

Brackett, E.M. (1984). *The risk approach in health care.* World health organization public health paper No. 76. Geneva.

Brownlee, J. (1922). *The use of death rates as a measure of hygienic conditions.* Medical Research Council, Special Report Series No. 60. His Majesty's Stationery Office, London.

Commission on Health Research for Development. (1990). *Health research: Essential link to equity in development.* Oxford University Press, New York.

Council for Economic Planning and Development. (1988). *Population projections for the year 1986 throughout 2030.*

Council for Economic Planning and Development. (1990). *Taiwan statistical data book, 1990.* Taipei, Taiwan.

Council for Economic Planning and Development. (1990). *Urban and regional development statistics, Republic of China.*

Crimmins, E.M., Saito, Y., & Ingegneri, D. (1989). Changing in life expectancy and disability-free-life expectancy in the United States. *Population and Development Review*, 15:235-267.

Department of Health. (1991). *Public health in Taiwan area, Republic of China.* Department of Health, Executive Yuan, Taipei, Taiwan, R.O.C.

Dever, G.E.A. (1984). *Epidemiology in health services management.* Aspen Systems Corporation, Rockville, Maryland.

Dougherty, C.J. (1988). *American health care: Realities, rights, and reform.* Oxford University Press.

Easterbrook, G. (1987). The revolution in medicine. *Newsweek*, January, 26.

Easterlin, R.A. (1991). The economic impact of prospective population changes in advanced industrialized countries: An historic perspective. *Journal of Gerontology: Social Sciences*, 46(6): 5299-5309.

Evans, R.G. & G.L. Stoddart. (1990). Producing health, consuming health care. *Social Science and Medicine*, 31 (12):347-363.

Fries, J.F. (1989). The compression of morbidity: Near or far? *The Milbank Quarterly*, 67 (2):208-231.

Fries, J.F., Greer, L.W., & Levine, S. (1989). Health promotion and the compression of morbidity. *The Lancet*, March 4.

Gardner, J.W. (1989). On Leadership. New York, NY: Free Press.

Ghana Health Assesment Project Team. (1981). A quantitative method of assesing the health impact of different diseases in less developed countries. *International Journal of Epidemiology*, 10(1):73-80.

Jamison, D.T. & W.H. Mosley. (1990). Selecting disease control priorities in developing countries. In Jamison, D.T., & Mosley, W.H. (editors) *Disease Control Priorities in Developing Countries.* Oxford: Oxford University Press.

Kidder, L.H. (1981). *Research methods in social relations.* New York: Holt, Rinehart and Winston.

Kotler, P. (1982). *Marketing for nonprofit organization*, Second Edition. Englewood Cliffs, NJ: Prentice Hall.

Lalonde, M. (1974). A new perspective on the health of canadians. *Health and Welfare*, Ottawa, Canada.

Measham, A.R. (1991). *Forward to disease control priorities in developing countries.* D.T. Jamison & W.H. Mosley (Ed.). The World Bank.

Ministry of Interior. (1989). *1988 Taiwan-Fukien Demographic Fact Book.* Republic of China, Taipei. Taiwan, R.O.C.

National Center for Health Statistics. (1989). *Vital and health statistics: Data systems of the national center for health statistics.* United States Public Health Services.

Olshansky, S.J. (1991). Trading off longer life for worsening health: The expansion of morbidity hypothesis. *Journal of Aging and Health*, 3(2):194-216.

Peggy, R.S. (1979). The Ethnographic Paradigms. *Administrative Science Quarterly*, 24:534.

Reynolds, J. & K.S. Gaspari. (1985). *Cost effectiveness analysis.* PRICO Monograph Series, Methods paper 2.

Romeder, J.M. & McWhinnie, J.R. (1977). Potential years of life lost between ages 1 and 70: An indicator of premature mortality for health planning. *International Journal of Epidemiology*, 6 (2):143-151.

Russell, L.B. (1986). *Is prevention better than cure?* Brookings Institute, Washington, DC.

Rustein, D.D., Berenberg, W., Chalmers, T.C., Child, C.G., Fishman, A.P., & Perrin, E.B. (1976). Measuring the quality of medical care—A clinical method. *New England Journal of Medicine*, 294 (11):582-588.

Schultz, T.W. (1981). *Investing in people: Th economics of population quality.* Berkeley, CA: University of California Press.

Stycos, J.M. (1981). A critique of focus group and survey research: The machismo case. *Studies in Family Planning*, 12 (12):450-454.

Vilnus, D. & S. Dandoy. (1990). A priority rating system for public health programs. *Public Health Reports*, 105 (5):463-470.

ADAPTATION AND LIFE SATISFACTION OF NATIVE MIGRANTS IN URBAN TAIWAN

Kao-Chiao Hsieh

I. INTRODUCTION

In recent decades, industrial and economic development in Taiwan had caused changes in social and economic structure, and led to large population concentrations in cities or industrial towns. Taiwanese society as a whole is in transition. Whether urban or rural, whether a dominant group or a minority group, whether the elite or the populace, all have been impacted by changes and have experienced life crisis and adaptation problems.

The native people (or the mountain people) are a minority group in Taiwan. Traditionally, they were a small, isolated, and self-sufficient society, bound by an unique set of ideas and social norms. Their lifestyle, economic production, kinship, and social organization were integrated by a belief system into a strong social unity. How the mountain people adapt to the changing industrial society is a challenge for societal development.

Research in Human Capital and Development, Volume 7, pages 29-51.

ISBN: 1-55938-132-9

The mountain people moved to Taiwan island much earlier than Han people (or the Chinese) did (around 1500 to 1700 A.D.). They originally lived in the basin and swamp-land of the western plain. Later on, because of the Han people's emigration to Taiwan, they were forced to move to thc remote mountain areas. Thereafter, many fights among tribes, and interior conflict and expansion within tribes, dispersed the aboriginal groups throughout the mountain areas, and created their present pattern of settlement. The mountain people include nine tribes: Tayal, Amis, Bunun, Rukai, Paiwan, Pyuma, Tsou, Thao, and Saisiat. Each of them occupied an area and formed an independent tribal society. Now, there are about 310,000 of them (1.5% of total Taiwan population) scattered in the mountain areas of twelve counties.

Until the Ming and Ching dynasties (1386-1911 A.D.), when the Chinese largely emigrated to Taiwan from the mainland China, the aborigine tribes did not have much contact with one another. However, under the impact of the dominant Chinese culture or group, the loosely connected tribes bonded together and became a united mountain society for preserving their tradition. The mountain society hardly changed during the colonial period of Japanese sovereignty (1895-1945), because the Japanese authority delimited the aborigine settlements as a mountain reservation and isolated them from the outside world. As a result, the mountain people's culture and lifestyle remained largely intact (Hsu, 1988).

After Taiwan's restoration to China in 1945, a mountain policy was enacted by the Taiwan Provincial government to protect the mountain people and to develop the mountain society. Along with Taiwan's overall socioeconomic development, the mountain society showed an important growth. From 1967 to 1985, household income increased from NT$24,000 to NT$267,000; the percentage of population who received a higher education increased from 0.15 percent to 1.97 percent; and the infant mortality rate decreased from 37 in 1976 to 14 in 1986 per thousand. Compared to Taiwan as a whole, per capita income of mountain people is only 38 percent of Taiwan's per capita income, the percentage of higher educational people differs by six percentage points from that of Taiwan. These figures show that the development of mountain society has been great, but it still lags far behind the dominant ethnic group. Thus, the mountain people have a more difficult time in adaptating to the larger Taiwan society.

Nevertheless, changes in the mountain society have taken place under the impact of interior growth and external pressures. First, a self-government system established by the Taiwan Provincial Government in the mountain areas not only separated politics from social organization and religious belief system, but also destroyed the traditional social associations (Taipei County Records Committee, 1988, p. 84). As a result, the cultural mechanism of social control in mountain society has lost its ground, and became a disruptive factor in its social organization.

Second, the intrusion of a market and money economy on the mountain society destroyed their traditional lifestyles of farming, hunting, and fishing, and even the self-supporting idea in which every family believed. The domestic and captured animals were no longer viewed as the offerings of ceremonies and worship; goods and labor were no longer exchanged according to social network. Their values now are expressed in money rather than culture. It disrupts the persistence of social organization and religious ceremonies in the mountain society (Yu, 1989).

Third, the developing of mountain resources and roads by the government opened up the closed mountain society, which enabled the influx of many tourists and businessmen of Han people in the mountain areas. They not only took away natural resources and cultural items from the mountain people, but also created economic deprivation, a distorted value system, and a deviant behavior for mountain society (Hwang & Liu, 1989). Thus, the native people developed a consumer orientation, which dealt a terrible blow to the traditional culture.

Although the mountain people had contact with outside culture during the period of Japanese rule, they did not actively respond to it, and the chance for modernization was thus lost. Recently, the replacement of an old and usual tool, idea, or style of behavior by a new one has occurred in the mountain society; but for such changes to have a modernizing impact on the society, there has to be a large-scale reorganization of the social and economic structure to accommodate the presence of another cultural group. That is, it is necessay for the mountain society to change completely to fully integrate into the dominant society (McElroy & Townsend, 1985). Thus far, however, the mountain society has not reached this stage of development, because they themselves can not produce a self-developing dynamic force from within and to initiate the desired change and control over the environment (Hsu, 1988; Lee, 1983). While the traditional culture no longer offers native people an effective way of life to overcome the problems created by the new environment; the native people also do not have the competence to use knowledge to create their own culture. Thus, the mountain society has encountered many social problems.

Since the 1960s, Taiwan's industrial and economic development has created a prosperous life, particular in urban areas. Whereas the impoverished agricultural life of the mountain people has not improved very much, and the felt needs have risen without satisfaction. A sharp contrast pushes the native people to leave their homeland and pull them toward cities. The number of out-migrants, particularly the young and the better educated people, is increasing more and more in mountain society.

Because of an isolated cultural pattern and a dark brown skincolor, the urban migrants from the mountain society have become an ethnic group called "urban natives." A majority of them do not have much education or special skills, therefore, they engage in unskilled labor works and change jobs often. It is appropriate to call them a kind of "urban nomadic peoples" earning a living by moving around the various jobs on the bottom of occupational structure.

Most urban natives grew up in the mountain areas, they only contacted and interacted within a small group of people, and they were all familiar with each other. In addition, they lacked modern knowledge and techniques with which to perform a meaningful work role, and to participate in the cultural activities of the urban community. Their lives in cities are full of unfamiliarity and insecurity (Fu, 1987), thus, they tend to live in their own small world. On the other hand, the Han people have a stereotyped attitude toward the native people, and call them "fan ah" (barbarian) which means a man with characteristics such as foolish, idle, ignorant, drinking, and so forth (Chen, 1987). This has resulted in the Han people having a disrespectful and unfriendly attitude toward the native people whom they regard as inferior. In short, the discrimination of Han people and the lower socioeconomic status of the native peoples interact to create an unfavorable circumstance within which urban natives must make an adaptation.

Recently, the problem about the adaptation of native people to urban conditions has attracted a great deal of attention. Much research on this problem has been carried out, some of which has explored the adaptation pattern of urban natives (Chang, 1974; Lee, 1978), whereas others have investigated the living conditions of urban natives (Lin, 1980, 1983; Wu, 1988). During the 1980s, when adequate adaptation in the lifestyle of mountain society had not yet happened, the native people became disillusioned and frustrated in accommodating to the dominant urban culture, and some individuals attempted to revitalize their culture and to reaffirm their ethnic identity. These movements somewhat reduced the psychological stress of rapid change. Whether they can successfully cope with the problems remains a question.

Cities are stressful places to live, pushing many people beyond normal limits of life, and the native migrants are no exception. They are relatively rigid in adapting to city ways and changing their beliefs, thus, they show more difficulty in adapt to urban environment. The main question we are concerned with is how the urban natives can adjust to urban conditions and create a satisfactory life. This paper attempts to explore this question.

II. NATIVE MIGRANTS AS AN ETHNIC GROUP IN CITIES

Only recently, a large population of the native people left their hometown for other counties and cities, thus creating a minority group of native people in urban areas.

Emigration Growth

Since the 1960s, the mountain society has lost a large population through emigration, which includes both long-distance and short-distance moves. The former are those who moved across the boundary of a county, the latter are those who just moved within the county. In 1971, the population of mountain people lost 1,650 (male 539; female 1,111) in long-distant migration and 3,205 (male 1,523; female 1,682) in short-distant migration. In 1986, the population of mountain people again lost 2,224 (male 909; female 1,315) in long-distant migration and 1,791 (male 723; 1,068) in short-distant migration.

From 1971 to 1986, the number of long-distant emigrants increased 35 percent (male 69%; female 18%), that of short-distant emigrants decreased 44 percent (male 53%; female 37%). Even so, the number of emigrants from the mountain society remained large, particularly the long-distant emigrants. It may show that the more the mountain people moved out the more they moved toward the large cities. The number of females in both categorics of migration, particularly long-distant emigration, is more than that of male. During the past fifteen years, the mountain society has lost a great deal of population and more than half of those leaving were female.

But how many mountain people who moved to cities are unknown? According to Wang's estimate (1987), the number was very small before 1960. Only 615 of the native people lived in cities in 1961. Since then, this number has grown rapidly. From the household registration data, it was estimated that more than 25,000 of the natives lived in the urban areas in 1987. Indeed, this figure is understated, because many native people stayed in cities but did not formally change their address in the household registration system. According to Tu's estimate (1985), about 25 percent (83,000) of the native population lived in cities, that is, one of every four native people lived in cities.

Native Migrants Appeared in Urban Areas

After World War II, during the reconstruction era of Taiwan, there was little change in the geographic distribution of the native people. Even as late as 1960, most of the native people still lived in the mountain areas, predominantly in rural areas.

Beginning in 1970s, many native people moved from the mountain to the Han people's society, especially to the large cities where they provided a cheap source of labor, forming the necessary human capital for the development of Taiwan industry. Migration of the mountain people was further spurred by the gradually decline in agricultural production, and increasing income differences between the mountain people and the Han people. The migration trend continues into present, and still remains large.

The overwhelming reality is that in the past fifteen years the mountain society has been transformed from a principally rural people to an urbanized minority group in Taiwan. The proportion of native people living in major cities continues to increase. If the status of increasing urban natives are not improved, the prospects of urban development will be obscured. Therefore, an understanding of the adaptation of the native people to urban conditions is essential.

Adaptation To Urban Life

The native people in urban Taiwan are a minority group. Not only is their population a smaller proportion, but also they have special physical or cultural traits which are held in low esteem by the dominant segments of the society. Because they lived in the mountain areas, relatively isolated from outside world, urban natives formed a self-conscious unit by the special traits which their members share.

Since Taiwan's development has been led by a technologically dominant cultural group, its prevailing culture is different from that which the native people have learned in the mountains. Thus, movement of the native people to Han people's society, particularly cities, will involve adjustment to a new sociocultural environment. Not only will they need to change or modify their culture and group relations which are incompatible with urban life, but they also need to acquire the cultural traits and social relationships that will help them survive and develop in an urban environment. This adaptation is not just change by substitution. According to McElroy and Townsend (1985, p. 382), to become a modern urban dweller is to experience reorganization, rearrangement of priorities, and a new set of values and felt needs. Therefore, change is necessary for the native people to play their role more effectively and to integrate themselves into urban life.

However, integration into the dominant society is not an easy task. Not only does the minority desire absorption into the dominant society, but the majority also wants to accept them. If social rejection exists in the dominant society, the minority group will produce a self-rejection to identify with the predominant culture (Kitagawa, 1965).

The culture that urban Taiwan has produced includes a set of values and norms which emphasize competition, achievement, economic success, rationality, and hardwork. Contrarily, the native culture stresses cooperation, noncompetition, religious belief, and fatalism. Native people's heritages are at variance with urban Taiwan culture. It is possible for the native people to be caught in a dilemma, for instance, they want educational and employment opportunities and at the same time want to live according to the native ways that make it difficult to take advantage of such opportunities.

The ideology native people hold about the nature and goals of migration also influence the dilemma. For example, involuntary migrants will experience much more stress, difficulty, and rejection than voluntary migrants do; the migrants who intend to stay in cities will more easily adapt to urban ways than those who do not (Philpott, 1970).

However, the effect of the subjective consciousness of migrants is related to the social and cultural environments of urban society. Compared with other Taiwanese, the native people are relatively recent newcomers to the urban scene and, most important, they are to a varying degree a deprived minority, encountering problems of acceptance and adjustment. Until very recently, they have been dismissed as unimportant or marginal to the mainstream of urban Taiwan.

With the development of industry and democracy, pluralism became an important element in Taiwan's urban culture. It implies that Taiwan society tolerates racial, cultural, linquistic or religious differences. This pattern not only reduces stress on the integration of the native people into urban society, but also provides a wider space for the natives to preserve their ways of life. Indeed, Taiwan creates a favorable atmosphere to assimilate the native people into its social and economic fabric. Even so, certain factors existing in urban Taiwan still operate on the process of assimilation

Residential Segregation

An important aspect of assimilation is the degree to which migrant groups are spatially isolated from the mainstream of the society (Massey, 1981). Residential segregation is not only important as an indicator of assimilation in its own right, but also has implications for other dimensions of sociocultural integration that are highly related to propinquity, for example, inter-marriage (Gordon, 1964; Leiberson, 1963).

People living in segregated areas tend to develop different lifestyles and to perceive people as different and to act differently toward other persons than they do toward people who live within their own area. This social and cultural isolation will be reinforced by intensive interaction among others within the same locale. Thus, the more people are segregated, the more they interact in a way that reinforces their minority values and lifestyle (Wilson & Schutz, 1978).

The residential segregation of native people in urban Taiwan is not so significant. They have not been deliberately relegated to specified areas of the city by law or social tradition such as race in the United Staes or Caste in India. However, social and economic forces influence the residential distribution of native migrants in cities. Most native migrants prefer to live with members of their own group, thus, they settled and maintained different neighborhoods. Certain neighborhoods developed a ghetto-like settlement. Some native migrants illegally set up their squatter settlements, others just temporarily stayed in construction places where they worked. These neighborhoods or squatter settlements offered the native migrants an organized, often tightly knit sociological unit, where many of the subcultural elements such as language, childrearing patterns, leisure patterns and others persisted.

Familism and Intermarriage

The traditional family in the mountain societies was altered by migration. Most of the native people who migrated to cities were not single but married, and their spouse and children usually accompanied them in migration. Family obligation thus did not disappear, but kinship became focused increasingly on the nuclear family.

Many migrants are tied to their mountain relatives by visits and remittances. This pattern serves as a safety valve for the impoverished life of old parents in the hometown and for the migrants struggling in the city. On the other hand, the single young migrants easily shuttled back and forth between city and mountain, which interfered with holding stable city jobs and further slowed the development of an urban culture.

Because the native people lived in quite isolated mountain areas, they frequently married only within their groups. Recently, this marriage pattern has been disrupted by intermarriage. More and more native people, especially women, have married Han people. For instance, the young, native women who married retired soldiers are a common case. This has created a disproportionate sex ratio (over 120) in the group aged 25-44 in mountain society. This assimilation of some natives through intermarriage opened up other types of assimilation (Gordon, 1964).

Occupational Segregation

The fact that people in different occupations tend to have different incomes, educations, and lifestyles prompts them to choose housing in certain areas. The result of this is a segregation of occupational groups within certain geographical areas, because of the tendency of certain ethnic groups to be concentrated within certain occupations. This also led to ethnic segregation, and was a source of conflict.

But what is the factor which creates occupational segregation for minority groups? According to Banfield's arguement (1974, pp. 61-63), it is not the effect of race, but rather that of class. In contrast, according to Jenks' analysis (1972, pp. 190-191), there are external factors which affected the ability or capacity of ethnic groups to achieve occupational equality.

A key factor affecting the future of the migrants group in urban-industrial society is social mobility. The process of migrant assimilation is fundamentally one of social mobility (Piore, 1979), and the degree of social integration tends to increase with class (Massey, 1981). In assessing the prospects for the migrants, an understanding of their social mobility and class status is therefore essential.

According to a survey on economy and the quality of life of the native peoples (Department of Civil Affairs, 1985), the occupations in which the native people are engaged do not differ much between city and mountain. The main difference is one of degree rather than kind. The native people in the mountain areas converged on agriculture and related areas; the native migrants in cities focused on manufacture, construction, and transportation. Most native migrants in cities are labor workers, with only a few in white-collar occupations. In this sense, migration to the native people means geographic mobility but not social mobility.

Social Discrimination

The Han people have long held a stereotyped attitude toward the native people which has led to discrimination against them. Recently, many efforts made by government and society have made progress toward alleviating some of the prejudices and misconception about this group. However, discrimination has not completely disappeared, but lingers on in the minds of the Han people.

At the same time, there is a deliberate policy of assimilation, which has not paid much respect for native people's culture and language. For most native people, the city has not benefited them much. Most are forced to live in slums or quatter settlements where they find themselves at a distinct cultural disadvantage.

In short, rural to urban migration is potenially stressful for any population, but especially in the case of ethnic minority groups, because it involves a change in culture. Change may disrupt the order of a person's life. In order to survive and develop, the native migrants must try to cope with this situation. How to deal with change or problem and reach an adaptation to the urban environment has no general rule that requires special techniques. It depends on what the native migrants are used to, what the native migrants expect, and whether the native migrants have been able in the past to expand their capacity to respond adequately to the stressors of the city (McElroy & Townsend, 1985).

Residential segregation, family life, occupational segregation, and social discrimination are among the most powerful forces impacting on the life satisfaction of ethnic minority group. Because not all adjustments guarantee the satisfaction of each individual, for some native migrants the effect is positive and for others it is negative. The degree of life satisfaction depends on how native migrants response to the stressors. Life satisfaction which native migrants acquired in turn influences how they perceive the stress and make further adjustments. Adjustment and life satisfaction thus form a circular process.

III. METHOD AND SOURCE OF DATA

This study attempts to examine the adaptation of native migrants to the conditions of urban life, but not to describe the native minority group as a whole. The individual is the unit of observation. In 1989 a native migrant sample was taken from the native people who lived in Taipei and Kaohsiung metropolitan areas. This is the source of data for the study.

Where to locate the sample is a key problem of investigating migrants. Fortunately, the household registration system which is well established in Taiwan provides us with a useful sampling framework. From the household rosters, which identified the native people in cities, a sample of 900 household units was randomly drawn. However, the roster does not precisely reflect where the migrants really lived. Too many empty households made it difficult for us to achieve the expected sample size, even when substitute samples were used. The final sample size we obtained was 731 units, in each of which the household heads were interviewed.

Among the interviewed native migrants, 58 percent are male and 42 percent female; their average age is 37 years old; 80 percent of them are married, 9 percent single, and ll percent other; 46 percent of them achieved elementary education, 18 percent junior high education, 16 percent senior high education, and only a few had higher levels of education; 64 percent of them engaged in manufactures, 12 percent clerical work, 10 percent personnel services, 5 percent agriculture, 4 percent management and administration, 4 percent salesworkers, and 0.3 percent professional; 9 percent of them have lived in cities for more than 30 years, 19 percent 10-20 years, and 68 percent moved to cities after 1970. These figures briefly describe the characteristics of the native migrants studied.

The data were collected through a structured interview survey. The questionnaire included questions about migration experience, family life, occupation, social relationships and activities, changes in lifestyle, adjustment for stress, and life satisfaction. Analytically, a principal component factor analysis was used to simplify scale items of adjustment and life satisfaction, and to extract from them the manipulatable dimensions to describe the migrants' adaptation. However, in order to observe the response of interviewees to each item in the dimension, percentage analysis is also undertaken. In addition, multi-regression analysis was used to identify the factors which are significantly related to adjustment and life satisfaction.

IV. RESEARCH FINDINGS

Adjustment of Urban Natives to Stress in Urban Life

In this investigation, the question: "When you meet with stress or an undesirable event, how do you solve it or adjust to it?" was used to measure adjustment. Fourteen variables were used to measure this dimension. Because adjustment has multiple approaches, the technique of principal

Table 1. Factor Analysis and Percentage Distribution of the Variables in the Measurement of Adjustment

		Distribution				
	Factor loading	*Percentage*				*No*
Dimension and variable	*coefficient*	*Never*	*Occasional*	*Often*	*Always*	*Answer*
Positive way of adjustment.						
1 Confer with family members, relatives or friends about a solution	.46204	6.0	33.0	45.1	14.8	1.1
2 Accept it, since it already occurred	.62880	9.4	31.9	41.7	15.2	1.8
3 Look it from another direction	.63596	8.8	42.0	39.1	6.7	3.4
4 Do my best to divert attention to a meaningful thing and activity	.70361	7.8	33.4	48.6	8.2	2.1
5 Cool down, then face the problem	.75811	3.1	27.6	54.7	12.3	2.2
6 Solve it by one's own ability	.63735	4.8	19.8	48.4	23.9	3.0
Explained variance = 22.1%						
Negative way of adjustment						
1 Don't believe that it is occurred	.60731	40.9	40.8	10.1	4.4	3.8
2 Reduce annoyance by smoking, drinking or drug	.60822	51.6	39.0	5.7	1.9	1.8
3 To hide the matter	.43630	23.4	54.2	15.2	4.7	2.6
4 Absent-mind and unable to concentrate thinking	.40029	27.4	54.0	14.1	1.6	2.9
5 To blame the matter on other	.71771	38.0	47.3	10.3	1.5	2.9
Explained variance = 14.8%						

Note: $N = 731$.

component factor analysis was used to derive factors or components from the variables. However, the analysis emphasizes the correlations of the variables with the components rather than their total variance. This resulted in four factors that explain 53 percent of the original variance. Because of the large explained variance, the first and second factors were taken to show the dimensions of adjustment in the study and factor loading coefficient over 0.4 were used to determine those variables to be included in each factor. The results are shown in Table 1. The variables included in the first factor show a common pattern of response to stress; that is, the native people sought adequate strategies to solve the problem but not to escape it. Thus, we called this dimension a positive way of adjustment. In the sense, the people can effectively use their resources to solve their problems and satisfy their personality needs.

On the other hand, the variables in the second factor indicate that another common pattern of response to stress is that the people rather escape the reality or blame others. We called this dimension a negative way of adjustment.

As shown earlier, the adjustment of native migrants to stress in the urban environment involves both positive and negative ways. But how do the native people use them? As shown in the percentages of the column of positive adjustments (Table 1), 60 percent of the respondents often dealt with problems through discussions or exchanging opinions; 57 percent of the respondents often accepted the reality or diverted their attention to more meaningful activities, 67 percent often cooled down, then faced the problem; and 70 percent used their own abilities to solve the problem. From these figures, it is clear that among the positive ways of adjustment, depending on one's own ability is the most popular, to cool down and face the problem next, and discussion third.

As for negative ways of adjustment, 14 percent of the respondents often denied the matter, 8 percent often reduced annoyance by smoking, drinking or using drugs; 20 percent often hide the matter; 16 percent were unable to concentrate their thinking;and 12 percent blamed others. Among those negative factors, hiding the matter is most popular, an absent-mind and unable to concentrate thinking next, and to deny the matter third. Overall these data clearly indicate that only a small portion of native migrants often used the negative way to adjust to stress. Both positive and negative ways were used by the native migrants to adjust to stress or to solve problems in urban life, but most people often used the positive way and most people only occasionally used the negative way.

Life Satisfaction of Urban Natives

In order to study the adaptation of native migrants to the urban environment, we used fifteen items or variables to construct a life satisfaction scale. The technique of principal component analysis was again applied to handle the empirical data, and again the variables with a factor loading coefficient over 0.4 were included in each dimension. The results are shown in Table 2. Two factors were identified. In the first factor, the variables clearly involve the native migrants with others. So we named this set of variables "social life" satisfaction variables. On the other hand, the second factor included variables that referred to a kind of mood, so we called this set of variables "psychological life" satisfaction variables.

Table 2. Factor Analysis and Percentage Distribution of Variables in the Measurement of Life Satisfaction

				Distribution	
	Factor loading	*Percentage*			*No*
Dimension and variable	*coefficient*	*Yes*	*No*	*Uncertainty*	*Answer*
Social life satisfaction					
1 Thing is better now than that was in hometown	.47107	66.3	10.9	21.3	1.4
2 I am happier now than was in hometown	.70930	49.5	15.7	32.8	1.9
3 Compared to other people my age in hometown, I make a good appearance	.49684	53.2	12.0	33.5	1.2
4 The present is one of my best time of my life	.74011	33.1	24.5	40.8	1.6
5 I get along with my family members now	.58909	57.6	11.2	28.6	2.6
Explained variance = 19.2%					
Psychological life satisfaction					
1 Most things I do now are boring or monotonous	.40447	25.7	49.4	23.0	1.9
2 I feel whatever I perform is good	.52514	34.5	18.7	44.3	2.5
3 I am often unhappy with Han people's criticism	.69648	54.7	26.8	16.4	1.9
4 Compared to other native people in cities, I often feel unhappy	.45181	9.2	65.7	22.8	2.1
Explained variance = 10.4					

Note: $N = 731$

Even though the adaptation achieved by native migrants in the urban environment can be classified into the categories of social life and psychological life, there remains the question as to what extent satisfaction has been achieved in each area of life. As shown in the percentages of social life in Table 2, it is found that except for the variable about the present being the best time of my life, most of the respondents said that they did things better, earned a better life, made a good appearance, and got along with family members better now than they did in their hometown. Nevertheless, one-fifth to one-third of the respondents, particular in the variable about the best time of my life, are not sure whether they have a better social life or not. Only a small portion of the respondents said no. Generally speaking, most native migrants did achieve a satisfied social life.

As regards psychological life, 66 percent of the respondents said they didn't often feel unhappy in comparison with the native peers in cities, only a few felt so; 49 percent of the respondents said the thimgs they do are not boring; 27 percent were not unhappy with Han people's criticism, 55 percent being unhappy; and 34 percent felt whatever they performed was good, 19 percent did not feel that way. Generally speaking, less than half of the native migrants achieved a satisfied psychological life. However, the fact that over half of the respondents said they often felt unhappy with Han people's criticism may suggest that social discrimination is an important obstacle in the development of adaptation in the psychological life of native migrants.

In short, life satisfaction the native migrants acquired by adequate adjustment varies with life dimensions. More native migrants have a satisfied social life rather than a satisfied psychological life. Social discrimination may be accountable for the difference.

The Effects of Social Factors on Adjustment and Life Satisfaction

Based on theoretical knowledge, the variables in regard to migration experience, family life, occupation, social activities, living arrangement and way of life are selected from our data as independent variables for adjustment and life satisfaction. The technique of multiple regression analysis is used to determine the significant variables which may affect adjustment and life satisfaction. The results are shown in Table 3.

Ten variables are significantly related to the positive way of adjustment. These are having more knowledge about cities, living in cities longer, having more visits from family members from ones hometown, a permanent job, an unfavorable attitude toward intermarriage, a feeling that urban life is better, a modern value orientation, no change in lifestyle, a shorter waiting period for feeling well physically and mentally, or a preference for hometown.

As for the negative ways of adjustment, the seven significant variables are having less knowledge about cities, having not got what expected, having been brought up in a traditional way, having been more visits from family members in one's hometown, being more satisfied with ones income, having experienced social discrimination, or not attending church.

As shown in Table 3, many variables are found to be significantly related to life satisfaction. In the aspect of social life, the significant variables are the length of living in cities, family members with first migration, present income, discrimination in the city, despised by Han people in the community, ownership of house, urban life, change in drinking habit, value orientation, and waiting period for feeling well physically and mentally.

Table 3. Beta Coefficients of a Multiple Regression Analysis with Adjustment and Life Satisfaction of the Native Migrants in Cities as the Dependent Variables Respectively

Independent variable (*in separated equation*)	*Adjustment* (*no*=0, yes=1)		*Life satisfaction* (*yes*=0, no=1)	
	Positive	*Negative*	*Social*	*Psycho*
Migration experience				
1 Understanding of cities (yes=0, no=1)	−.1900***	.1243**	.0846	.0240***
2 How many times did you since you first left home?	.0603	−.0760	.0707	.0755
3 Upon arriving in cities, do you get what you have first? (yes=0, no=1)	.0993	−.1127*	.0564	.0919
4 How long have you lived in cities?	−.1294**	−.0431	.1467**	.0725
Family life				
1 How your parents bring (tradition=1 to modern=6)	.0100	−.2648*	−.1184	.1753*
2 How many times your family members in home town come to visit you.	.2097*	.2027*	−.0344	−.1288
3 Your families moved with you in migration	−.0703	−.1433	.2686**	.0002
4 Send money to your family members in hometown (yes=0, no=1)	−.0967	.0101	.0948	.1148
5 How often your hometown's relatives and friends come to visit you.	−.0004	.0364	−.1626	−.2781**
Occupational life				
1 The present job is better than that in hometown (worse=1, same=2, better=3)	−.1228	.0156	.0374	−.0689
2 The present job is permanent (yes=0, no=1)	−.2523**	−.0211	.1298	.0428
3 There are the native in your work place (yes=0, no=1)	−.0565	.1394	.0720	.0237
4 How many times you change jobs since you left home	−.1065	.0593	.0428	−.0166
5 You satisfy with the present income (1=very satisfied to 5=very unsatisfied)	.1581	−.2623**	.2208**	.2581**
Social life				
1 You agree with inter- (score 1 to 5=very disagree)	.1578**	.0491	−.0112	.1684**
2 There is social discrimination in Taiwan society (yes=0, no=1)	−.0171	.1996**	.0292	−.1340*
3 How often you attend cities	−.0850	.2713***	.0292	−.1340*
4 How often you participation community activities	.0627	−.0345	−.0444	−.2100**
5 How often you are despised in cities (never=1, casual=2, often=3)	−.0467	−.0460	.2554**	−.2491**

(*continued*)

Table 3. Continued

Independent variable (in separated equation)	Adjustment (no=0, yes=1)		Life satisfaction (yes=0, no=1)	
	Positive	Negative	Social	Psycho
Living arrangement				
1 You are despised by Han people in your community (yes=0, no=1)	−.1045	.1376	−.1874**	−.1653**
2 How often you interact with your neighbors	.0220	.0642	.0310	−.1298*
3 You own the house (yes=0, no=1)	.0003	.0616	.1431**	.0326
4 Urban life is better than rural life (worse=1, same=2, better=3)	.3210***	−.1168	−.3613***	−.1468*
5 Your neighbors are the native people (yes=0, no=1)	.1318*	−.0878	−.0748	.0663
Changes in way of life				
1 You changed drinking habit (less=1, same=2, more=3)	.1517	.0193	.2085*	.0335
2 How much you change lifestyle (much=1, little=2, same=3)	.2278*	.0667	.0682	.1075
3 What is your value orientation (tradition=0, modern=1)	.2304**	.0684	−.4452***	−.2215*
4 How long you wait for feeling well physically and mentally	−.2146*	−.0521	.2313**	.2833**
5 Now you love hometown in particular (yes=0, no=1)	−.3244***	−.1165	−.0411	−.0450

Note: * p = 0.05,
** p = 0.01,
*** p =0.001

As for psychological life, it was found that if the native migrants have such social characteristics as having been brought up in a traditional way, receiving more visits from relatives and friends in hometown, a satisfied income, a favorable attitude toward intermarriage, no social discrimination, participation in community activities, not despised by the people in the urban life, not despised by Han people in the community, a better urban life, a modern value orientation, or a shorter period for feeling well physically and mentally, then they tend to have a psychological satisfaction with life.

Effect of Adjustment on Life Satisfaction

As a person attempts to deal with problems, he will initiate a series of changes or adjustments in the relationship between himself and the environment. An adequate adjustment will lead to life satisfaction.

As shown in Table 4, social life as a dependent variable in regression analysis has beta coefficients of −0.14760 with the positive ways of adjustment and

Table 4. Beta Coefficients of Regression Analysis with Life Satisfaction as the Dependent Variable and Adjustment as the Independent Variable

	Life Satisfaction	
Adjustment	*Social Life*	*Psychological Life*
Positive ways	−.14760	−.25222
Negative ways	−.18719	−.17564

Note: All beta coefficients are at the significant level of less than 0.05

−0.18791 with the negative ways of adjustment effect life satisfaction, and the effect of negative ways is more important than that of positive ways.

As for psychological life, the beta coefficients with positive and negative ways of adjustment are -0.25222 and -0.17564 respectively. This indicates that both positive and negative ways of adjustment affect psychological life satisfaction, with the effect of positive ways being more important than that of negative ways.

As shown in the analysis, both positive and negative ways of adjustment used by the native migrants to deal with stress or problems in urban life effect life satisfaction or adaptation, but positive ways of adjustment are more important to psychological life satisfaction and negative ways are more important to social life satisfaction.

Some of the major findings may be summarized as follows. (1) The native migrants used both positive and negative ways to adjust to stress in urban environment. with positive ways, being used more often than negative ways; (2) Generally speaking, most native migrants achieved a satisfied social life, but a smaller portion of them achieved a satisfied psychological life. This seems to indicate that it is easier to achieve a satisfied social life than a satisfied psychological life; (3) Many social factors influence the native migrants' ways of adjustment to urban stress. The important factors for positive ways are more knowledge about cities, more visits from family members in hometown, a permanent job, a better urban life, not much change in lifestyle, a modern value orientation, a shorter waiting period for feeling well physically and mentally, and a preference for hometown. The more important factors for negative ways are having been brought up in a traditional way, more visits from family members in hometown, satisfied with income, without attending church, and not despised by Han people in the community; (4) Many social factors were found to effect life satisfaction. The important factors related to a satisfied social life are moving with family members in migration, satisfied with income, no discrimination in urban life, a better urban life, no change in drinking habits, modern value orientation, and a shorter waiting period for feeling well physically and mentally. As for a satisfied psychological life, the important factors are more visits from relatives, no discrimination in urban life, modern value orientation, and a shorter waiting period for feeling well physically and mentally; and (5) Finally, the ways the native migrants used to adjust to stress in urban environment have much affect on their life satisfaction. Both positive and negative ways of adjustment can achieve a satisfied social and psychological lives, but positive ways are more important to a satisfied psychological life and negative ways are more important to a satisfied social life.

V. EXPLANATION AND DISCUSSION

The findings from our data imply certain ideas and problems which need to be explained and discussed.

1. As noted above, the native migrants used both the positive and negative ways to adjust to stress or problems they encountered in the urban environment. Both of them led to life satisfaction. We usually tend to think of negative ways as a negative effect, because the term bears on the denying of fact and a conflict mood. In fact, the problems the people encountered vary in nature and extent. Each may require special coping techniques during a period of adjustment. For individuals to remain reasonably satisfied over the course of life, they must undergo slight change in the ways they think of themselves or their environment. But modification or change in a stressful environment can assume different forms. As far as techniques are concerned, adjusting is neutral in nature, and their effects depend on if they fit the nature of the problem which needs to be solved. Thus, they can be either positive or negative. If the adjusting way, whether positive or negative, can solve problems or eliminate stress, it can lead to satisfaction in life. Otherwise, both of them result in frustration. Even though the negative ways of adjustment can produce a satisfied effect, it may also incur anxiety and disturbance. That may be the reason why most native migrants use it only occasionally.

2. In the adjusting process, the social characteristics a person possesses significantly influence whether he uses positive or negative ways. As shown in our data, such social characteristics as more knowledge about cities, living in cities longer, more visits from family members in hometown, a permanent job, a better life, no change in lifestyle, modern value orientation, shorter waiting period for feeling well physically and mentally, and preference for hometown, tend to lead the native migrants to use positive ways of adjustment. And the characteristics like less knowledge about cities, brought up in a traditional way, more visits from family members in hometown, satisfied with income, social discrimination, and not attending church, tend to lead the native migrants to use negative ways of adjustment. In contrast, except for the variable about visits from family members in ones hometown, which not only gives

the native migrants social support but also prevents them from developing social relationships in cities, the social characteristics which are related to the positive or the negative ways are quite different. It may be inferred from this that the more social integration the native migrants have, the more they tend to use the positive ways of adjustment; the less social integration the native migrants have, the more they tend to use negative ways of adjustment. In this sense, the integration unnecessarily excluded the original way of life. In short, both modification and preservation in way of life occurred in the adjusting process, and contributed to the special coping techniques used; how the native migrants use an adjusting strategy will depdend on their cognitive development and the problem encountered.

3. Most native migrants achieved a satisfied life, but social life is more satisfactory than psychological life. This is because psychological satisfactions are rooted in social factors as well as in internal psychological needs (Hendricks & Hendricks, 1977, p. 151). In this sense, a satisfied social life contributes to a satisfied psychological life.

In recent decades, the development in Taiwanese society has greatly increased productivity, job opportunities, incomes and overall standards of living; however, for the mountain society, development has been slower and they have experienced many problems like poverty, unemployment, and lower education. Many factors pushed the native people to leave their hometown, and they were pulled toward cities. Most of them were young and in good health, and voluntarily emigrated for a better life in cities, so they were in a better position to accommodate to the new environment.

There are many jobs available in the cities, particularly labor and semi-skilled, and the native migrants easily can get a good paying job and live a better life, then quickly settle down in the city. On the other hand, migration may break down the families and causes a disruption in social network. But as shown in our data, most native migrants moved with their family members, particularly wife and children. Some of those who did not bring families in migration get them together as soon as they settled down. Further, improvements in transportation now make it more convenient for the migrants and their family members or friends in the hometown to visit each other. Therefore, the native migrants have not been deprived of their demand for attachment the lack of which could produce an emotional and social loneliness in the cities. These societal circumstances in urban Taiwan can be a source of positive influence which are capable of increasing the problem management capacities for the migrants.

The mountain culture may be among the most powerful forces impacting on satisfaction. Traditionally, the aborigine tribes in Taiwan were organized by clan and territory: an aborigine society might have a clan group and a territorial group, but both of them might or might not coincide. A territorial group may not exclude other clans or tribes; its purpose is to protect from invasion or attack by outside forces in certain areas. This organization may be capable of satisfying the requirements of urban life. On the other hand, the clan and the extended family was emphasized in the mountain society, but they were rather limited to economic production, defense and religious rites. As for family life, emphasis was placed on the nuclear type of family, that is, the couple and children or parents. Thus, family life centered on individuals, then extended outward for a large family. The large family and small family coexisted in the mountain society. However, in order to meet the requirement of nomadic life, the small family could easily separate from the large family and become an independent family anytime. As a result, the small or nuclear family prevailed in many aborigine tribes such as Tayal, Paiwan, Yamis, and Rukai. The children formed their own family immediately after marriage (Chiang, 1986, p. 498). This kind of family life coincides with the urbanized Taiwanese.

Certain cultures may also be a source of negative influence. In the mountain society, some religious beliefs, are fused in economic and social activities, which may conflict with modern economic activities. Being strictly obedient to taboos will result in a negative effect which can produce psychological pressure and a disruption in adaptation, for instance, stopping work at a long mourning. Nevertheless, their belief system comprises myths, ceremonies and rites, and its core is spirits—gods and ghosts—which still powerfully influence ones actual life. This belief system may be a strong force impacting on life satisfaction, but whether positive or negative is unknown.

For a long time now, there has been discrimination against the native people in Taiwan. Although this attitude has weakened with Taiwan's socioeconomic development, it has not disappeared. For instance, the cheaper labor provided by the native migrants in economic activities may suppress or work against the discrimination, but there is no such force to reduce the stress in social activities. Thus far it can be the most powertful source of negative influence.

As shown in our evaluation of societal circumstances, more positive forces than negative forces significantly influence the lives of native migrants. As a result, most native migrants are able to achieve a satisfied life.

4. Many social forces contributed to a satisfied social life as well as a satisfied psychological life. The factors contributing to satisfactory social life and psychological life are not clearly separated. The factors particularly related to social life are family members with migration, a better urban life, and no change in drinking habits. They may show that as the native migrants adjusted to the stress on the urban environment, they get satisfaction from family life and social gatherings, which are the important feature of their cultural life. The Han people usually see the native's drinking as bad behavior, but it is just the Han people's prejudice against the native people. Indeed, drinking can be an important factor related to the native people's life satisfaction in the urban environment. As for psychological life, the major factors here are more visits from hometown relatives and friends, a favorable attitude toward

intermarriage, and participating in community activities. It is shown that a satisfied psychological life depends on social participation. In addition, being satisfied with ones income, modern value orientation, shorter waiting period for feeling well physically and mentally, no discrimination in cities, and not despised by Han people in communities, significantly influence both social life and psychological life. They may indicate that income, social discrimination, value orientation, and a waiting period for feeling well physically and mentally are the most important sources of life satisfaction. Particular in the waiting period for feeling well physically and mentally, if this period can be shorter, the migrants will more easily attain satisfaction or adaptation. This author has tested this hypothesis in another study on social adaptation of urban migrants (Hsieh, 1985).

5. Adjustment involves both positive and negative ways. Even though both of them can lead to a satisfied life, they will make different contributions to different aspects of life. Because the negative ways of adjustment may lead to anxiety and disturbance, they may not be an adequate way to be used in achieving psychological life satisfaction. Contrarily there are many conflicting circumstances in social life, perhaps negative ways will work better in this situation. Although the positive ways of adjustment increase psychological burden less, they may not effectively deal with the uncertain circumstances, so they may work better in psychological life than social life.

VI. CONCLUSION

The adjusting process is a normal part of life and happens to any population, but adjusting ways vary individually and culturally. As we found from the data in this research, the native migrants used both positive and negative ways to adjust to stress in an urban environment, but the positive ways of adjustment were used more often. However, which way of adjustment the native migrants used is significantly impacted by their social characteristics. As shown in our data, the social factors that influence positive ways or negative ways are different, but most important is the problem of social integration. Therefore, the more the native migrants have a social integration, the more the native migrants use the positive ways of adjustment; the less social integration the native migrants have, the more they use the negative ways of adjustment.

While it was found from our data that most native migrants have achieved a satisfied life in cities, there is a different degree of satisfaction in social and psychological dimensions of life, specifically, social life is more satisfied than psychological life.

There are many powerful social forces affecting life satisfaction. Some social factors, for example, family migration, better urban life, and social gatherings are particularly important to social life satisfaction; other social factors, for example, interaction with relatives and friends in hometown, participation in community activities, and a favorable attitude toward intermarriage especially contribute to psychological life satisfaction. In the sense, social factors, like internal factors, are the base of psychological life.

However, many social factors have a positive effect on social and psychological dimensions of life. Most important of these are income, social discrimination, value orientation, and waiting period for feeling well physically and mentally. Thus, it may be concluded that the more the native migrants acquired a satisfactory income, they did not suffer from social discrimination, had a modern value orientation, and waited a shorter period for feeling well physically and mentally, the more they attained both social and psychological life satisfactions.

Whatever ways of adjustment the native migrants use to adapt to an urban environment seems to be impacted by the positive or negative sociocultural circumstances which prevail in urban Taiwan society. Even though both of them can lead to a satisfied life, they will make different contributions to different aspects of life. Since the negative ways of adjustment may incur anxiety and disturbance, they may not be used to achieve a psychological life satisfaction. Contrarily, there are many conflict situations in social life; perhaps negative ways may work better in these situations. Although the positive ways of adjustment increase psychological burden less, they may not effectively deal with conflict situation, so it may work better in psychological life than social life.

REFERENCES

Benfield, E.C. (1974). *The Unheavenly City Revisited* (pp. 61-63). Boston: Little, Brown.

Chang, M.-K. (1989). The preservation and development of aboriginal cultures in the development of national park. In *Report on the Planning of Lan-Yu National Park*. Taipei: Institute of Ethnology, Acadeia Sinica.

Chang, H-C. (1974). The investigation of migrants adaptation in Taipei city. *Journal of Sociology*. Department, N.T.U.

Chen, I-M. (1987). Do you understand him? *Time Weekly Magazine*, No. 476, Taipei.

Chiang, L-Y. (1986). *The Study of Aboriginal Family in Taiwan*. Taipei: Chien-Hua Publisher Co.

Department of Civil Affairs, T.P.G. (1985). *A Survey on the Economy and Life Quality of Taiwan Aborigine*. Taichung.

Fu, Yang-Chih. (1987). The socio-economic status and socio-psychological state. A paper presented in the Conference for Urban Welfare Problem and Development in a Changing Society. Taipei: Bureau of Social Affairs, Taipei Municipal Government.

Gordon, M. M. (1964). *Assimilation in American Life* (p. 276). New York: Oxford University Press.

Hendricks J. & C. D. Hendericks. (1977). *Aging in Mass Society*. Cambridge, MA: Winthrop Publishers.

Hsieh, K-C. (1985). *Urban Migration and Social Adjustment: A Case Study of Kaohsiung City.* Taipei: Chi-Liu Publishers Co.

Hsu, M-C. (1988). The cultural identification movement of Taiwan native people. A paper presented in the Conference for New Social Movements in Taiwan. National Ching-Hua University.

Hwang, Mei-Yin. (1987). Urban adaptation and human rights of the aboriginal migrants. In Chinese Human Rights Association, (Eds.), *Traditional Socio-Cultures and Human Rights of Taiwan Aborigines.* Taipei: Ta-Chia Publishers.

Hwang, M.-Y. & P.-H. Liu. (1989). National Lang-Yu ecological and Ya-meei cultural study center. In *Report on the Planning of Lan-Yu National Park.* Taipei: Institute of Ethnology, Academia Sinica.

Jenks, C. (1972). *Inequality* (pp. 190-191). New York: Basic Books.

Kitagawa, D. (1965). Assimilation or pluralism? In A. M. Rose & Carolin B. Rose (eds.), *Minority Problems.* Harper & Row.

Lieberson, S. (1963). *Ethnic Patterns in American Cities.* New York: Free Press.

Lee, I-Y. (1978). *The Modernized Adaptation of Aborigine Tribes in Cities.* Institute of Ethnology, Academia Sinica.

Lee, I-Y. (1983). *Report on Research and Evaluation of the Aboriginal Administration and Policy.* Institute of Ethnology, Academia Sinica.

Lin, K-P. (1980). *Survey on Living Conditions of Aboriginal Inhabitants in Taipei Metropolitan Area.*

Massey, D.S. (1981). Dimensions of the new immigration to the United States and the prospects for assimilation. *Annual Review of Sociology*, (7): 57-85.

McElroy, A. & P. K. Townsend. (1985). *Medical Anthropology in Ecological Perspective.* London: Westview Press.

Philpott, S. B. (1970). The implications of migration for sending societies: some theoretical considerations. *Migration and Anthropology: Proceedings of the. 1970 Annual Spring Meeting.*

Taipei County Records Committee. (1988). *The Annals of Taipei County.* (7) Folkway.

Tu, Y-S. (1986). How much we understand the aborigine tribes' life. *Social Welfare.* Bureau of Social Affairs, T. M. G.

Wilson, R. A. & A. Schutz. (1978). *Urban Sociology.* Englewood Cliffs, NJ: Prentice-Hall.

Wu, H-C. (1988). *A Study on the Rural-Urban Migration and Life of A-Mei Tribe.* Taipei: Institute of Geography, National Taiwan Normal University.

Yu, K-H. (1989). The preservation and development of Ya-Meei cultures. *Report on the Planning of Lan-Yu National Park.* Institute of Ethnology, Academia Sinica.

THE IMPACT OF CHRONIC DISEASES ON QUALITY OF LIFE AMONG THE ELDERLY IN TAIWAN

Jersey Liang, Shwu-Chong Wu,
and Ching-Yeh Chiang

I. INTRODUCTION

The significance of quality of life has been increasingly recognized in both basic and applied research related to health, health care, and aging. Outcomes of diseases, clinical trials, and treatments are now frequently defined in terms of behavioral and psychosocial consequences in addition to survival and biomedical parameters. This recognition is underscored by the observation that treatments given to patients with chronic conditions account for the majority of health care expenditures in societies with an aging population (Rice, Hageson, & Kopstein, 1985). The objectives of health care are therefore to influence socially and individually relevant health and quality of life (Ware, 1984). Accordingly, measures of the behavioral and psychosocial impact of diseases are critical in evaluating the causes and consequences of changes in

Research in Human Capital and Development, Volume 7, pages 53-68.

ISBN: 1-55938-132-9

individual and population health. In addition, these outcomes are meaningful to and highly valued by patients. Knowledge of the impact of diseases on quality of life is particularly useful in assessing the effects of health policies and programs, in allocating resources to underserved segments of the population, and in projecting demand for health services (Stewart, Greenfield, Hays, Wells, Rogers, Berry, McGlynn, & Ware, 1989).

Ware and his associates have provided a useful framework describing the impact of disease on quality of life (Stewart et al., 1989; Tarlov et al., 1989; Ware, 1984). Conceptualized as distinct and heterogenous entities, diseases are assumed to influence four aspects of quality of life including personal functioning, mental health, general health perception, and role functioning. Personal functioning is defined as the capacity to perform tasks of daily living including self-care, mobility, and other physical activities. Mental health consists of psychological distress and well-being. The former refers to psychiatric symptoms, whereas the latter denotes a sense of satisfaction and happiness. General health perception or self-reported health status encompasses an individual's evaluation of personal health in terms of diseases, personal functioning, and mental health. It is a powerful predictor of individual differences in health and illness behavior and survival. Finally, role functioning refers to the health-related capacity to perform significant social roles including formal employment, school work, or homemaking.

There have been numerous studies of the behavioral and psychosocial consequences of diseases. As observed by Stewart and her associates (1989), most earlier studies focused on a single disease, without taking into account the impact of other co-existing conditions. The conceptualization of quality of life was relatively underdeveloped. Most samples were small and nonrepresentative, and comparison groups were often not available. Recently, significant progress in the study of disease impact on quality of life has been made. Several studies, involving large representative samples, multivariate analyses, the assessment of the effects of co-morbidity, and improved conceptualization of quality of life, have emerged (e.g., Guralnik, LaCroix, Everett, & Kovar, 1989; Seeman, Guralnik, Kaplan, Knudsen, & Cohen, 1989; Stewart et al., 1989; Verbrugge, Lepkowski, & Inmanaka, 1989).

While significant progress has been made in research concerning the impact of diseases on quality of life, the current literature is limited in several aspects. First, most investigators have relied on a single-equation approach, and only direct effects can be estimated. Although the interrelationships among various chronic diseases and other factors are recognized, the causal linkages among them have rarely been explicitly specified and examined. Consequently, indirect effects are often overlooked and misleading conclusions may result. In addition, in most previous studies, measurement errors were not adjusted when parameter estimates were derived. This can lead to biased estimates.

Second, most studies of the relationships between chronic diseases and disability among the aged were based on data collected in the United States and other western developed nations (Guralnik et al., 1989; Manton, 1990; Seeman, et al., 1989; Verbrugge et al., 1989). Research utilizing data obtained from non-western cultures can yield important insights concerning the generalizability of previous findings. Should the results from western and non-western societies diverge from each other, this may suggest that important factors are omitted from the current analytical framework and/or the existence of alternative causal mechanisms depending on the cultural context.

This present research examines the impact of some 12 chronic diseases on two major dimensions of quality of life: functional status and self-rated health. Data for this study came from the 1989 Survey of Health and Living Status of the Elderly in Taiwan which involved a probability sample of 4,049 respondents age 60 and over in Taiwan. Direct as well as indirect effects of chronic diseases on the quality of life were estimated by utilizing a structural equation approach.

II. MODEL SPECIFICATIONS

The impact of chronic diseases on quality of life was analyzed within the context of two structural models which differ in the specifications of chronic conditions. In the first model (M_1), 13 chronic conditions are specified in order to assess their relative effects on functional status and self-rated health. In the second model (M_2), chronic conditions are measured by a single-indicator composite which is a count of total number of conditions. In M_2, the combined effect of all chronic conditions on the quality of life can be assessed.

Figure 1 presents a diagram of the proposed disaggregated model. In order to simplify the figure, only linkages among the latent variables are presented. Measurement specifications associated with the latent variables are omitted. In Figure 1, the ξs (xis) refer to the latent exogenous variables whereas ηs (etas) refer to the latent endogenous variables. The βs (betas) and γs (gammas) refer to structural coefficients or direct effects associated with ηs and ξs. The notations used here are in accordance with the LISREL conventions suggested by Jöreskog and Sörbom (1988).

According to M_1, chronic diseases have direct effects on the quality of life which consists of functional status and self-rated health. In particular, 13 types of chronic conditions, $\eta 1$ to $\eta 13$, are specified. These include arthritis, stroke, high blood pressure, diabetes, circulation trouble, heart trouble, respiratory disease, digestive disease, skeletal disease, eye disorder, visual impairment, hearing impairment, and others. In addition, self-rated health ($\eta 15$) is also directly affected by functional status ($\eta 14$). Finally, all chronic conditions, functional status, and self-rated health are affected by three exogenous

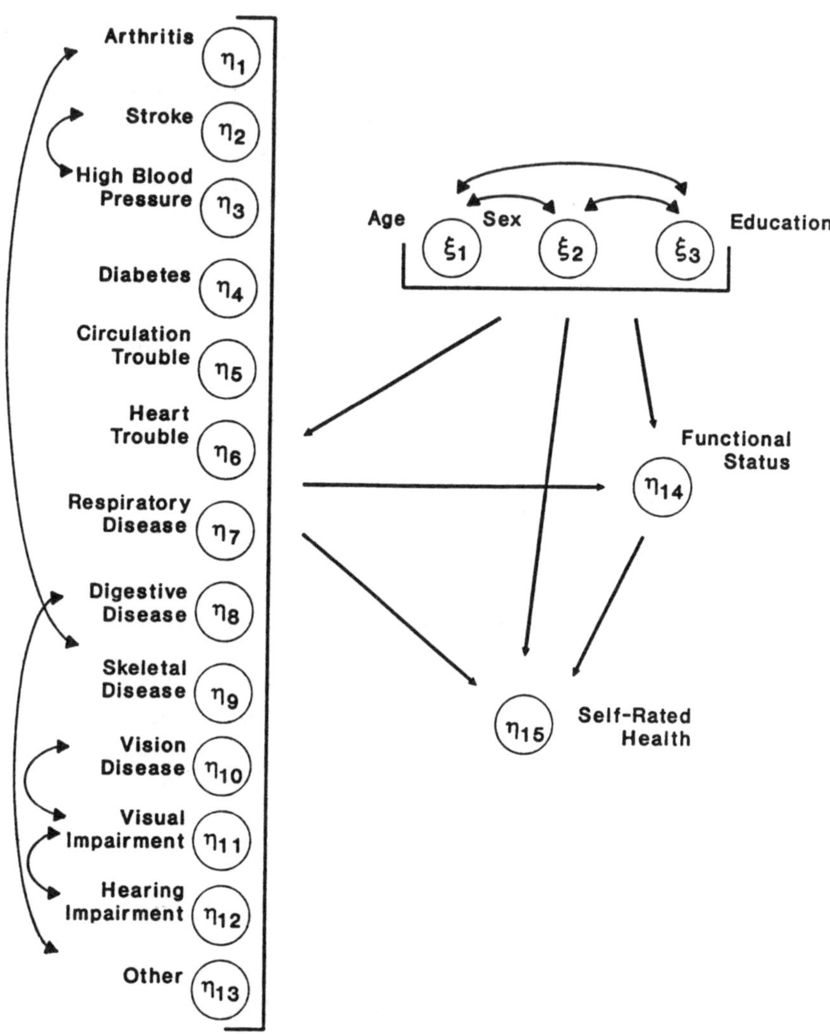

Figure 1. The Disaggregated Model of Self-Reported Physical Health

variables: age (ξ1), sex (ξ2), and education (ξ3). The rationale for these specifications can be found in earlier works by Ware (1984), Liang (1986), and Liang, Bennett, Whitelaw, & Maeda (1991).

Within M_1, correlations among all 13 chronic conditions were initially assumed. However, only five pairs of statistically significant correlations

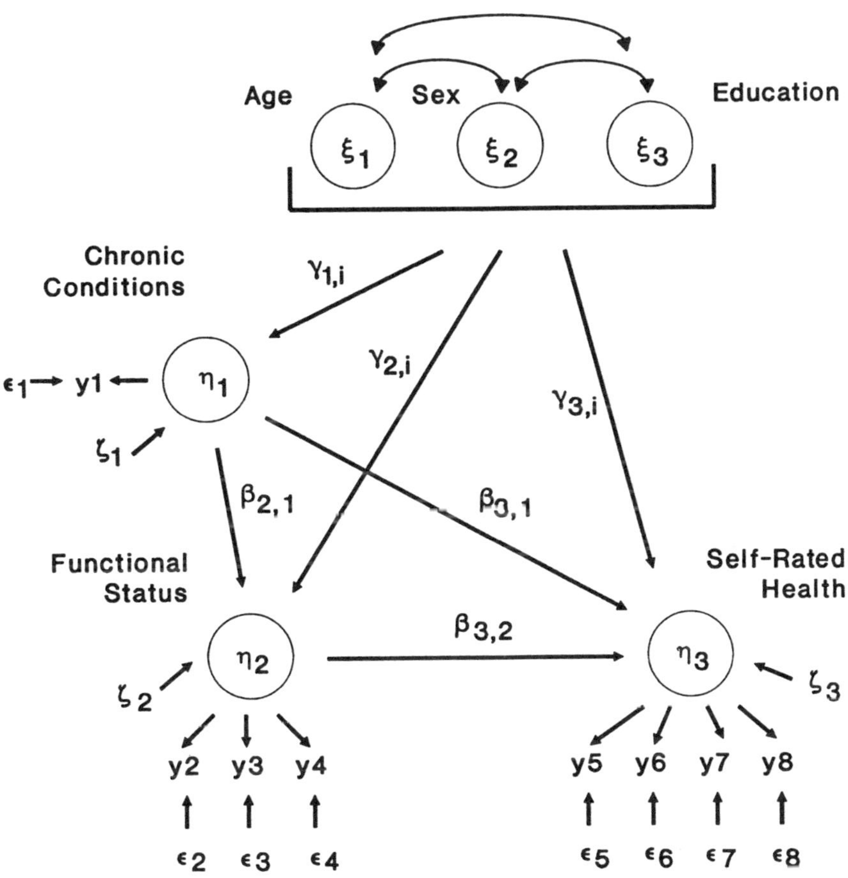

Figure 2. Composite Model of Self-Reported Physical Health

among the chronic conditions were identified on the basis of preliminary analyses. Whereas the correlations involving (1) arthritis and skeletal disease, (2) vision disease and visual impairment, and (3) stroke and hypertension are not surprising, the co-prevalence between (a) digestive disease and other chronic diseases, and (b) visual and hearing impairments are difficult to explain.

Figure 2 presents a diagram of M_2 in which chronic diseases are specified as a composite of 13 types of conditions. In comparison with M_1, this model is considerably simplified, and enables one to estimate the overall effects of diseases on the quality of life.

III. DATA AND METHODS

Survey Design

Data for this research came from the 1989 Survey of Health and Living Status of the Elderly in Taiwan. This survey involved a national sample with 4,412 respondents aged 60 and over, selected through multi-stage probability sampling procedure. The first stage consisted of a stratified sample of the different types of administrative units (referred to generically as townships). Blocks (lins) in the selected townships served as clusters in the second stage. Each stage was selected proportional to population size. Two respondents were selected systematically from the register in each selected lin. Selected respondents who were not residing at their register address were interviewed at their current location, anywhere in Taiwan.

Personal interviews were conducted to collect data covering background and marital history, household composition and social support, health, occupational history, activities and general attitudes, residence history, economics and financial well-being, and emotional and instrumental support. Overall, the 4,049 completed interviews constitute a response rate of 91.8 percent. Given that measures of self-rated health were analyzed in the study, proxy respondents were excluded. After excluding proxy interviews, the remaining 3,736 respondents constituted the total sample of this research.

Measurement

Chronic conditions were mostly measured by self-reports of medically confirmed diseases. In total, 13 types of conditions were included. Seven diseases were dummy coded. They were arthritis, high blood pressure, diabetes, circulation trouble, heart trouble, respiratory problems, and stroke. Eye disorder was assessed by a simple count of "yes" responses to cataract, glaucoma, and other eye diseases. Similarly, digestive disease was a composite of liver or gall bladder problems and ulcer or gastrointestinal, or other digestive tract disorders. Skeletal disease was a composite of spur formation or sciatica pain, broken bone, and missing limbs. Visual and hearing impairments were measured by 5-point scales of one's self-assessment of those abilities. Finally, the category of "other conditions" was measured by the summation of the presence of thyroid disease, high blood cholesterol, anemia, constipation, kidney disease, prostate trouble, other urinary tract disorders, and skin disorders. Reliabilities of self-reported chronic conditions were assumed to be .64 on the basis of previous research (Elinson, 1988).

Functional status was indexed by activities of daily living (ADL), instrumental activities of daily living (IADL), and physical fitness. ADL was measured by one item, "difficulty in bathing." IADL was a composite of five items: shopping, managing money, using the telephone, doing heavy work in or around the house, and taking a bus or train. Physical fitness was a composite of 7 items including: climbing 2-3 flights of stairs, walking about 200-300 meters, lifting or carrying 25 lbs, crouching, reaching up over one's head, using fingers to grasp or handle, and standing or being on one's feet for about 2 hours.

Self-rated health was measured by four indicators including (1) self-evaluation of present health, (2) comparison of present health with previous health, (3) comparison of one's health with those of one's peers, and (4) general health satisfaction. All items were coded such that a high score reflects poorer health.

The three exogenous variables, age, sex, and education, were measured by self-reported single indicators. Age and education were measured in years. Sex was coded as a dummy variable. According to the estimates derived from the 1970 U.S. Census (U.S. Bureau of Census, 1975) and our own sensitivity analysis, reliabilities for age, sex, and education were fixed at .8, .9, and .7 respectively.

Data Analysis

The proposed models were evaluated by using LISREL 7 (Jöreskog and Sörbom, 1988). As a widely used statistical software for structural equation modeling, LISREL involves a confirmatory factor analytic model that simultaneously deals with measurement errors and causal specifications. In addition, data analyses were replicated to minimize the capitalization of chance. Specifically, the total sample was randomly divided into four subsamples. One subsample was analyzed first for exploratory purposes to develop a model of acceptable fit. The analysis was subsequently replicated by using the other three subsamples. Thus, in addition to the statistical significance tests, convergent findings from multiple replications further reinforce one's confidence in the robustness of the results.

After excluding cases with missing data on any one indicator involved in the model evaluation, the effective sample size ranged from 1,820 to 1,827. Table 1 presents descriptive statistics for the total sample ($N = 3{,}736$) and effective sample ($N = 3{,}647$) used in the analyses. The characteristics of the total sample differ little from those of the effective sample. Thus, biases due to the selective effects of missing item data are not plausible.

IV. FINDINGS

Table 2 presents the standardized maximum likelihood estimates and measures of fit associated with the desegregated model. Three measures were applied

Table 1. Descriptive Statistics for Items in the Analysis for Total and Effective Sample

Item	*Total Sample* ($N = 3736$)	*Effective Sample* ($N = 3647$)
Age		
Mean	68.53	68.52
SD	6.43	6.34
Sex		
% female	42.3	42.4
Education in years		
Mean	3.18	3.87
SD	54.51	4.58
Arthritis		
% yes	29.6	29.7
Stroke		
% yes	3.0	3.0
High blood pressure		
% yes	26.2	26.2
Diabetes		
% yes	8.0	8.1
Circulation trouble		
% yes	19.0	19.1
Heart trouble		
% yes	21.6	21.9
Respiratory disease		
% yes	17.9	18.2
Digestive disease		
% yes	27.6	27.9
Skeletal disease		
% yes	25.2	25.4
Vision disease		
% yes	40.9	40.9
Visual impairment		
% very or quite well	60.2	60.1
Hearing impairment		
% very or quite well	76.4	76.3
Other disease		
% yes	38.6	38.8
Present Health		
% excellent or very good	39.6	38.4
Health compared to others		
% better or about the same	80.3	80.3
Health compared to last year		
% better or about the same	57.5	57.4
Satisfaction with health		
% very or completely satisfied	45.8	45.7
ADL difficulty		
% no	96.3	96.4

(*continued*)

Table 1. Continued

Item	*Total Sample* ($N = 3736$)	*Effective Sample* ($N = 3647$)
IDAL difficulty		
Mean	1.51	1.50
SD	2.89	2.87
Fitness Difficulty		
Mean	2.62	2.62
SD	4.04	4.01
Condition composite		
Mean	2.83	2.85
SD	2.30	2.30

in assessing the overall fit of the model. With 166 degrees of freedom, the likelihood ratios in all four subsamples vary from 664.13 to 737.81, indicating a probability of less than .001. These reflect a poor fit of the model to the data in all four subsamples.

Given that the likelihood ratio is very sensitive to sample size, measures of fit adjusted for sample size are more appropriate. Two such measures are the Goodness-of-Fit Index (GFI) and Adjusted Goodness-of-Fit Index (AGFI) devised by Jöreskog and Sörbom (1988). AGFI is GFI adjusted for the degree of freedom (Bollen, 1989). The GFIs and AGFIs vary from .865 to .930. These are considered to be of reasonable goodness-of-fit by most standards. Thus, the fit of the desegregated model is supported by these overall fit measures from the four subsamples.

Parameter estimates are consistent with the measurement specifications associated with functional status and self-rated health (M_1). Specifically, all estimates of factor loadings on functional status and self-rated health are statistically significant at the .05 level, and are in the expected direction.

With reference to the causal linkages among exogenous variables (i.e., age, sex, and education), the results of chronic conditions, functional status, and self-rated health, can be summarized as follows. First, stroke, disorders of circulatory system, and visual impairment have been shown to have a significant effect on functional impairment. Relatively speaking, stroke tends to have the largest effect, followed by visual impairment and circulatory disease. Whereas the effects of stroke and visual impairment on functional impairment are statistically significant in all four samples, the effect of circulatory disease is significant in three out of the four subsamples. Second, arthritis, high blood pressure, digestive disease, eye disorder, hearing impairment, and diseases in the "other category" fail to show a statistically significant effect on functional status in at least three out of the four subsamples. Third, evidence concerning the effects of diabetes, heart disease, respiratory disease, and skeletal disease is inconclusive in that their effects were significant in only two out of the four

Table 2. Standardized Maximum Likelihood Estimates and Measures of Fit for the Disaggregated Model of Self-Reported Physical Health

	Sample 1 (N=920)	*Sample 2* (N=907)	*Sample 3* (N=903)	*Sample 4* (N=917)
Effect (βs) *of Chronic conditions* (η_1 - η_{13}) *on Functional Status* (η_{14}):				
η_1 Arthritis	.000+	.059+	.035+	.042+
η_2 Stroke	.275	.358	.428	.212
η_3 High Blood Pressure	.011+	−.064+	−.025+	−.032+
η_4 Diabetes	.039+	.098	.075	−.012+
η_5 Circulation Trouble	.099	.162	.080	.049+
η_6 Heart Trouble	−.020+	.019+	.090	.114
η_7 Respiratory Disease	.021+	.146	.089	−.001+
η_8 Digestive Disease	.015+	−.003+	−.030+	.004+
η_9 Skeletal Disease	.150	.134	.030+	.062+
η_{10} Vision Disease	−.080+	−.097+	−.087+	−.075+
η_{11} Visual Impairment	.350	.326	.270	.275
η_{12} Hearing Impairment	.010+	−.021+	.040+	−.063+
η_{13} Other	−.004+	.041+	.043+	.104
Effect (βs) *of Chronic Conditions* (η_1 - η_{13}) *on Self-rated Health* (η_{15}):				
η_1 Arthritis	.059+	.125	.083	−.015+
η_2 Stroke	−.004+	.064+	.100	.005+
η_3 High Blood Pressure	.072	.035+	.061+	.111
η_4 Diabetes	.086	.123	.060+	.138
η_5 Circulation Trouble	.203	.143	.058+	.100
η_6 Heart Trouble	.127	.174	.270	.166
η_7 Respiratory Disease	.159	.124	.097	.176
η_8 Digestive Disease	.143	.082	.090	.160
η_9 Skeletal Disease	.074+	.075	.096+	.074+
η_{10} Vision Disease	−.010+	−.083+	−.087	.000+
η_{11} Visual Impairment	.129+	.271	.301	.270
η_{12} Hearing Impairment	.109+	.122	.042+	.100+
η_{13} Other	.122	.142	.092	.104
Effect (β) *of Functional Status* (η_{14}) *on:*				
η_{15} Self-rated Health	.378	.327	.299	.289
Effect (γs) *of Age* (ξ_1) *on*				
η_1 Arthritis	.053+	.082+	−.015+	.041+
η_2 Stroke	.042+	.027+	−.049+	.061+
η_3 High Blood Pressure	.092	.056+	−.116	.007+
η_4 Diabetes	.003+	.064+	−.075+	−.060+
η_5 Circulation Trouble	.166	.190	.017+	.116
η_6 Heart Trouble	.075+	.064+	−.034+	.094
η_7 Respiratory Disease	.115	.023+	.051+	.143
η_8 Digestive Disease	−.047+	−.006+	−.054+	.030+
η_9 Skeletal Disease	.078+	.027+	.005+	−.009+
η_{10} Vision Disease	.186	.179	.090+	.134
η_{11} Visual Impairment	.293	.321	.184	.262
η_{12} Hearing Impairment	.501	.402	.293	.367
η_{13} Other	.157	.168	−.005+	.093
η_{14} Functional Status	.321	.251	.275	.350
η_{15} Self-rated Health	−.190	−.169	−.131	−.193

(*continued*)

Table 2. Continued

	Sample 1 (N=920)	*Sample 2* (N=907)	*Sample 3* (N=903)	*Sample 4* (N=917)
Effect (γs) *of Sex* (ξ_2) *on*				
η_1 Arthritis	.161	.131	.117	.174
η_2 Stroke	−.026+	−.036+	−.027+	−.052+
η_3 High Blood Pressure	.097	.143	.075+	.178
η_4 Diabetes	.124	.122	.131	.105
η_5 Circulation Trouble	.090	.117	.127	.225
η_6 Heart Trouble	.124	.172	.129	.196
η_7 Respiratory Disease	−.133	−.102	−.082+	−.061+
η_8 Digestive Disease	.140	−.056+	.021+	.038+
η_9 Skeletal Disease	.194	.187	.098	.148
η_{10} Vision Disease	.115	.095	.186	.212
η_{11} Visual Impairment	.175	.160	.075+	.172
η_{12} Hearing Impairment	.049+	−.012+	.086+	−.059+
η_{13} Other	.041+	.103	.003+	.005+
η_{14} Functional Status	.108	.108	.130	.083
η_{15} Self-rated Health	.047+	−.038+	−.001+	−.035+
Effect (γs) *of Education* (ξ_3) *on*				
η_1 Arthritis	−.208	−.178	−.212	−.147
η_2 Stroke	.018+	−.047+	−.084+	.033+
η_3 High Blood Pressure	−.045+	.069+	−.037+	.052+
η_4 Diabetes	−.068+	.034+	−.046+	−.036+
η_5 Circulation Trouble	−.253	−.175	−.176	−.118
η_6 Heart Trouble	−.134	−.053+	−.113	−.168
η_7 Respiratory Disease	−.214	−.138	−.126	−.135
η_8 Digestive Disease	−.118	−.123	−.068+	−.152
η_9 Skeletal Disease	−.123	−.083+	−.125	−.108
η_{10} Vision Disease	−.030+	.005+	−.048+	−.032+
η_{11} Visual Impairment	−.363	−.434	−.503	−.356
η_{12} Hearing Impairment	−.230	−.259	−.316	−.213
η_{13} Other	−.143	−.058+	−.156	−.163
η_{14} Functional Status	−.028+	.018+	−.001+	−.085+
η_{15} Self-rated Health	.017+	.032+	.010+	−.031+
Residual Variances and Covariances Ψs *of First-Order Factors* (ηs)				
Ψ (1,1)	.902	.921	.925	.926
Ψ (2,2)	.997	.997	.993	.992
Ψ (3,3)	.976	.981	.980	.973
Ψ (4,4)	.974	.984	.973	.982
Ψ (5,5)	.873	.891	.936	.900
Ψ (6,6)	.947	.955	.961	.896
Ψ (7,7)	.937	.980	.980	.957
Ψ (8,8)	.954	.987	.992	.969
Ψ (9,9)	.922	.945	.966	.955
Ψ (10,10)	.947	.959	.945	.931
Ψ (11,11)	.678	.575	.648	.703
Ψ (12,12)	.654	.733	.797	.801

(*continued*)

Table 2. Continued

	Sample 1 (N=920)	*Sample 2* (N=907)	*Sample 3* (N=903)	*Sample 4* (N=917)
Ψ (13,13)	.946	.949	.975	.959
Ψ (14,14)	.481	.460	.520	.583
Ψ (15,15)	.447	.443	.466	.488
Ψ (3,2)	.309	.262	.284	.228
Ψ (9,1)	.258	.251	.358	.267
Ψ (11,10)	.296	.338	.360	.269
Ψ (12,11)	.241	.265	.316	.332
Ψ (13,8)	.335	.321	.296	.239
Measures of Fit				
χ^2 (df=166)	664.13	718.76	737.81	721.91
Probability	.000	.000	.000	.000
GFI	.930	.926	.919	.923
AGFI	.884	.876	.865	.873

Note: To conserve space, only the parameter estimates associated with latent structural models are presented. All items are significant at the .05 level except those marked by a plus (+) sign.

subsamples. In addition to chronic conditions, both age and sex have a statistically significant effect on functional status, whereas education makes little difference. Specifically, older individuals and women are more likely to suffer from functional impairment. In total, some 42 to 54 percent of variance in functional status is explained by M_1.

Seven chronic conditions have a significant effect on self-rated health in at least three out of four subsamples (Table 2). These include diabetes, circulatory disease, heart disease, respiratory disease, digestive disease, visual impairment, and disease in the "other category." This is consistent with the notion that the presence of chronic conditions has a direct bearing on the individual's self-rated health. On the other hand, stroke, hypertension, skeletal disease, and disease of vision do not have a statistically significant effect on self-rated health in at least three out of the four subsamples. The effect of arthritis on self-rated health is inconclusive.

In all four subsamples, functional status has a sizable effect on self-rated health. Given this effect, effects of chronic diseases on self-rated health need to be further explicated. Although stroke does not have a direct effect, it nevertheless exerts an indirect effect on self-rated health via functional status. Circulatory disease and visual impairment influence self-rated health both directly and indirectly. In addition, age, but not sex and eduction has a significant effect on self-rated health. That is, when chronic diseases and functional status are held constant, older individuals tend to rate their health to be better (Table 2). As a whole, 51 to 56 percent of the variance in self-rated health is explained by the disaggregated model.

Table 3. Standardized Maximum Likelihood Estimates and Measures of Fit for the Composite Model of Self-Reported Physical Health

	Sample 1 (N=920)	*Sample 2* (N=907)	*Sample 3* (N=903)	*Sample 4* (N=917)
Effect (βs) of Chronic Condition (η_1) on:				
η_2 Functional Status	.343	.431	.345	.335
η_3 Self-Related Health	.535	.489	.514	.521
Effect (β) of Functional Status (η_2) on:				
η_3 Self-Related Health	.345	.350	.337	.261
Effect (γs) of Age (ξ_1) on:				
η_1 Chronic Condition	.121	.145	−.035+	.065+
η_2 Functional Status	.384	.301	.310	.390
η_3 Self-Rated Health	−.096	−.070	−.092	−.075+
Effect (γs) of Sex (ξ_2) on:				
η_1 Chronic Condition	.168	.162	.143	.210
η_2 Functional Status	.129	.104	.094	.074
η_3 Self-Rated Health	.052+	−.010+	−.002+	−.020
Effect (γs) of Education (ξ_3) on:				
η_1 Chronic Condition	−.116	−.052+	−.083+	−.088
η_2 Functional Status	−.118	−.151	−.162	−.158
η_3 Self-Rated Health	−.098	−.135	−.148	−.167
Residual Varinaces (Ψs)				
Ψ (1,1)	.925	.939	.965	.929
Ψ (2,2)	.605	.581	.694	.627
Ψ (3,3)	.391	.427	.438	.495
Measures of Fit				
χ^2 (df=33)	133.36	190.78	141.75	130.12
Probability	.000	.000	.000	.000
GFI	.974	.963	.972	.975
AGFI	.949	.926	.944	.950

Note: To conserve space, only the parameter estimates associated with the latent structural model are presented. All estimates are significant at the .05 level except those marked by a plus (+) sign.

What are the effects of age, sex, and education on the presence of chronic conditions? Age is a significant predictor of the presence of circulatory disease, disease of vision, visual impairment, and "other" diseases (Table 2). Women are more likely to suffer from arthritis, hypertension, diabetes, circulatory disease, heart disease, respiratory disease, skeletal disease, eye disorder, and visual impairment. Persons with higher education are less likely to suffer from arthritis, circulatory disease, heart disease, respiratory disease, digestive disease, skeletal disease, visual impairment, hearing impairment, and other conditions. With the exception of visual and hearing impairments, the amount of variance in chronic diseases explained by age, sex, and education has been less than 10 percent. Explained variance in visual and hearing impairments ranges from 19 to 36 percent.

The combined effect of all chronic conditions on health related quality of life is also examined within the composite model (Figure 2). The results associated with this model are presented in Table 3. The model (M_2) is supported by the results both in terms of the overall goodness-of-fit and parameter estimates. According to Table 3, chronic conditions exert a statistically significant direct impact on both functional status and self-rated health even when age, sex, and education are taken into account. Relatively speaking, chronic diseases have a greater direct effect on self-rated health than that of functional status. The amounts of explained variance in chronic conditions, functional impairments, and self-rated health in M_2 are approximately 7, 35, and 55 percent which are similar to their counterparts in M_1.

V. DISCUSSION

This study contributes to a further understanding of the effects of chronic diseases on quality of life. Findings from the present research in many respects are similar to those based on data collected in the United States (Stewart et al., 1989; Verbrugge, et al., 1989). With reference to the relative impact of diseases on disability, the substantial effects of stroke and visual impairment and the rather minor effects of hypertension, vision disease, and diabetes are consistent with the findings reported by Verbrugge et al. (1989) and Stewart et al. (1989). The significant effects of age and sex on disability in addition to those of chronic conditions were also reported by Verbrugge and her associates. Accordingly, the above observations can now be generalized to data derived from Taiwan, a non-western society significantly different from the United States.

There are however some differences between the findings of this research and previous research. The statistically significant effects of sociodemographic characteristics and many other chronic conditions on disability reported by previous investigators (Stewart et al., 1989; Verbrugge et al., 1989) were not substantiated by the present research. A possible explanation for this difference lies in the difference in sample size. The samples used by Stewart et al. (1989) and Verbrugge et al. (1989) involved some 9,000 and 16,000 individuals respectively, whereas the sample size of this study is only 4,000, and each subsample involved only some 900 respondents. Given that no regression coefficients were reported in the previous studies, direct comparison is difficult. However, the relative importance of the effects of diseases on disability derived from this study is similar to those reported previously.

The present research also differs from previous studies in terms of the amount of variance explained in disability. The explained variance reported by Stewart et al. and Verbrugge et al. was about 23 or 24 percent, while from 42 to 54 percent of variance in disability is explained in M_1. This is likely to be due to the fact that measurement errors were not adjusted in previous studies.

According to the present analysis, seven chronic conditions have a significant and direct effect on self-rated health (Table 2). These include diabetes, circulatory disease, heart disease, respiratory disease, digestive disease, visual impairment, and disease in the "other category." On the other hand, stroke, hypertension, skeletal disease, and disease of vision do not have a statistically significant effect on self-rated health, and the effect of arthritis on self-rated health is inconclusive. These findings are similar but by no means entirely consistent with those reported by Stewart et al. (1989). In addition, M_1 and M_2 explained substantially more variance in self-rated health (51 to 56%) than that in health perception (29%) as reported by Stewart et al. (1989).

As only the effects of diseases on disability and self-reported health were examined in this study, several directions for further analyses may be suggested. First, additional analyses involving other dimensions of quality of life such as mental health and social role performance may be undertaken. Although the effects of diseases on multiple dimensions of quality of life were analyzed by Stewart et al. (1989), these dimensions were treated as independent from one another, and the structural linkages among them have not been examined. The explication of these linkages and comparative research involving data from different cultures may contribute to further knowledge regarding the effects of chronic diseases.

Second, it would be interesting to analyze the interaction effects due to comorbidity by using data from different societies in addition to western developed nations. Interaction effects due to two or more coexisting chronic conditions were examined by some investigators (Stewart et al., 1989; Verbrugge et al., 1989). Because these effects were examined almost always within the context of single equations instead of an explicitly specified structural model, such analyses were limited to the interactive effects involving specific pairs of diseases, whereas other interactive effects involving a given disease and many other diseases and covariates were overlooked.

Third, almost all recent large-scale studies of the impact of chronic diseases were cross-sectional in design. Consequently, dimensions of quality of life, particularly morbidity and mortality, cannot be conceptualized as outcomes of the invididual's health conditions at an earlier time. In view of the substantial differences acorss individuals in trajectories of change in health and the fact that morbidity and mortality are critical dimensions of quality of life, longitudinal analyses of the impact of diseases are imperative. Longitudinal studies of the impact of diseases have been rare. One exception is the study undertaken by Seeman et al. (1989) in which baseline morbidity show significant associations with 17-year mortality, the development of new conditions, and the onset of depression. However, in their formulation, diseases were modeled by a single composite, making the relative effects of various chronic diseases less clear.

Finally, better conceptualization and measurement of chronic diseases are needed. Specifically, multiple indicators of diseases including self-report, diagnoses made by health professionals, and physical measures should be considered. In addition to the presence of a given disease, the severity of disease needs to be taken into account.

ACKNOWLEDGMENTS

This research was supported under Grant R01 AG08094 by the U.S. National Institute on Aging and by matching funds provided by the Chinese National Department of Health and the Taiwan Provincial Department of Health. Ken Bollen and Neal Krause have made useful comments on issues related to data analysis. The assistance provided by Joan Bennett, Cathy Fegan, Scott Montgomery, and C.K. Shaw is gratefully acknowledged.

REFERENCES

Bollen, K.A. (1989). *Structural Equations with Latent Variables*. New York: John Wiley & Sons.

Elinson, J. (1988). Defining and measuring health and illness. In K.W. Schaie, R.T. Campbell, W. Meredith, & S.C. Rawlings, (Eds.), *Methodological Issues in Aging Research*. New York: Springer Publishing Company.

Guralnik, J.M., LaCroix, A.Z., Everett, D.E., & Kovar, M.G. (1989). Aging in the eighties: The prevalence of Comorbidity and its association with disability. *Advance data from vital and health statistics*. No. 170. Hyattsville, MD.

Jöreskog, K.G. & Sörbom, D. (1988). *LISREL 7: A guide to the program and applications*. Chicago, IL: SPSS Inc.

Liang, J. (1986). Self-reported physical health among aged adults. *Journal of Gerontology* 41, 248-260.

Liang, J., Bennett, J., Whitelaw, N., & Maeda, D. (1991). The structure of self-reported physical health among the aged in the United States and Japan. *Medical Care* 29: 1161-1180.

Manton, K. G. (1990). Mortality and morbidity. Pp. 64-90 in R.H. Binstock & L.K. George (Eds.), *Handbook of aging and the social sciences*. New York: Academic Press.

Rice, D.P., Hogeson, T.A., & Kopstein, A.N. (1985). The economic costs of illness: A replication and update. *Health Care Financing Review* 7, 61-80.

Seeman, T.E., Guralnik, J.M., Kaplan, G.A., Knudsen, L., & Cohen, R. (1989). The health consequences of multiple morbidity in the elderly: The Alameda County Study. *Journal of Aging and Health* 1: 50-66.

Stewart, A.L., Greenfield, S., Hays, R.D., Wells, K., Rogers, W., Berry, S.D., McGlynn, E.A., & Ware, J.E. (1989). Functional status and well-being of patients with chronic conditions: Results from the medical outcomes study. *Journal of American Medical Association* 262, 907-913.

Tarlov, A.R., Ware, J.E., Greenfield, S., Nelson, E.C., Perrin, E., & Zubkoff, M. (1989). The medical outcomes study: An application of methods for monitoring the results of medical care. *Journal of American Medical Association* 262, 925-930.

U.S. Bureau of Census. (1975). *1970 Census of population and housing. Evaluation and research programs. Vol. II: Accuracy of data for selected population characteristics as measured by the 1970 CPS-Census Match.* PHC(E)-II. Washington, D.C.: Government Printing Office.

Verbrugge, L.M., Lepkowski, J.M., & Inmanaka, Y. (1989). Comorbidity and its impact on disability. *Milbank Memorial Quarterly* 67, 450-484.

Ware, J.E. (1984). Conceptualizing disease impact and treatment outcome. *Cancer* 53, 2316-2326.

STRUCTURAL CHANGES OF THE ELDERLY POPULATION AND HEALTH

Ming-cheng Chang and Hui-sheng Lin

I. INTRODUCTION

Taiwan's net reproduction rate (NRR) fell to 1.0 in 1983, 0.89 in 1985 and to 0.84 in 1988. In 1964, when the island-wide family planning program was promoted, the total fertility rate was 5.10 and the net reproduction rate was 2.27. The sustained fertility rate was 6.55 and the net reproduction rate was 2.82. Taiwan completed the fertility aspect of the demographic transition during the 20 years after the intensive family planning program was implemented.

Along with the fertility transition in Taiwan, the central concern related to population problems is gradually shifting from high fertility to other issues, especially population aging. As this picture of our demographic future has come into clear focus in recent years, it has stimulated anxiety about long-term socioeconomic implications. In particular, a central concern of government, professionals, and researchers is the issue of the dependencies of older people and what policies or measures should be formulated in order to meet their needs.

Research in Human Capital and Development, Volume 7, pages 69-91.

ISBN: 1-55938-132-9

Planning for the future health demand requires knowledge of the present and related data about possible changes in demographic and socioeconomic situations in the future, and health data as well. Using plausible population projections together with results of the 1989 Survey of Health and Living Status of the Elderly in Taiwan, this study illustrates the impact of structural changes of the elderly on the future demand for health care in Taiwan.

II. FUTURE PROJECTIONS OF POPULATION

In 1988 Taiwan's population of 19.7 million was growing at the rate of 1.2 percent per annum in spite of a total fertility rate (TFR) of 1.84 or below replacement-level fertility. It is understandable that Taiwan's temporarily young age structure resulting from formerly higher fertility levels is responsible for this phenomenon. Once the age structure becomes stationary, Taiwan's population will reach zero growth and then produce a negative growth rate. How long will it take? Various population projections constructed with the aid of the component method provide an adequate answer.

Table 1 displays alternative population projections for Taiwan based on various plausible assumptions about fertility and mortality.[1] Roughly, they show that the population will grow by 4.2 to 6.1 million during the next 32 to 42 years. The amount of population growth is likely to be less important from an economic and social view point than the changes in age structure which have been discussed in several recent studies. (Chang, 1987; Freedman, 1986).

A net reproduction rate (NRR) of 0.9 with a constant age-specific birth rate at the 1988 level and slightly declining mortality yields the "high" results among the projections shown. The population stops growing close to 2030—after about 42 years—at a total of 25.8 million, after having added about 6.1 million people.

In Taiwan, it is likely that population growth in the near future will be at a lower rather than a higher projected level, because the TFR fell to abut 1.7 in 1986 and 1987. The increase in the fertility level in 1988 was entirely due to the "dragon year" effect.

Another reason for expecting a continued decline for some time into the future is due to structural changes under way today. For example, the educational distribution of women of childbearing age is changing rapidly. Sixty one percent of the birth cohort of 1950-1954 had only a primary education, but for some time now virtually all primary school graduates have been going on to junior and senior high school and the proportions going on to higher education are also increasing rapidly. This means that, even if age-education-specific fertility rates remain unchanged, fertility will fall because of the changing educational distribution. In the period from 1966 to 1980, 24 percent

Table 1. Population Projections for Taiwan

Year	Population (millions)	Birth rate (per 1000)	Death rate (per 1000)	Rate of Natural Increase (per 1000)	Percent of Population			Dependency ratio (%)	
					Under 15	*15-64*	*65 +*	*young*	*old*
1988	19.79	17.24	5.14	12.10	28.23	66.16	5.61	42.67	8.48
High									
1990	2026	17.00	5.46	11.53	27.22	66.72	6.06	40.80	9.08
1995	21.36	15.94	5.88	10.06	24.53	68.25	7.22	35.94	10.58
2000	22.38	15.14	6.22	8.92	22.22	69.65	8.13	31.90	11.67
2010	24.18	13.41	7.02	6.38	20.64	70.00	9.36	29.49	13.37
2020	25.33	11.71	8.31	3.40	18.38	68.61	13.01	26.79	18.96
2030	25.85	11.32	10.62	0.69	17.01	64.64	18.35	26.31	28.39
2040	25.50	10.62	13.84	−2.85	16.69	62.38	20.93	26.76	33.55
2050	24.53	10.50	14.85	−4.34	16.20	61.05	22.75	26.54	37.26
Medium									
1990	20.25	16.73	5.46	11.26	27.20	66.74	6.06	40.76	9.08
1995	21.27	14.88	5.89	8.98	24.21	68.544	7.25	35.32	10.58
2000	22.12	13.41	6.27	7.14	21.30	70.47	8.23	30.23	11.68
2010	23.44	11.99	7.21	4.78	18.54	71.81	9.65	25.82	13.44
2020	24.14	10.06	8.67	1.39	16.45	69.89	13.66	23.54	19.54
2030	24.02	9.19	11.35	−2.16	14.61	65.64	19.75	22.26	30.09
2040	22.99	8.72	14.83	−6.10	13.95	62.93	23.22	22.20	36.96
2050	21.31	8.35	16.85	−8.50	13.55	60.26	26.19	22.49	43.46

(continued)

Table 1. (Continued)

Year	Population (millions)	Birth rate (per 1000)	Death rate (per 1000)	Rate of Natural Increase (per 1000)	Percent of Population			Dependency ratio (%)	
					Under 15	15-64	65 +	young	old
Low									
1990	20.25	16.73	5.46	11.26	27.20	66.74	6.06	40.76	9.08
1995	21.27	14.88	5.89	8.98	24.21	68.54	7.25	35.32	10.58
2000	22.13	13.48	6.27	7.21	21.31	70.47	8.23	30.24	11.68
2010	23.40	11.29	7.22	4.07	18.39	71.94	9.67	25.56	13.44
2020	23.86	8.94	8.76	0.18	15.41	70.78	13.81	21.77	19.51
2030	23.39	7.61	11.63	−4.01	12.91	66.81	20.28	19.32	30.35
2040	21.82	6.37	15.55	−9.18	11.37	64.17	24.46	17.72	38.12
2050	19.48	5.44	18.32	−12.88	9.88	61.46	28.66	16.08	46.03

Note: Additional population growth until zero growth is attained (millions): High, 6.1; medium, 4.4; low, 4.2.
Basic assumptions: Life expectancy at birth for the three projections will rise from 71.1 for men and 76.1 for women in 1988 to 74.7 for men and 79.5 for women by 2011. Total fertility rate stays at 1988 level of 1,837 for high assumption; for medium assumptions, it falls to 1,698 by 1995 and to 1,600 by 2000; for low projection, TFR falls to 1,698 by 1995 and to 1,400 by 2020, and to 1,100 by 2050.

Source: Projections of the population of the Taiwan area, Republic of China, 1988-2030," prepared by the Manpower Planning Department, Council for Economic Planning Development, Executive Yuan, Republic of China.

of the decline in the total fertility rate was a result of changes in the educational distribution rather than in the age-education-specific marital fertility rate (Liu, 1983). We have calculated that the projected changes in age/educational distributions expected between 1984 and 1994 would produce a 9 percent decline in the total fertility rate without any further decline in age/education-specific fertility rates.

It is also true that the more poorly educated and rural sectors of the population have, after a lag of six to eight years, reached the lower rates of the more urban and better educated strata. In 1987 the total fertility rate of the rural townships was 23 percent higher than that of Taiwan's large cities, but the rural total fertility rate of 1.89 in 1987 had been the fertility rate of cities only six years ago. The lag behind the Taipei rate has been only a few years longer, and we estimate that the Taipei total fertility rate for 1989 was below 1.50. There is also a small potential for fertility decline if there is a further decrease in the small remaining number of women who are not practicing contraception and want more children.

Changes in fertility preferences should continue to result in lower fertility for at least a while. The recent decline in the numbers preferring three children and the increase in the numbers preferring two is likely to continue, especially since the number satisfied with one son continues to increase. Furthermore, in 1985 Taipei couples had preferences 0.3 points below that for Taiwan as a whole, and in the past Taiwan has reached the Taipei level after a lag of a few years (Change, Freedman, & Sun, 1987).

The increasing practice of contraception that accounted for the rapid fall in fertility over the last 25 years is no longer an independent factor in the future situation.

However, there continues to be some reasons to expect a leveling-off of the fertility decline. There is still very little evidence of the preferences for one child that has become so marked in Western societies. Even among young wives only 3 percent indicated a preference for one child in 1985. This is no doubt affected by the continued, if diminishing, preference for sons.

The increasing number of women who work in the economic sector before marriage, and after marriage as well, might be expected to reduce family size preference. Because effective birth control is almost universal, downward shifts in preferences are likely to be realized in actual fertility changes.

On the basis of the above considerations, it is likely that fertility will continue to decline for some time. But how far it will decline and whether and when it will level off is still an open question. Our expectation is that our future fertility rates might fluctuate before reaching zero population growth. For example, in the Dragon Year of 2000, our new prediction might soon be followed by an unpredicted baby boom if fertility repeats the same pattern in the last Dragon Year in 1988. Our future demographic trends need not be linear, but unquestionably the TFR will continued to fall. As such, our preferred medium projection assumes a decline in the total fertility rate from the 1988 level of 1.84 to a level of 1.6 by 2000, with a leveling-off of fertility at that point. This assumption accommodates a virtually certain moderate decline in total fertility rates, but does not accept more radical declines of total fertility rates to 1.4 by 2020 and to 1.1. by 2050 as posited in the "low" official projection. All three projections assumes modest additional declines in mortality, a factor that affects population growth relatively little, since mortality rates are already very low and further declines will affect only the older population beyond the reproductive ages.

The medium population projection produces a near zero-growth level by the year 2022, in about 34 years, and adds about 4.4 million to the 1988 population. On the other hand, the more radical low assumption produces a near zero-growth population of around 23.9 million in about 2020, with a projected decline in the rate of natural increase to 0.2 per thousand per annum by 2020, to about −4.0 per thousand per annum by 2030, and to about −12.9 per thousand per annum by 2050. This is certain if the net reproduction rate of less than 1.0 continues indefinitely.

The declines in fertility and mortality in Taiwan will result in the aging of the population. At zero population growth, there will be a major shift in the relative numbers of young (under 15) and old (over 64) dependents, moving from a young/old ratio of almost 5 to 1 in 1988 to about 1 to 1.1 from a high projection, and to about 1 to 0.9 for a low projection (Table 1).

For the inter-country comparison, we consider the population age 60 years and above the aged. As shown in Table 2, the increase int he number of the elderly may not alter the age profile significantly. Under the "medium" projections, the proportion is expected to rise from 9 percent to 19.5 percent in 2020, due to the shrinking of the more recent cohorts. The old dependency ratio is conventionally computed to illustrate the relative sizes of the elderly to the working age population (Table 1).

III. STRUCTURAL CHANGES OF THE ELDERLY

Using the medium projections, the future sex-age structure of the elderly population can be examined further. Please note that the projections presented in this section and throughout this report do not imply certainty about future events. By the year 2030, they represent forecasts based on continued patterns from the past and assumptions about future trends in mortality in a closed population. In other words, the projected sex age structure of the elderly population at any point from now to zero growth is solely determined by the survival rate of each related birth cohort in the base population.

Table 2. Projected Population by Sex and age in Taiwan 1988-2030

	1988	*1990*	*1995*	*2000*	*2010*	*2020*	*2030*
60-64	38	36	32	29	30	33	26
65-69	27	27	28	26	22	27	25
70-74	17	18	19	20	20	17	21
75-79	13	12	11	13	14	11	16
80+	9	10	10	10	14	13	14
	100	100	100	100	100	100	100
N	799,333	865,699	1,040,262	1,241,115	1,660,145	2,581,876	3,378,440
Mean age	69.31	69.36	69.50	69.78	70.47	69.82	70.93

Source: Medium Projections of Table 1.

Table 2 displays the sex-age distribution of the elderly age 60 and over in 1988 and gives a glimpse into the future. Over the next two decades, there will be a trend towards an increasing proportion of the very old among the aged population in Taiwan. The mean age and the share of the very old (those age 75+) in the old population (60+) is projected to consistently rise until the year 2010. However, after the year 2010 the proportion decreases from 29 percent in 2010 to 24 percent in 2020. This is due to the fact that most of the soldiers who migrated from Mainland China to Taiwan before 1949 will pass away and the proportion will drop to that of the year 2010 in which life expectancy at birth was assumed to stop rising.

Similarly, the aging process among the elderly was found for either males or females. It should be noted that unlike most of the countries in the world, the sex ratios among the elderly are over 100 during the period from 1988 to 2000 (Table 2). Again, this is entirely due to the effect of soldiers who migrated from the Mainland China to Taiwan before the communists took over in 1949. These soldiers are currently age 60 and above. Their effect on the sex ratio is reflected on each five-year age group of people older than 60. The situation will normalize in 2020.

Educational Structure

The educational structure of the elderly in Taiwan can be projected by using a cohort approach. To do this, data on sex-age educational structure for those aged 20 and above in 1988 in Taiwan, derived from population registers, were used. With the exception of age cohort 20-24, most people have completed their educational career. It can be viewed as a fixed status. As such, the future educational compositions of the elderly were profiled by applying the projected sex-age structure of the elderly to the fixed educational status of corresponding birth cohorts.

As illustrated in Table 3, the elderly population of today received the bulk of its formal education before World War II when educational opportunities

Table 3A. Projected Educational Distribution of Elderly in Taiwan (In percentages)

Education	*1985*	*1990*	*1995*	*2000*	*2005*	*2010*	*2015*	*2020*	*2025*
				Age 60-64					
Less than primary	45	36	36	38	23	12	8	4	2
Primary school	32	40	44	41	47	47	41	23	13
Junior high	8	10	9	7	10	12	13	26	33
Senior high or more	14	14	11	13	20	29	38	47	52
Total %	100	100	100	100	100	100	100	100	100
N	602082	704813	730645	762384	783641	979274	1437063	1642886	17251102
				Age 65-69					
Less than primary	—	46	36	36	38	23	12	8	4
Primary school	—	32	39	44	41	47	47	41	23
Junior high	—	8	10	9	7	10	12	13	26
Senior high or more	—	13	14	11	13	20	29	38	47
Total %	100	100	100	100	100	100	100	100	100
N	451912	530178	639771	667619	701986	724606	911789	1337251	1528838
				Age 70 and over					
Less than primary	—	65	30	51	46	44	39	31	23
Primary school	—	22	26	31	35	36	39	42	41
Junior high	—	4	6	7	8	7	8	9	10
Senior high or more	—	9	10	12	11	12	14	18	25
Total %	100	100	100	100	100	100	100	100	100
N	567609	697804	902681	1152414	1359878	1537905	1690598	1958939	2532352

Table 3B. Projected Educational Distribution of Males in Taiwan
(In percentages)

Education Level	*1985*	*1990*	*1995*	*2000*	*2005*	*2010*	*2015*	*2020*	*2025*
				Age 60-64					
Less than primary	30	21	24	25	12	6	4	2	1
Primary school	39	45	49	47	50	45	37	17	10
Junior high	11	13	11	9	12	13	15	29	36
Senior high or more	19	20	17	19	27	36	44	51	53
Total %	100	100	100	100	100	100	100	100	100
N	352159	409517	388493	373470	385064	484179	707325	807643	849080
				Age 65-69					
Less than primary	—	30	21	24	25	12	6	4	2
Primary school	—	39	45	49	47	50	45	37	17
Junior high	—	11	13	11	9	12	13	15	29
Senior high or more	—	19	20	17	19	27	36	44	51
Total %	100	100	100	100	100	100	100	100	100
N	226495	304761	365795	348854	337908	351071	443875	648116	739895
				Age 60 and over					
Less than primary	42	34	30	29	24	19	13	10	7
Primary school	34	39	42	43	45	45	42	34	26
Junior high	8	10	10	10	11	11	12	18	24
Senior high or more	16	18	17	18	20	25	32	39	43
Total %	100	100	100	100	100	100	100	100	100
N	855580	1067096	1232835	13411302	1426078	1581690	1941312	2397180	2749088

(continued)

Table 3B. (Continued)

Education Level	*1985*	*1990*	*1995*	*2000*	*2005*	*2010*	*2015*	*2020*	*2025*
				Age 65 and over					
Less than primary	49	42	34	30	29	24	19	13	10
Primary school	31	34	39	42	43	45	45	42	34
Junior high	6	8	10	10	11	11	12	18	
Senior high or more	13	16	18	17	18	20	25	32	39
Total %	100	100	100	100	100	100	100	100	100
N	503421	657579	844342	967832	1040014	1097511	1233987	1549537	1900008
				Age 70 and over					
Less than primary	—	49	42	34	30	29	24	19	13
Primary school	—	31	34	39	42	43	45	45	42
Junior high	—	6	8	10	10	10	11	11	12
Senior high or more	—	13	16	18	17	18	20	25	32
Total %	100	100	100	100	100	100	100	100	100
N	276926	352818	478547	618978	702106	746440	790112	901421	1160113

Table 3C. Projected Educational Distribution of Females in Taiwan

Education Level	*1985*	*1990*	*1995*	*2000*	*2005*	*2010*	*2015*	*2020*	*2025*
				Age 60-64					
Less than primary	67	56	49	51	33	17	11	6	2
Primary school	23	32	39	36	45	49	44	28	16
Junior high	4	5	6	6	9	11	12	23	30
Senior high or more	6	6	56	7	13	23	33	44	52
Total %	100	100	100	100	100	100	100	100	100
N	249923	295236	342152	388914	397577	495095	729738	835223	876022
				Age 65-69					
Less than primary	—	67	56	49	51	33	17	11	6
Primary school	—	23	32	39	36	45	49	44	28
Junior high	—	4	5	6	6	9	11	12	23
Senior high or more	—	6	6	5	7	13	23	33	44
Total %	100	100	100	100	100	100	100	100	100
N	179002	225417	273976	318765	364078	373535	467914	689135	788943
				Age 60 and over					
Less than primary	77	70	63	59	52	42	31	23	17
Primary school	16	22	27	30	34	39	41	36	31
Junior high	3	4	5	5	6	7	9	13	18
Senior high or more	4	5	5	6	8	12	20	27	35
Total %	100	100	100	100	100	100	100	100	100
N	719608	865699	1040262	1241115	1419427	1660095	2097838	2581876	3037204

(*continued*)

Table 3C. (Continued)

Education Level	*1985*	*1990*	*1995*	*2000*	*2005*	*2010*	*2015*	*2020*	*2025*
				Age 65 and over					
Less than primary	82	77	70	63	59	52	42	31	23
Primary school	12	16	22	27	30	34	39	41	36
Junior high	2	3	4	5	5	6	7	9	13
Senior high or more	4	4	5	5	6	8	12	20	27
Total %	100	100	100	100	100	100	100	100	100
N	469685	570403	698110	852201	1021850	1165000	1368400	1746653	2161182
				Age 70 and over					
Less than primary	—	82	77	70	63	59	52	42	31
Primary school	—	12	16	22	27	30	34	39	41
Junior high	—	2	3	4	5	5	6	7	9
Senior high or more	—	4	4	5	5	6	8	12	20
Total %	100	100	100	100	100	100	100	100	100
N	290683	344986	424134	533436	657772	791465	900486	1057518	1372239

were more limited than in recent decades and when the economic structure of the country put less emphasis on schooling. As a result, a great majority of the elderly age 60-64 received less than primary and primary school education respectively in Taiwan as a whole. A similar situation was found for males and females. However, there are significant differences in educational attainment by sex within the older population.

The strides made by this country in providing for universal education, fostering and rewarding college education, and increasing educational opportunities for women and minorities are reflected in the projected rapid increase in educational attainment by the older population in the future when people educated after World War II join the ranks of the older population. For example, the proportion of the elderly people age 60-64 who received at least a senior high school education was 14 percent in 1990 which will increase to 47 percent in 2020. Furthermore, although educational attainment of the female elderly population, was less than that for the male population the gap will narrow somewhat in the next few years and will decrease further in the next century.

IV. HEALTH CARE AND IMPLICATIONS OF THE STRUCTURAL CHANGES

As Newman and Anderson (1974) pointed out, the estimation of society's need for health services and facilities depends on many factors including at least the following: (1) mortality and morbidity patterns; (2) organization of the health and medical care system; (3) demographic processes related to the size and composition of the population; and (4) patterns of health service utilization. Because this paper deals with the effect of the aging of the aged population on health care and medical demand in Taiwan, only morbidity patterns and the last two factors are considered in this section.

The last factor regarding the need for health services and facilities refers to health services utilization. Utilization is viewed as reflecting the demand for health and medical services, where demand may be a result of illness, perception of illness, or the interaction of illness and social processes. If there are increasing trends in the utilization of health services (holding other factors constant), efforts must be made to increase medical manpower and supporting facilities. When trying to achieve this goal, it is important to understand demographic and social factors related to future health and medical demands in order to plan for the development of medical facilities and personnel.

In order to demonstrate the effect of the structural changes of the elderly on health care and demand, data for this research were derived from the 1989 Survey of Health and Living Status of the Elderly in Taiwan. This survey involved a national sample with 4,412 respondents age 60 and over, selected through a multi-strata probability sampling procedure. Overall, the 4,049 completed interviews constitute a response rate of 91.8 percent. Measures of self-rated health care are analyzed in this study.

As we will observe, the health statistical data derived from the 1989 Taiwan aging survey indicate that age, sex, and education play an important role in determining health and disability status, mobility, and health services utilization. This implies that the demographic and social picture described in the previous section has profound implications for health services. To examine the impact of the structural changes of the elderly on the future demand for health care, a static components methodology, which implies (1) the rates regarding health and disability status, mobility, and health services utilization by age, sex, and/or education remain unchanged over the projection period, and (2) the structural changes of the elderly are determined exogenously, was used. The projected sex-age structure was applied to the cross-sectional health data to examine the effects of the structural changes on health demand. We realize full well that this procedure involves considerable conjecture and it may promote controversy regarding future morbidity patterns.

Health Status

Table 4 gives the elderly respondents' self-evaluation of their health status by sex and age in Taiwan in 1989. Contrary to popular opinion, a great majority of the elderly view their health positively. For both sexes, about 75 percent of elderly people described their health as excellent, very good, or good; only 21 percent reported that their health is fair or poor.

As expected, there is a general deterioration in reported health status with advancing age. The proportion of old people claiming to be in good health declines with advancing age. Furthermore, the health status of men is consistently better than women in each age group.

An important aspect of health status particularly as it relates to need for assistance from others, is ability to move about. In Table 5 information is presented on this aspect. Overall, only 7.6 percent of the elderly are reported to have foot problems restricting activity and 9.5 percent are reported to have difficulty walking 200-300 meters indicating that most of elderly persons can get around the home without difficulty. Although, as expected, there is a steady decline in mobility with age, even among those age 80 +, about 70 percent are able to get around the house without help. As compared with elderly women, elderly men seem to have a little more foot problems which restrict activity. However, in terms of walking 200-300 meters, older women have more difficulty than older men. The sex-age pattern is generally existing for this aspect of disability.

Table 4. Self-Assessment of Health by Sex and Age for Persons 60 Years and Older in Taiwan, 1989

Age	*Excellent*	*Very good*	*Good*	*Fair*	*Poor*	*NA*	*Total* %	*Total* N
				Both Sexes				
60-64	19.5	24.7	34.7	16.5	2.9	1.8	100.0	1,562
65-69	19.3	19.1	38.5	17.3	3.8	1.9	100.0	1,129
70-74	13.2	19.5	38.8	20.1	3.8	4.5	100.0	711
75-79	10.1	19.4	39.3	19.7	6.2	5.3	100.0	417
80+	7.4	13.5	33.5	21.3	7.4	17.0	100.0	230
Total	16.7	21.1	36.9	17.9	3.9	3.5	100.1	4,049
				Male				
60-64	24.5	25.2	32.8	12.8	2.5	2.1	100.0	981
65-69	25.2	21.4	37.1	11.1	3.1	2.2	100.0	650
70-74	17.6	22.4	36.8	15.4	3.0	4.9	100.0	370
75-79	11.1	22.7	41.5	13.5	6.8	4.3	100.0	207
80+	9.9	15.3	29.7	20.7	7.2	17.1	100.0	111
Total	21.7	23.0	35.3	13.2	3.4	3.5	100.1	2,319
				Female				
60-64	11.0	23.9	37.9	22.5	3.4	1.2	100.0	580
65-69	11.3	16.1	40.5	25.7	4.8	1.7	100.0	479
70-74	8.5	16.4	41.1	25.2	4.7	4.1	100.0	341
75-79	9.0	16.2	37.1	25.7	5.7	6.2	100.0	210
80+	5.0	11.8	37.0	21.8	7.6	16.8	100.0	119
Total	9.9	18.5	39.1	24.3	4.6	3.6	100.1	1,730

Chronic Conditions

The pattern of illness and disease in Taiwan has changed from acute to chronic conditions which are now the more prevalent health problems for elderly persons. There has also been a change in the pattern of wellness within an individual's lifetime. As individuals grow older, acute conditions become less frequent and chronic conditions become more prevalent. Cross-sectional data from the 1989 Taiwan aging survey have shown that the likelihood of suffering from a chronic illness increases somewhat with age. A great majority of elderly persons have at least one chronic condition. Multiple conditions are fairly common among older persons.

To illustrate the age effect on the increases in chronic conditions, three major chronic diseases were chosen for this purpose. As shown in Table 5, arthritis and rheumatism is clearly a very common condition, with higher prevalence rates among elderly women than among elderly men. The next common condition is heart trouble which affects more than one-fifth

Table 5. Persons Suffering from Certain Disabilities, and/or Specific Health Problems by Sex and Age, Taiwan, 1989

	60-64	65-69	70-74	75-79	80+	Total
	Both Sexes					
Disability:						
Foot problem restricting activity	3.2	5.4	8.2	16.1	30.9	7.6
Difficulty walking 200-300 metres	4.9	6.6	11.7	17.0	35.2	9.5
Health problem:						
Arthritis or rheumatism	28.4	31.1	32.1	29.6	34.3	30.2
Heart trouble	20.3	21.9	22.3	22.0	26.1	21.6
Diabetes	8.2	9.0	9.8	5.8	6.5	8.4
Number of cases	1,562	1,129	711	417	230	4,049
	Male					
Disability:						
Foot problem restricting activity	3.6	5.7	8.1	17.4	36.9	7.7
Difficulty walking 200-300 metres	3.7	5.2	8.7	17.4	30.6	7.4
Health problems:						
Arthritis or rheumatism	23.6	23.8	26.5	24.1	28.8	24.5
Heart trouble	16.4	16.1	18.4	21.2	23.4	17.4
Diabetes	6.6	5.6	8.1	3.8	7.2	6.4
Number of cases	981	650	370	207	111	2,319
	Female					
Disability:						
Foot problem restricting activity	2.6	5.0	8.2	14.8	25.2	7.4
Difficulty walking 200-300 metres	6.7	8.5	15.0	16.7	39.5	12.3
Health problems:						
Arthritis or rheumatism	36.3	40.9	38.1	34.7	39.5	38.0
Heart trouble	27.1	29.7	26.7	22.8	28.5	27.3
Diabetes	11.1	13.6	11.7	7.6	5.9	11.1
Number of cases	580	479	341	210	119	1,730

of the elderly and the similar sex differential as arthritis was observed for this health problem. As compared with arthritis and heart trouble, diabetes is somewhat less common, but still more than 8 percent of elderly persons suffered from this disease and the prevalence was higher for females than for males. With the exception of diabetes, in general, the prevalence of arthritis and heart trouble tended to increase with advancing age.

Age and Sex Effects on the Prevalence of Disabilities and Health Problems

As described in the previous sections, the poor health status and the prevalence of most disabilities and specific health problems tended to increase with the advance of age, and differed among the male and female elderly. Therefore, it can be expected that the future aging of the aged population in Taiwan will lead to the increase of the absolute and relative size of the elderly suffering from certain disabilities and health problems. On the other hand, the decreases in the future sex ratios will reduce the overall prevalence of disabilities, but lead to the increase of the prevalence rates of various health problems. Applying projected changes in sex and age structure of the elderly to the micro health statistical data at static status shown in Tables 4 and 5, one can obtain the sex and age effects on the health status and the prevalence of disabilities and specific health problems.

Table 6 displays age and sex effects on rates for self-assessment of health status as "fair," and "poor," and disability/specific health problems. As expected, in general, the aging of the aged population will lead to the worsening of the overall health status of the elderly, which in turn affects the increases in the prevalence of disabilities and specific health problems. For example, the proportion with fair and poor health was 23 percent in 1989, which increases to 24.4 percent in 2010. Similarly, during the corresponding period, the proportion with foot problems which restricts activity and with arthritis increases from 7.6 percent and 30.2 percent in 1989 to 10.4 percent and 30.7 percent in 2010 respectively. On the other hand, with few exceptions, the proportion with poor health and the proportion with poor health and the prevalence of most disabilities and specific health problems increase with decrease in sex ratios.

Because the health situation of elderly persons with lower educational level is generally poorer than that of higher educated elderly, lower educated elderly are more likely to utilize health services than higher educated elderly. As indicated in Table 8, the proportion of elderly persons ever visiting hospital, clinic, pharmacy, drug store of Chinese medicine, flock medicine or temple during the past one year was higher among lower educated elderly than among higher educated ones. However, the higher educated elderly are more likely to utilize modern medical services than lower educated ones. With few exceptions, the proportion ever visiting public and private hospital or clinic during the past one year tended to be higher among higher educated elderly than among lower ones, especially for those age 70 and above (Table 9). Similarly, higher proportion of hospital stay was observed among the higher educated elderly persons. This indicated that the demand for better medical care is greater for higher educated elderly. Probably, education is a proxy of income.

As discussed previously, the education of future cohorts will differ appreciably from those of their predecessors. Level of educational attainment will increase and substantially higher proportions will have completed at least some senior high or above education. As this result, other things being equal, it can be expected that a rising level of education attainment will be increasing

Table 6. Age and Sex-Ratio Effects on Rates for Self-assessment of Health "Fair," and "Poor," and Disability/Specific Health Problems
(In percentages)

	1989	*1990*	*1995*	*2000*	*2005*	*2010*	*2015*	*2020*	*2025*	*2030*
				BOTH SEXES						
				Age Effect						
Health "fair" and "poor"	23.0	23.3	23.6	23.9	24.3	24.4	24.1	23.9	24.1	24.5
Foot problem restricting activity	7.6	8.2	8.6	9.,3	10.1	10.4	9.8	9.5	9.5	10.3
Difficulty walking 200-300 metres	9.5	10.2	10.7	11.4	12.2	12.5	11.9	11.6	11.7	12.4
Arthritis or rheumatism	30.2	30.4	30.5	30.6	30.7	30.7	30.5	30.6	30.7	30.8
Heart trouble	21.6	21.7	21.8	21.9	22.1	22.1	22.0	22.0	22.0	22.1
Diabetes	8.4	8.3	8.3	8.3	8.2	8.1	8.1	8.2	8.3	8.2
60+ N(100,000)	17.8	19.3	22.7	25.8	28.5	32.4	40.4	49.4	57.9	64.0
%	100.0	104.2	122.5	139.2	153.4	174.7	217.7	266.2	312.0	345.2
				Sex-Ratio Effect						
Health "fair" and "poor"	23.0	23.1	23.5	24.1	25.1	25.1	24.8	24.6	24.7	25.0
Foot problem restricting activity	7.6	8.1	8.5	9.2	10.0	10.3	9.7	9.4	9.4	10.1
Difficulty walking 200-300 metres	9.5	10.2	10.8	11.7	12.5	12.8	12.2	11.8	11.9	12.6
Arthritis or rheumatism	30.2	30.4	30.7	31.0	31.6	31.6	31.5	31.6	31.6	31.6
Heart trouble	21.6	21.9	22.2	22.5	23.0	23.0	22.8	22.8	22.9	22.9
Diabetes	8.4	8.4	8.4	8.5	8.6	8.5	8.6	8.7	8.7	8.5

AGE EFFECT

					Male					
Health "fair" and "poor"	17.2	17.5	17.9	18.5	19.2	19.4	19.0	18.6	18.6	18.9
Foot problem restricting activity	7.7	8.3	9.0	10.1	11.3	11.7	10.8	10.2	10.1	10.9
Difficulty walking 200-300 metres	7.4	7.9	8.6	9.6	10.5	10.8	10.0	9.5	9.5	10.2
Arthritis or rheumatism	24.5	24.2	24.4	24.6	24.7	24.8	24.6	24.5	24.6	24.7
Heart trouble	17.4	17.5	17.7	18.1	18.4	18.4	18.1	17.9	18.0	18.2
Diabetes	6.4	6.3	6.3	6.3	6.3	6.3	6.4	6.4	6.4	6.3
60+ N(100,000)	9.8	10.7	12.3	13.4	14.3	15.8	19.4	23.6	27.5	30.3
%	100.0	104.3	120.5	131.1	139.4	154.6	189.8	230.4	268.7	295.7
					Female					
Health "fair" and "poor"	30.0	30.0	30.1	30.2	30.5	30.4	30.2	30.2	30.4	30.7
Foot problem restricting activity	7.4	7.9	8.0	8.3	8.8	9.1	8.7	8.7	8.7	9.4
Difficulty walking 200-300 metres	12.3	13.1	13.3	13.5	14.2	14.6	14.2	14.0	14.2	14.9
Arthritis or rheumatism	38.0	38.0	38.0	38.0	38.0	37.9	37.8	38.1	38.1	38.0
Heart trouble	27.3	27.3	27.4	27.3	27.2	27.2	27.2	27.4	27.4	27.2
Diabetes	11.1	10.9	10.9	10.9	10.7	10.6	10.6	10.8	10.8	10.6
60+ N(100,000)	3.0	8.6	10.4	12.4	14.2	16.6	21.0	25.8	30.4	33.8
%	100.0	104.0	125.0	149.1	170.6	199.5	252.1	310.3	365.0	406.0

Table 7. Elderly Persons Suffering from Specific Health Problems by Age and Education, Taiwan, 1989 (In percentages)

Education	*60-64*	*65-69*	*70+*	*Total*
		Heart Disease		
Less than primary	23.3	25.3	22.9	23.7
Primary school	18.1	17.8	26.5	19.9
Junior high	19.1	20.7	22.0	20.2
Senior high or more	16.5	17.2	17.7	17.0
Total %	20.2	22.2	23.1	21.8
		Circulation trouble		
Less than primary	19.5	21.1	25.8	22.7
Primary school	17.6	15.6	20.2	17.6
Junior high	14.2	13.4	21.7	15.5
Senior high or more	21.5	17.2	20.0	19.9
Total %	28.1	31.2	31.9	30.3
		Urinary tract		
Less than primary	4.4	5.3	6.0	5.4
Primary school	2.5	4.5	6.0	3.8
Junior high	1.4	2.4	6.7	2.8
Senior high or more	2.0	2.3	7.9	3.4
Total %	3.2	4.5	6.2	4.6
		N		
Less than primary	676	631	994	2,301
Primary school	518	270	235	1,023
Junior high	141	82	60	283
Senior high or more	200	128	90	418
Total %	1,535	1,111	1,379	4,025

Table 8. Proportion of Elderly Persons Ever Visiting Hospital, Clinic, Pharmacy, Drug Store of Chinese Medicine, Flok Medician or Temple During the Past One Year, Taiwan, 1989 (In Percentages)

Education	*60-64*	*65-69*	*70+*	*Total*
Less than primary	88.4	87.7	88.0	88.0
Primary school	86.3	88.1	87.0	87.0
Junior high	81.6	90.7	84.8	85.2
Senior high or more	82.3	80.5	85.7	82.7
Total %	85.8	86.5	87.3	86.6
		N		
Less than primary	493	520	918	1,931
Primary school	475	278	247	1,000
Junior high	125	86	66	277
Senior high or more	300	236	223	759
Total %	1,393	1,120	1,454	3,967

Table 9. Physician Visit and Hospital Stay by Age and Education, Taiwan, 1989 (In percentages)

Education	*60-64*	*65-69*	*70+*	*Total*
Ever visited public or private hospital/clinic during the past one year				
Less than primary	73.4	75.4	74.0	74.5
Primary school	73.3	73.3	77.9	74.4
Junior high	74.6	76.5	83.1	77.0
Senior high or more	72.6	75.8	83.1	75.8
Total %	73.8	75.0	75.7	74.8
Ever stayed in hsopital during the past six months				
Less than primary	10.1	12.4	9.4	10.4
Primary school	9.5	7.8	10.6	9.3
Junior high	6.4	12.2	13.3	9.5
Senior high or more	10.5	14.8	14.4	12.7
Total %	9.6	11.5	10.1	10.3
N				
Less than primary	676	631	994	2,301
Primary school	518	270	235	1,023
Junior high	141	82	60	283
Senior high or more	200	128	90	418
Total %	1,535	1,111	1,379	4,025

the demand for better medical care. As such, the costs of medical care for the elderly in Taiwan in the future may be multiplied considerably more by the greater demand for higher quality health services among higher educated elderly and by rising per capita costs of high-technology health care than by the rapid increase in the number of the elderly.

CONCLUSION

Recent demographic transition from high to low birth and death rates in Taiwan suggests a negative rate of population growth after about 2020, and dramatic changes in the age structure of the future population. A study by Chang (1988) indicated that there will be a rapid growth of prevalence of sickness, length of stay in hospital, and financial resources required for medical services which is partly attributable to an increase in the overall population from now to zero growth of the Taiwan's population. But, to a greater extent, it is attributable to an increase in elderly persons age 65 and above and the aging of patients among the total population.

On the other hand, as discussed in this paper, the structural changes of the elderly in terms of age, sex, and educational attainment in the future will reinforce the health demand in Taiwan. In the next two decades, the aging among the elderly is proceeding both for males and females. Furthermore, the sex ratios will be decreasing and normalizing until the year 2020. In addition, the educational characteristics of future cohorts will also differ appreciably from those of their predecessors. Level of educational attainment will increase and substantially higher proportion will complete at least some senior high or above education. Since the poor health status, the prevalence of most disabilities and specific health problems, physician visit and hospital stay tended to increase with advancing age, with sex differentials in most conditions among elderly persons, the changes in sex-age structure will have an important impact on health demand in the future in Taiwan. Moreover, higher educated elderly seems more likely to use modern medical facilities and changes in educational composition will also have an effect on health demand.

Evidence from this study seems to suggest that educational modernization for the future elderly in Taiwan will be increasing the demand for better medical care. Taiwan is now actively preparing health insurance for all people by 1994 and producing larger numbers of health personnel equipped to provide and thus to generate further demand for high-technology health care. Government policy is, in principle, to foster the best possible services for the population. The health budget does not yet adequately reflect this goal. The findings from this study provide some basic information for government to consider health planning for the elderly in Taiwan.

ACKNOWLEDGMENTS

The authors wish to thank Mr. Lai-chiu Chow and Miss Shu-ywe Jenq for their assistance of the computer programming.

NOTE

1. Our projections are based on the report "Projections of the Population of the Taiwan Area, Republic of China, 1988 to 2050," from the Manpower Department, Executive Yuan, Republic of China, 1989.

REFERENCES

Chang, M. (1987). From now to zero population growth and its economic and social implications: The case of Taiwan. The Proceedings of the Workshop on Comparative Study of Fertility Control Experiences in Republic of Korea and Republic of China, 3-10 November, 1986, Seoul, Korea.

Chang, M., R. Freedman, & T. Sun. (1987). Trends in fertility, family size preferences, and family planning practice: Taiwan, 1961-85. *Studies in Family Planning* 18(6), 320-338.

Chang, M. (1988). Population aging and health demand in the Taiwan area, R.O.C. Paper presented at the International Conference on Population Change and Health Care for the Elderly, held in Taipei, December 14-15.

Freedman, R. (1986). Policy options after the demographic transition: The case of Taiwan. *Population and Development Review*, 12(1), 77-100.

Liu, P.K.C. (1983). The role of education in fertility transition in Taiwan. Discussion paper 8302. Taipei: Academia Sinica, Institute of Economics.

Newman, J.F. & O.W. Anderson. (1974). Projections of health service personnel and facilities. In C.L. Erhardt & J.E. Berlin (eds.), *Mortality and Morbidity in the United States.* Cambridge, MA: Harvard University Press.

AGED CARE IN PERSPECTIVE-QUO VADIS?

Tracey A. McDonald

I. INTRODUCTION

Throughout most discussions of the demands for resources required for the provision of health services to any group of citizens, rarely does the discussion turn directly to nurses or nursing services. Despite this, nurses account for over half of the health care workforce and only nurses give direct holistic health services on a twenty four hour basis. Why are nurses so invisible in discussions about services, innovations, economics, and strategic planning? The reluctance of government representatives, physicians and administrators to use the word "nurse" is an indication that nursing is perceived by these groups as being either suspect or of little consequence—or are there deeper, more sinister reasons for the non-recognition of the amount and intensity of nurses' contribution to the health of the population?

Australian nurses are among the best clinicians in the world and to achieve this we have had to overcome enormous barriers to education and political recognition. Australian nurses are now better educated, and skilled in research and clinical analysis—and are better able than ever before to perform the

Research in Human Capital and Development, Volume 7, pages 93-112.

ISBN: 1-55938-132-9

complex health service that is nursing. Gerontic nurses specialise in the intellectually intricate art of emotional and physical support required by senior citizens. These clinical specialists have been quietly meeting the challenge of aged care in hospitals, nursing homes and in the community; and take seriously our advocacy role on behalf of senior citizens in seeking a fairer share of health resources and social acceptance of the value of older citizens.

A Brief Demographic Background

Across the continent of Australia, a land of comparative size to the United States of America, and most of which is hostile to rural or urban development, is a relatively small population of around 17 million people. Australia's dependence on immigration to compensate for our limited population, has resulted in a situation where one in five Australians was born overseas and people born in Europe account for approximately 70 percent of these overseas born Australians. (Australian Institute of Health, 1989)

Of the total population, 4.42 percent of males and 6.08 percent of females are age 65 and over (10.5 percent in all). The Commonwealth Commission for the Future (1987) expects that over the next 25 years, Australia's population will increase by about 25 percent (assuming a net gain in population due to immigration of between 50,000 and 100,000). Along with this increase, the proportion of Australians over 65 years is expected to increase to approximately 16 percent by 2021. There is no doubt that Australia's population is slowly aging. The Commonwealth Year Book of Australia (1985) sets the median age of the population (i.e., the age where half the population is older and half younger) in 1990 at 31.63 years compared to the 1981 median age of 29.61 years. In 2001 the median age is projected to be 33.44 years; in 2011 it will be 34.99 years; and in 2021 it will be 35.52 years.

The proportion of people age 65 and over has been steadily increasing since the early 1970s when there was also a decrease in fertility rates and an improved life expectancy. The combination of these trends has created a perception of a "greying" society, which various groups have sought to sensationalize—or manipulate, to add political support to claims for resources.

Wilson (1989) notes that in the 20 years to 1986, the number of persons over 65 rose from some 930,000 to about 1,650,000, that is, by some 75 percent. The relative importance of this development in the total population is of no great concern when in reality it means that the elderly population has only increased from approximately one in twelve in 1966 to about one in ten in 1986. Wilson further states that the dependency ratio of the population (i.e., those outside the age range of 15-64 and presumed to be the productive or economically active group) has seen an even slower increase over the period 1966-1986. In 1966 there were 4.4 people in the workforce for every elderly person, while in 1989 there were 4.9 people in the workforce for each elderly person.

In the international context, Australia is second only to Japan in the low proportion of population over age 65. In other countries such as Sweden and the United Kingdom the proportion of elderly are almost 50 percent higher than that in Australia. In these two countries, over the next 20 years there will be a downward trend in the proportion of senior population, ie.those over age 65. Even so, Australia's position in relation to these countries will not change substantially. By 2010, and taking into account the effects of immigration, Australia will have a similar proportion of seniors as will the United States. Japan will, in this period, see an accelerated growth in its elderly population, and Switzerland and France will also see an increasing trend, but to a lesser extent than Japan (Hugo, 1984).

While the increasing numbers of seniors in Australia's population is apparently not as alarming as popular literature would have us believe, changes within the elderly population are worthy of scrutiny within the context of dependency. The most rapidly increasing population group contains those Australians age over 75 years. Hugo and Wood (1984) estimate that between 1986 and 2001 the population age 65-74 will increase by 17 percent and the 75-84 group will increase by 98 percent. By the year 2011 Australia's population aged over 85 years will have increased in number by about 145 percent.

The increase in the older age groups of Australians has another interesting aspect. The older the age group, the more females there are compared to males. In 1986 in the 65-74 age group there were 1.4 females for every male; in the 75-84 age group there were 1.59 females for every male; and in the over 85 age group there were 2.73 females to every male. By 2001 the total group age 65 and over will feel the effects of an increase in male survivors, but in the older groups there will be even fewer males to every female than there are today (Wilson, 1989).

II. HEALTH NEEDS OF AUSTRALIA'S SENIOR POPULATION

The high proportion of senior females in the Australian population has resulted in some interesting health-related behaviour patterns. Women of all ages are more likely than men, to seek medical and other health services earlier in their illness or problem. This is particularly obvious from puberty to menopause, where the normal female physiology of menstruation and pregnancy has been medicalized to such an extent that women are conditioned to seek medical services for all physiology that does not correspond with that of males. The long term effects of this medical conditioning during youth, may explain why senior women continue this pattern of seeking medical intervention as a means of preventing health breakdown. It is possible that Kannegiesser's (1990) observation that "the ageing of our population alone is nearly doubling the cost of health care" and that the responsibility for dealing with the problem must not be left only to the "politicians, economists and doctors" is in fact a beginning of an important insight into the scope and complexity of present and future health care needs of seniors in Australia and in other comparable communities.

Much of the expense involved in existing methods and approaches to health services for people over 65 is related to the misinterpretation of normal physiology of older people. Few nursing and medical clinicians would argue that because of marked differences in physiology, children and babies must not be treated as small adults—but some of these clinicians will compare reactions and response times of quite old people to care and treatment, against the metabolic speed and physical capabilities of young adults. Still other clinicians frequently underestimate the physical resilience and intellectual strengths of seniors, with demoralizing results.

These observations do not, I realize, cast light on anything that is particularly startling or new. The large numbers of elderly people in the acute hospital system and in long term nursing institutions have been on the health cost agenda for some time now. But in discussions of this issue, emphasis is generally given to the economics of maintaining the current system of dealing with the health needs of those over 65 and not to the pursuit of viable alternative health service strategies. It appears that the public hospital system and other illness-oriented services have become self-propelling. Frail aged people who cannot find help in this maze are destined to fall back on their own resources or those of their families. Currently, approximately 4 percent of the aged population in Australia are in nursing homes while the majority are living in the community, where resources are scarce and access to professional nursing services is limited. Most economic predictions of health services assume that past and current approaches to the care of the aged will continue unchanged, and so prevent any fresh examination of viable alternatives to the present organization of health care, and aged care in particular. This situation reminds me of Irving Zola's story which he used to explain the dilemmas of modern health practice:

> You know, he said sometimes it feels like this. There I am standing by the shore of a swiftly flowing river and I hear the cry of a drowning man. So I jump into the river, put my arms around him, pull him to shore and apply artificial respiration. Just when he begins to breathe, another man cries for help. So back in the river again, reaching, pulling, applying, breathing and then—another yell for help. You know, I am so busy jumping in, pulling them to shore, applying artificial respiration, that I have no time to see who the hell is upstream pushing them all in! (McDonald & Avery, 1988).

Australians have traditionally given special reverence to medical 'solutions' for their health problems and there is no overwhelming necessity to reiterate the evolution of the medical orientation of our health system organization. However, medical solutions are increasingly expensive and with doubtful benefits to the elderly people who come seeking respite from the processes of normal ageing. I hasten to add, that these people certainly have a need for support, guidance and treatment—but is medicine with its focus on 'cure' the most appropriate and most cost-effective approach to meeting these needs?

In a recent survey (McDonald, 1989) conducted on the delivery of professional nursing services to recipients of War Veteran Pensions, entailing third-party reimbursement to nurses, the major problem areas and service needs were determined along with the major nursing functions involved in meeting those needs. The major areas of need were related to chronic illness and physical disability. The next major need related to emotional disability and the person's social and family relationships. This category was more common than the demand for physical treatment. Nursing services included emotional counselling, patient education, consultancy, advocacy and referrals as well as physical care and treatment. Acute illness and mental disability were not seen as significant problems, nor were social conditions a concern for most patients and their families.

These results correspond to another survey of community based nursing care given to 1109 people other than veterans (McDonald & Wilson, 1991). The majority of patients sampled were over 50 with the major groupings between 70-90 years of age. The largest age group was between 79-82. Forty-four percent of the sample were male and 56 percent female. The largest number (49%) lived with only one other person in the household. Mostly this was an elderly spouse. There are obvious implications for carer health and the possible effects of carer stress if professional nursing services are not available. The next largest number (23%) lived alone.

Of the sample, only 18 percent required no assistance or encouragement with physical care; while 32 percent of the sample were very dependent on others for activities of daily living. Twenty percent did not require any treatments and overall only 49 percent depended on nurses for medical treatments. Seventeen percent needed no emotional support or counselling. Thirty five percent were socially independent and only 6 percent were culturally dependent and unable to mix generally in society.

The traditional perception of nursing is that we give only physical care in the form of hygiene or treatments requested by physicians yet in this study it is clear that these tasks do not account for all of the nursing care services given. Nurses obviously give far more holistic health services than they are given credit for. Note also that the "free" services to patients and their families are not mentioned, for example, stress relief and counselling of carers; advocacy services with regard to day-to-day running of the household; consultancy services with physicians and other professionals; environmental safety checks in patient's houses and many others. Nurses generally and herontic specialists in particular, have been encouraged by administrators and other disciplines to trivialize these aspects of their services, yet these are fundamental aspects of grontic nursing. It is these services which enable senior citizens to remain independent and in their own homes.

The perception that our slowly aging population automatically translates into increased morbidity and escalating costs of heath services prompts the more hysterical commentators to predict that the day is fast approaching when we will be overrun by elderly, sick, disabled, and unproductive Australians and that this will seriously undermine the social and economic stability of our society! As noted earlier, Australia's population is slowly aging compared to other countries, and with aging comes some increase in chronicity. Increases in medical technology contribute to the survival of severely chronically debilitated elderly people who must be cared for in institutions such as nursing homes or hospitals. The current population of senior Australians have lived through world wars and depressions and have adopted lifestyles such as high cholesterol diets, alcohol and tobacco use, and stressful pursuits, which were not known to have negative effects on their future health. Compared to the current population of senior citizens, future groups of aged Australians are more likely to be healthier, better educated and more able to control those factors which contribute to health breakdown. The preventable nature of many of the health problems of older people is directly related to the quality of health support which may be available to them.

The survival of elderly people in terms of active healthy longevity is more a function of improved nutrition, better public health measures and the reduction of infections through advances in pharmacology—than a direct result of medical intervention. Ninety-six percent of senior Australians live at home and most of these own their homes. In New South Wales 74 percent of seniors own their own homes outright. The significance of this to financial well-being cannot be overstated. According to Kendig (1989) in the future, this level of home ownership is predicted to remain stable while the more educated and better prepared future aged groups will be more likely to have income from superannuation.

In the "Directions on Ageing in New South Wales" Report (Kendig, 1989) several health facts were compiled. It stated that:

1. The majority of older people have one or more chronic conditions but in most cases, this does not limit their daily lives. The major conditions are arthritis, incontinence, cardiovascular disease, osteoporosis, foot problems, sight problems, hearing problems and dementia and related disorders;
2. Health difficulties of people aged 65-74 years generally are similar to those of younger people. In advanced old age the prevalence of disease increases and individuals are more likely to experience multiple and interrelated pathology;
3. Many health difficulties are acute and episodic rather than chronic;
4. Injuries, particularly falls and broken hips are major causes of admission to institutions;

5. The majority of older people take two or more kinds of medication on a regular basis and risk adverse drug reactions;
6. As age increases so does the incidence of dementia. It is projected that the estimated 35,000 dementia sufferers in 1986 will increase to 62,000 by 2006;
7. Fifty-seven percent of older people had seen a medical practitioner in the month prior to interview and the use of medical, optical and oral services was not related to income. Income did have an effect on the use of dental and podiatry services. 1 in 10 respondents had been in hospital in the previous six months;
8. In 1986 utilisation of public hospital beds by aged people showed 33 percent of all hospital bed days were taken by people aged 70+ years (pp. 24-25).

In all of these statements and estimations there is a significant gap in the reporting of nursing input and nursing control over the care and services received. Gerontic nursing is both a specialty and a significant aspect of general nursing practice in the community and in acute hospitals. The sluggish recognition of the significance of gerontic nursing to the current and future servicing of the health needs of older people, can be attributed to the reluctance of competing disciplines to recognise that nursing is something other than a unified, simple, task related occupation. Just as medicine has specialties in paediatrics, geriatrics, operating room, endocrinology, and so forth, so there are nursing specialists in gerontology, operating room, education, midwifery, critical care, management, paediatrics, surgery, medicine, and so on. Nurses have not promoted themselves or their specialties as a general rule, and so have contributed to this lack of recognition among colleagues and indirectly, among the general public.

Physician Resistance to Alternative Models of Care

It is regrettable that there has been a consistent resistance by physicians to any attempt by nurses to project a true picture of what nursing is all about. Professor Clare (1990) himself a physician, believes that nurses may have pursued tertiary qualifications in order to increase their status, influence and monetary rewards and to move away from clinical nursing. He states that nurses seek status by mimicking physicians in an academic preparation away from patients, and that this has been a result of feminist influences among a predominantly female profession, against medicine which is predominantly male. Many nurses reading this will no doubt have heard similar comments from other medical representatives, but is this superficial mimicry the whole story behind developments in nursing and medicine?

The medical profession, to quote Dingwell (1990):

> is a predominantly upper class and male occupation marked by a variety of occupational theories, two of the most important of which provide for views of the 'doctor' as a technician, indifferent to co-operation, or as a generalised wise man, entitled to dominate any

> relationship. These need not be critical, however if other members of the team can act without support or are prepared to accept subordinate roles (Clare, 1990).

Claims by medical academics that they wish to become more involved in the teaching of nursing, are quite misleading in that medical associations in Australia failed to accept invitations by nursing to consult on joint developments in nursing, medicine and health service, and have preferred to influence public opinion in the tabloid press and within their own association ranks with a campaign of misinformation about nursing and the education of students of nursing.

Nursing Realities in Aged Care

Nurses generally, have not sought to project themselves on the wider screen as alternatives to medicine; nor have we promoted an image of nursing that is radical or self-serving. The hallmark of Australian nursing has been conservatism and quiet persistence in improving the art and skills of nursing and regaining control over those factors which have the potential to enhance or impede nursing practice. The prime objective of these efforts have been more cost-effective and appropriate nursing services rather than self-agrandisement.

In nursing homes, the majority of patient needs are met by nurses, yet nursing is strangely omitted from references to resource utilization or outcomes of care. Diers (1990) believes that admissions to nursing homes and hospitals are in fact referrals for nursing care. This clarifies the role and professional expectations entwined in the nurse-client contract for service. It also challenges any delusion that nursing is, or should be, controlled by anyone other than nurses. Piccone (1990) maintains that while physicians directly influence acute hospital resources, nurses directly manage and control these resources 70 percent of the time. Discharge of patients from acute care is a matter of collaboration between the medical, nursing and allied disciplines, based on either the patient's (or family's) ability to cope with the situation, or the availability of community nursing services.

In community health care, referrals are made to nurses from unrestricted sources and nurses take the responsibility for discharging patients from care. In some areas across Australia, primary nursing is well established in the community where nurses influence and manage all service resources and the focus of care is determined by nurses. The importance of nurses in community development has been recognised by the Australian government and has resulted in increased consultation with nurses regarding our agenda for health service development and the special needs of community groups such as senior citizens. Clearly the federal government is now looking to be innovative in the types of services to be developed, while at the same time maintaining protection of vulnerable groups.

III. IS OUR GOAL "HEALTH FOR ALL"? OR ONLY FOR SOME?

Six years ago, Dr. Halfdan Mahler, the then Director-General of the World Health Organization placed his trust in nurses as the force most capable of bringing health within the grasp of the world community because of the emphasis we place on caring rather than merely curing. He also recognized the political and professional barriers nurses would have to overcome to do this and recommended that nurses would:

> Need to be organized and equipped to break down resistance to change; to sustain the initial effort; and then to develop strategies and action plans (1985, p. 2-5).

In Australia part of the strategy towards achieving the World Health primary care goals has meant overcoming the blockades to access by nurses to education. The movement of nurses into higher education courses now allows for preparation for professional practice as independent, autonomous primary health workers who can practice within communities with an acute understanding of people and their health in terms of social context rather than concentrating on risk factors, illness and disease.

In 1994 the Australia's federal government will take over the funding of nursing courses from the various states. It will be funding a profession which many still view in 1970s terms. That is, a hospital oriented, para-professional group of shift-workers dependent on medical direction and control. Medical opposition to nursing access to tertiary education is as widespread in Australia as it has been in America and Britain. Physicians confidently state that they do not want to see nurses "over-educated" for a role which is, they believe, subordinate to medicine. Part of the physician resistance to nurse education is seen in their efforts to encourage the development of 'technicians' to replace various aspects of professional nursing roles. These moves have been rationalised in terms of the dubious merits of employing one expensive "pair of hands" (a registered nurse), when for the same cost you can hire two pairs of unqualified hands? Claims that such changes are sanctioned by the federal government's structural efficiency policies (i.e., that where possible a generalist should be used in place of a specialist) demonstrates how little is known about the extensive and holistic nature of nursing as generalists. This lack of information or interest in nursing has unfortunately led to unskilled labour being a prominent feature of aged care in Australian nursing homes.

Federal funding of unskilled labour to replace nurses in nursing homes and aged hostels is an example of initiatives aimed at reducing costs associated with aged care. At the present time, unskilled workers outnumber nurses in the aged care institutional sector. These workers undergo a basic skills course lasting a few days, and then are introduced into the aged care sector to work under the supervision of scarce registered nurses. This move trivializes nursing and threatens to fragment the profession. It has been defended from an accounting viewpoint, but the real cost is to the quality of life of elderly Australians caused by a dramatic reduction of access to professional nursing services. This fact seems to have been lost on the bureaucracy, and on the general public.

Access to nursing home care, which is a mixture of serviced accommodation and professional nursing services, is controlled by the federal government. Policies guiding admission to such care clearly direct that all other options be considered and pursued before a nursing home admission can occur. This aspect of the process is controlled by the Geriatric Assessment Teams located in each region. The result of their assessment determines whether seniors will be admitted to an aged care facility or remain in the community, If they are admitted to a nursing home, the category of dependency, to which federal funding is linked for 12 months (regardless of changes in health status) remains. A more accurate system would be based on more frequent nursing assessments of dependency and the intensity of nursing care required in terms of time and nursing expertise. Thus nursing homes could be funded for the actual nursing care given rather than the 'drought or flood' funding situation we have at present.

Women

Over the next ten to twenty years the numbers of women living alone is expected to increase. Hugo and Wood (1984) notes that the proportion of elderly women living alone is approximately double that of elderly men. In the 75 and over age group 35 percent of women live alone. It is also relevant to note that the numbers of elderly men who are married drops from 80 percent in the 65-69 age group to around 64 percent in the 75 and over age group. Corresponding figures for married women is a drop from 58 percent in the 65-69 age group to 24 percent in the older group. These figures have not made allowance for the future effects of an increasing divorce rate in Australia, or the large numbers of childless women. Men, therefore, can expect to have company in late age whereas women are less likely to have this comfort. The implications of these developments lie in the diminished opportunities available to elderly women now and in the future, for family support and care, at a time when they are increasingly prone to physical and social limitations through frailty.

The government's national agenda for women, issued by the Prime Minister's Department and the Office of the Status of Women (1988) appears to understand the needs and preferences of elderly women in Australia. The government recognises that this group can expect lifestyle restrictions and increased requirements for "medical, social and emotional needs" and expects that these will be met through the jointly funded Home and Community Care program. In reality, this program offers to elderly people, unskilled personal assistance and a financial disincentive for them to request professional nursing care. The rhetoric of "appropriate measures" and "more informed and rational choices about care services" pervades the Government's National Agenda for Women—but the issues of partial decentralisation of control of health care financing; and encouragement of the private sector to be innovative and supportive, are not yet considered by the bureaucracy to be viable concepts. So in a situation that is clearly dominated by the needs of elderly Australian women, which could be met in a humane and professional way by nurses, the government appears to be shying away from the convictions so beautifully stated in its press releases and pamphlets.

The New Public Health Concept

Australians have embraced the World Health Organization's concept of the "New Public Health." The philosophy underlying this movement reflects acceptance, by Australians, of the Canadian Lalonde Report (1974). Themes arising from the new public health concept include a belief that society exerts an impact on people and their behaviors; and therefore lifestyle is not always a matter of choice. In answer to the New Public Health enquiry "How can we prevent illness and promote health in the elderly?" the feasibility of people altering their lifestyles to improve health behavior patterns must be examined. This must also be considered in tandem with the generation of policies and strategic plans within the health sector and governments which will promote or inhibit any conditions necessary for such changes. Up until now government policies and initiatives were more often focused on diagnosed illness and disability, than on health promotion and this still exerts some influence on community health services which support a predominantly elderly clientele. Lennie and Owen (1989) perceived the practice of community health in Australia as:

> An illness focussed, paramedical, 'para-hospital', residual service providing mainly secondary and tertiary prevention—that is, early detection and treatment, and support for chronic conditions (p. 90).

and they stated that policy and funding emphasises acute hospital services. This reflects irrefutably, a trivialization of community health.

A possible motivation for this movement away from public health goals could be, that by linking into illness treatment rather than primary care and prevention, community health services in Australia have been able to secure a defined niche in the overall health system which it might otherwise not have.

Administrators and bureaucrats who set up and fund health care services call upon established illness-oriented organisational patterns rather than pursuing alternative strategies which would preserve and enhance health. If this trend toward medical focus and control continues it will move community and gerontic health care further away from primary care initiatives.

Access by Australia's Seniors to Health Care

Medicare, Australia's universal health insurance scheme was set up to provide all citizens with access to health services, without the stigma of being declared a pauper. Yet the many capitulations and adjustments made to the system to appease the medical profession have placed even these basic goals in question. Medicare has seen a chequered life since its origins as Medibank in 1975. Despite alterations by subsequent federal governments to this health insurance scheme, the primary purpose has remained the provision of health insurance to cover basic health care services for all. This federal scheme attempts to redistribute costs of health care across the range of incomes and across the spectrum of people and groups at risk of health breakdown. Medicare is funded through a progressive health insurance levy on all incomes exceeding approximately $7,000.00 and this automatically excludes those on welfare.

As with all policies, there are intended consequences and there are unintended consequences. The redistribution of health costs through the benefits structure can be examined in this light. Medical benefits are fixed to a schedule of fees and the benefit allowed is 85 percent of the scheduled fee, with patients paying physicians at least $3.00 per consultation, over and above the schedule fee and the profit margin set by each physician. The schedule of fees was determined in consultation with the medical profession and is tied to various economic indicators to maintain equity in value over time. Despite these arrangements Carney and Hanks (1986) observed that the continuing great consternation and debate among the medical profession, has been, and is aimed at undermining any government commitment to economic policies of health cost redistribution. While some medical patients are able to be bulk-billed, (i.e., reimbursement of 85 percent of the scheduled fee is made directly to the physician who waives the other 15 percent) others find that they must pay considerable amounts above the schedule fee if they are to have access to ordinary medical services. This is disappointing when we consider the past medical influence associated with the provision of health services and health insurance, and the fact that the system which is now anathema to physicians, is a product of their own making.

This issue has become so politicized in Australia, that access by the general public, and senior citizens in particular, to medical services is being limited by physicians in a deliberate attempt to force government alterations to health policy in favor of increases to medical income. McKnight (1990) reported a situation where the physicians of one small town in New South Wales responded to a call from the Australian Medical Association to cease bulk-billing and force patients to pay the full amount which they felt they were due for services. The hardship caused to aged people in that town is related to the fact that the nearest Medicare office is 32 kilometres away and the alternative of posting their claims would entail a delay of weeks before the rebate would be received, then more time before Medicare rebate cheques can be cleared by the banks. This is another example of elderly Australians being used as a political lever to influence health resources.

IV. NURSING CONTRIBUTION TO THE HEALTH OF ELDERLY AUSTRALIANS

Australian nurses have always provided professional health services in the most arid and undesirable areas of Australia. Nurses, with none of the enticements and added privileges offered to physicians in the outback, have always met the challenge and set up practice in these remote and needy areas. Unfortunately this has not been fully recognized by governments. Recently in one such area of Australia where nurses have for years provided community services to the aged, including community development programs and other nursing supports, a medical practitioner was considered for the position of health team leader even though he had spent most of his professional life dealing with the health problems of young active men. The reactions of the highly qualified and experienced nurses who were to be directed by this inexperienced and unqualified person were distressing to observe. With years of professional practice and proven skills in aged care and health services management, these nurses felt disempowered and frustrated. Many of these family women felt trapped, but they planned to continue working until they could find a way out of aged care. Others who were not constrained by family responsibilities planned to move from the area as soon as other employment could be found. Unfortunately, this type of scurrilous treatment of nurses is not confined to remote areas. It is also a feature of acute and long term care facilities.

Can We Expect Nurses To Continue To Meet These Challenges?

Claims of a nursing shortage were alive and well in Australia throughout 1990. At that time managers and physicians in my country blamed the absence of nurses in the public hospital system on the movement of nurses out of hospital-based apprenticeship-type training and into the tertiary education sector where clinical experience was not able to be controlled by administrators.

Another reason for the lack of nurses at that time was thought to be the comparatively low wages offered, and perhaps the lack of child-care facilities. Half a million dollars (Australian) was spent in New South Wales alone on an advertising campaign to attract people to study nursing and to attract nurses back to the public hospital system. In the 1989 Australian Bureau of Statistics report "Career Paths of Qualified Nurses in Australia," of the 332,900 qualified nurses in Australia in 1989, only 57 percent were working as nurses (Castles, 1989). Now in 1991, there is an oversupply of nurses! In just one year we have moved from shortage to glut in the nursing workforce because of changes in the health industry and no movement in the market. With hospital bed closures and an emphasis on economic rationalism driving the health sector, fewer employment opportunities exist. In the aged care sector (as well as in hospitals) registered nurses are being replaced by nurse aides and unskilled laborers. New graduates of nursing courses will have to compete for work in a severely depleted health sector and for those who are not successful in gaining employment as a registered nurse, the dangers of de-skilling are obvious. A nursing credential is rapidly becoming a stepping stone to such careers as air hostessing, alternative therapies and the military—leaving fewer nurses to meet the challenges.

Another interesting feature of Australian nursing is the decline in numbers of practicing senior nurses (only 16 percent of the workforce in 1989). Many of these nurses leave and enter alternative businesses which offer them greater personal rewards than nursing in the health care system. The loss of these senior nurses constitute a 'brain-drain' and a reduction of aged access to experienced nursing care.

V. QUO VADIS?

Where are we going with aged care? I believe that a viable solution can be found to deal with both the departure of senior nurses from the profession, and the poor access which elderly Australians have to primary care.

With a small change in policy and with the encouragement of government, experienced nurses would happily set up independent practice in the community. Several nursing entrepreneurs have already paved the way for this development and their clients are predominantly senior citizens who find that they have a greater need for the support and advice of nurses than for poly-medication.

Nurses in primary health practice emphasise prevention and health promotion as well as conservative treatment alternatives which call on the existing strengths of clients and their community. Barriers and resistance to these nursing developments is slowly waning as it becomes clear that nursing consultation and treatment is a more appropriate response to the health maintenance needs of the aged. But systemic barriers still exist that prevent widespread access by elderly people to such nursing services.

Consumer need for professionally qualifiedherontic nurses in both nursing homes and the community, has increased considerably following the introduction of selection criteria for institutional care. The resulting increase in dependency of the aged people receiving care subsidised by the government has necessitated a change in approach to the delivery of nursing care to the elderly. Despite this increase in demand, gerontic nurses remain an underutilized health resource.

The major deterrents to gerontic nursing practise have been policy decisions taken at federal government level which have restricted general access to community based nursing care. Only war veterans and their families and those who are able to pay for private health insurance can afford to receive private nursing care at home. Even under these two avenues, medical sanction is required before reimbursement will be made for the nursing service. The only other access people have to nursing care at home, is to pay the full professional fee without hope of even partial reimbursement.

The vast numbers of elderly people who do not fall within these selective categories of consumers, are restricted in access to community nursing services. As a result, nursing support is restricted to weekly or fortnightly visits, despite the level of care clients may need.

Whether as an intended consequence, or an unintended consequence of government policy, under these arrangements the federal government has underwritten restrictions to nursing practice and tied nurses into a situation of direct conflict with medicine if we are to be able to provide adequate nursing services to the aged.

The cost of alternatives to providing professional nursing care to elderly people at home can be measured in admissions to hospitals and nursing homes with a concomitant loss of quality of life and independence. The fastest growing sector of our population are the very old, who while not at their physical peak, are not automatically in need of invasive and interventionist medical treatment. Many of the maladies of age require nursing care and support, with a constant monitoring of health and situation so that strategies to promote health and quality of life are possible. Certainly in acute illnesses or acute relapses of chronic conditions, medical consultation will be required, but the major service needs of the elderly are those which nurses are especially able to fulfil.

Credentialed gerontic nurses are even better able to deal with the limitations of age. Nursing's holistic approach to care of clients and their support networks, gives credence to quality of life over and above professional preferences in treating for a cure. This is the basic difference between caring and curing as well as being the fundamental difference in the professional approaches of nurses and physicians.

For those who remain at home (approximately 96 percent of the total elderly) the government undertakes to provide a wider range of care options to allow the aged to choose the type of care they should have. But in reality the range of care is limited, and linked to medically biased assessments of illness rather than health promotion and maintenance, or community development. Under existing arrangements, even meals-on-wheels is a matter of medical referral!

Access to nursing care and domiciliary benefits is also a matter controlled by the medical profession's decision to refer patients for nursing, and this is underwritten by the federal government in its health insurance regulations.

It is imperative that nurses receive full recognition under Medicare and private health insurance, so that Australian nurses can begin to influence the course of health-care economic policy and decisions and contribute to the battle against spiraling medical costs. The government and the public must be made aware of the benefits accruing from nurses in independent practice and the economic futility of channelling yet more funding into high cost and low return medical technology at the expense of less glamorous services and projects which will reduce the potential need for such esoteric medical procedures.

With developments in tertiary Australian nursing education which support nurses in their progress to doctoral level, it is understandable that there is a tendency for medical graduates to become territorial and defensive as the capacity of nurses to deliver services more relevant to the needs of an ageing population, become more widely accepted. But this territorial trend is not unique to Australia.

Nurses in Maryland, undertook a successful campaign, with the support of The American Association of Retired Persons (as discussed in Wold, 1979, pp. 118-121) and pensioner groups, to bring about changes in reimbursement policies which limit access to other than medical care. In USA the long battle against the systematic restriction of nursing practice and access to nursing services is similar to the campaign which is now underway in Australia. Already members of Australian citizen associations such as the Retired Miners and Senior Citizens are concerned that they have no direct access to professional nursing services and are lobbying authorities to have this reversed.

Economic Positions

Cost-effectiveness is a double edged sword in the argument for direct third-party reimbursement for nursing services. The sheer numbers of nurses in Australia, show up on a simple balance sheet as an enormous cost to health care. Misuse of data such as this has in the past been a favorite pastime of those who seek to constrain nursing growth. Australian nurse economists are currently researching and reviewing the cost-effectiveness of our practice and evaluating the productivity of nursing roles and specialties.

There has been little research conducted on the cost of nursing care compared to the cost of medical care. This is probably a result of the severe delineation of medical and nursing roles in institutions, as well as the widespread practice of attributing nursing inputs to the credit of the physician nominally in charge of the patient. In an area where comparison between the two is available, nursing care can be shown to be more cost-effective than physician care. The cost of nurse-midwifery care has been shown by Reid and Morris (as quoted in Tom, 1982) as being no more costly and possibly less costly, than traditional obstetric care. They put this effect down to the lower use of technological interventions by nurses unless in emergencies, compared to increased cost associated with routine use of technology by physicians. They also mention that nurses are more likely to initiate non-traditional and more natural procedures which, though they may increase the time involved, reduce the incidence of complications overall.

In the gerontic field then, there is no reason to expect that the trend would be any different. Nursing procedures and approaches that call on traditional nursing protocols and alternative health strategies to which elderly people are more able to relate, would reduce the need for the expensive poly-pharmacology which so dominates the physicians approach to the effects of ageing. Gerontic nurses call on people to take responsibility for their own health and happiness and should this entail a rejection of treatments and procedures, gerontic nurses are able to redesign sensitive nursing care strategies in consultation with the patient and the family. How different this approach is from the short, episodic appearances of the physician who has little interest in strategies which involve time or patient control over progress.

Independent practice and independent management are quite different concepts and have different implications for nursing roles and responsibilities. Varney (as quoted in Tom, 1982) claims that independent management calls on the practice of nursing within protocols which define nursing practice and provide for medical consultation and referral where necessary. On the other hand independent practise can mean nursing without formalized protocols for physician back-up.

The implications for nurses wishing to practice in either of these paradigms, lie in the physician resistance to the concept of any model of autonomous nursing practice that threatens the traditional medical posture of superiority over nurses, as well as the more dangerous threat to the commercial monopoly and control of health resources by the medical fraternity.

There are many alternative nursing practice modes that could be encouraged and that would flourish in Australia. Autonomous practice is one; health maintenence group practice is another; collaborative practice is yet another. The possibility of collaborative practice,however, is unlikely in Australia where physicians have for generations restricted, controlled and patronised nurses. But collaborative practice has been successfully set up in California where laws have had to be altered to cope with the scope and complexity of nursing practice. In that State, nursing is described as:

> those functions, including basic health care, which help people cope with difficulties in daily living which are associated with their actual or potential health or illness problems or the treatment thereof which require a substantial amount of scientific knowledge or technical skill (Tom, 1982, p. 264).

According to Kelly and McGarrick (1984) expanded nursing practice has been recognized in Missouri as legitimately overlapping medical practice in some areas where nursing practice and standardized procedures have been established and accepted by the profession. Expanded nursing practice in Australian hospitals has been limited to tasks that are pragmatically geared to the glut or lack of other resources. In the community context, however, nursing practice has been developing across all nursing specialties, and in particular, in the gerontic nursing. The number of nurses in private practice is increasing and consumer demand for these services is rising.

Nurses have a particular talent for cost-containment, and this, coupled with our flexibility and adaptability to change and technological developments, are the basis of the nursing thrust toward providing professional nursing services to the aged and infirm who are living at home, and to the provision of increasingly sophisticated care in the non-institutional setting. It is now apparent that we must validate our autonomous roles by gaining the recognition and remuneration that will encourage nursing development along this path. As this is achieved, economic constraints to patient choices of services will be removed and nurses will consolidate their function as essential first-line providers of health care. While nurses are kept outside this system, the escalating costs of medical services will continue unchecked.

The huge economic advantages to Medicare of available independent nursing services without double servicing through physicians, will lie in the creation of a healthy climate of business competition in the private sector (something that invariably causes market prices to fall) and the beneficiaries of such a trend would be those who are now forced to seek inappropriate health services because of anomalies in our health insurance arrangements and the Australian taxpayer.

VI. CONCLUSION

The most effective response to the health needs of a slowly aging Australian population is the encouragement of professional nurses to take a leading role in the delivery of appropriate lifestyle support services rather than a continued over-emphasis on interventionist and invasive medical treatment. The generations of bureaucratic and medical discouragement of nursing developments will not easily be overcome and nurses will have to be enticed to become entrepreneurs and risk-takers. In answering the ancient question "Quo vadis?" I believe that with the support of nursing colleagues and the general public, we can provide a viable alternative to the costly and depersonalising aged care systems and neglect that currently exist.

REFERENCES

Australian Institute of Health 1988. (1989). *Australia's health*. Biennial Report. Canberra: AGPS. p. 9.

Carney, T. & Hanks, P. (1986). *Australian social security law, policy and administration*. Melbourne: Oxford University Press.

Castles, I. (1989). *Career paths of qualified nurses in Australia: March to July 1989*. Australian Bureau of Statistics. Canberra: AGPS.

Clare, A. (1990). Health care management by consensus—Myth or reality? *Australian Health Review*, 12, 6-18.

Commonwealth Commission for the Future. (1987). A greying Australia. *Future*, 6, 26.

Commonwealth of Australia. (1985). *Year Book Australia 1985*. Canberra: AGPS

Diers, D. (1990). What casemix means for nurses: The USA experience. *Nursing and Casemix Conference*. Sydney.

Dingwell, R. (1990). Problems of teamwork in primary care. In Clare, A. (Ed.), *Health care management by consensus–Myth or reality?* Australian Health Review, 12, 4.

Hugo, G. (1984). *The ageing of ethnic populations in Australia with special reference to South Australia*. Occasional Paper in Gerontology, 6. Melbourne: National Research Institute of Gerontology and Geriatric Medicine.

Hugo, G., & Wood, D. (1984). *Ageing of the Australian population: Changing distribution and characteristics of the aged population*. Department of Immigration and Ethnic Affairs, Canberra: AGPS.

Kannegiesser, H. (1990). Future health options. *Directions in Government*, May 41-43.

Kelly, M., & McGarrick, T. (1984). Nursing negligence in collaborative practice: Legal liability in California. *Law, Medicine and Health Care*, 12, 6.

Kendig, H. (1989). *Directions on Ageing in New South Wales*. Printed and distributed by the Office on Ageing, Premier's Department, NSW Premier's Department. Sydney: AGPS.

Lalonde, M. (1974). *A new perspective on the health of Canadians: A working document*. Report to the Canadian Minister of National Health and Welfare. Ottawa: Information Canada.

Lennie, I., & Owen, A. (1989). Preface to the second edition of Australian Community Health Association. *Review of the community health program* Second edition. Sydney: Australian Community Health Association.

Mahler, H. (1985). *World health organization news release*.

McDonald, T.A. (1988). *Report: Recommendations to the Department of veteran's affairs for restructuring nursing service to veterans*. Sydney: Primary Nurse Practitioners Society.

McDonald, T.T.A. & Wilson, M.G.A. (1991). *The health atlas of the Illawarra: Wollongong, Kiama & Shellharbour*. Illawarra Healthy Cities Project. Wollongong: Illawarra Area Health Printer.

McDonald, T.A., & Avery, A. (1988). Private enterprise nursing: An augmentation of nursing roles. Australian Nurse Teacher's Society 3rd Annual Conference. Sydney.

McKnight, D. (1990). AMA calls on NSW doctors to stop bulk-billing fees. *The Sydney Morning Herald*. May 3.

Office of the Status of Women. (1988). *A say, a choice, a fair go*. Department of the Prime Minister. AGPS: Canberra.

Piccone, D. (1990). *The lamp*. Sydney: NSW Nurses Association.

Tom. S. (1982). Nurse-midwifery: A developing profession. *Law, Medicne and Health Care*, 10, 266.

Wilson, M.G.A. (1989). The greying of Australia through the 1990's. Pp. 3-5 in McDonald, T. (Ed.), *Ageing–The challenge for the 1990's*. Wollongong: University of Wollongong Press.

Wold, S.J. (1990). *Commuity health nursing: Issues and topics 1990*. Connecticut, Appleton & Lange.

PART II

LIFE STYLE AND HEALTH

THE STUDY OF SOCIAL LEARNING AND SOCIAL BONDING VARIABLES AS PREDICTORS OF CIGARETTE SMOKING BEHAVIOR AMONG NINTH-GRADE MALE STUDENTS IN TAIPEI, TAIWAN, THE REPUBLIC OF CHINA

Ching-Mei Lee and Lorraine G. Davis

I. INTRODUCTION

In the Republic of China (ROC), cigarette smoking tends to be a gender-linked phenomenon. Cigarette smoking is becoming popular among male adolescents in spite of the widespread knowledge that smoking is harmful. Several studies indicated that the smoking rate among junior high school students in Taipei was between one-fourth and one-fifth (Chen, 1987; Chen, 1985; Huang, 1981;

Research in Human Capital and Development, Volume 7, pages 115-134.

ISBN: 1-55938-132-9

Huang, 1982). Conversely, many fewer female students in the same age smoked cigarettes, with the smoking rate being around one twentieth (Chen, 1987; Huang, 1981). C.C. Chen showed that 34.9 percent of the ninth-grade male students had smoked cigarettes and 7.9 percent were current smokers. S.C. Huang's study demonstrated that among the ninth-grade male student group, 33.7 percent reported having smoked cigarettes. S.C. Chen's study indicated that 42.2 percent of the ninth-grade male students had smoked cigarettes.

This study attempted to assess the effects of social learning and social bonding variables on smoking behavior among male youth. The study is of particular importance at the present time because foreign tobacco companies have been allowed to market their products in the ROC much more freely since January 1987. One immediate result was that the volume of foreign tobacco imported into the ROC drastically increased. Between January 1 and October 31, 1987, 447,000 boxes of foreign tobaccos were imported. This amount is 22 times greater than the amount imported during the whole year of 1986 (Union Press, 1987). One primary marketing strategy used by those companies is designed to target adolescents. For example, the tobacco manufacturers use youths as models in poster and magazine advertisements, sponsor disco dance parties and music events, and distribute free samples of cigarettes at those events (Chen, 1988). Therefore, it is very important for schools and communities to explore factors contributing to smoking and to develop educational programs to help prevent adolescents from becoming smokers. The results of the study might facilitate a greater understanding of adolescent smoking behavior and hence be used in the development of effective antismoking interventions.

Social Learning Theory

Sutherland and Cressey's (1960) differential association theory has offered a powerful explanation for deviant behavior. Burgess and Akers (1966) reintegrated Sutherland and Cressey's differential association theory with behavioral reinforcement theory to develop a theory of deviant behavior that has been referred to as Social Learning Theory or Differential-Association-Reinforcement Theory. Akers, Krohn, Lanza-Kaduce, and Radosevich (1979) hypothesize that the possibility of deviant behavior would increase in the following situations: (a) when there is greater exposure to deviant models rather than to nondeviant models (imitation); (b) when there is more association with deviant than with nondeviant norms, peers, and adults (differential association); (c) when deviant behavior is differentially reinforced over nondeviant behavior (differential reinforcement); and (d) when there are more positive or neutralizing definitions of deviance than negative definitions. Akers et al. (1979) propose a process which specifies the interrelationships among the concepts. In this process, differential association with different groups occurs first. These groups provide the social contexts in which exposure to definitions, imitation of models, and social reinforcement for deviant or conforming behavior can occur. The definitions are learned through imitation and social reinforcement by members of the groups with whom one is associated and serve as discriminative stimuli for behavior. The definitions, in interaction with the imitation of behavioral models and the anticipated reinforcement, produce behavior.

The explanatory power of Akers' Social Learning Theory has been assessed on both drug use (Akers et al., 1979) and cigarette smoking (Krohn, Skinner, Massey, & Akers, 1985). Akers et al. also demonstrated that differential association was the most powerful explanatory component in terms of alcohol and marijuana use, with imitation being the weakest explanatory component.

Social Bonding Theory

Hirschi's Social Bonding or Social Control Theory recounts a process in which the bonds tying adolescents to conventional society are broken or weakened, freeing them from conventional social duty and making them more likely to conduct delinquent behavior (Krohn, Massey, Skinner, & Lauer, 1983). According to Hirschi, the mechanism of Social Bonding Theory is produced through the influence of four components that bond the person to conventional society: (a) attachment to conventional others, (b) commitment to conventional goals and activities, (c) involvement in conventional activities, and (d) beliefs in conventional norms.

Hirschi's Social Bonding Theory has been tested by researchers in the fields of drug use (Akers & Cochran, 1985) and cigarette smoking (Krohn et al., 1983). Krohn et al. also demonstrated that, among the social bonding indicators, beliefs in conventional norms and commitment to education had the strongest constraining effect on adolescent cigarette smoking.

The main purpose of the study was to predict cigarette smoking status among ninth-grade male Chinese students using Akers' Social Learning Model and Hirschi's Social Bonding Model. More specifically, the research initially explored cigarette smoking behavior of the student respondents. Next, several family status variables, Akers' Social Learning Model, and Hirschi's Social Bonding Model were used to predict cigarette smoking status. Finally, a comparison was made to evaluate the explanatory power of the social learning and social bonding models in predicting student's smoking status. The dependent variable smoking status was assessed on a 5-point continuum, ranging from never smoking, experimentally smoking, ex-smoking, occasionally smoking, to regularly smoking.

II. METHODOLOGY

Population and Sampling

The population of the study consisted of the ninth-grade male students enrolled in public junior high schools in Taipei during the 1988-1989 academic year. The population included about 20,000 male students in 55 public junior high coed schools and male schools in Taipei. Multistage cluster sampling method with stratification was used to choose the sample. In the first stage, public junior high school was the sampling unit. All public junior high coed schools and male schools in Taipei were stratified by size of school (large or small) and geographic location (east, west, north, or south). Large schools referred to schools that had more than 15 ninth-grade male classes, with small schools referring to those having 15 or fewer ninth-grade male classes. Then 11 schools were randomly selected from 55 public junior high coed schools or male schools in Taipei. In the second stage, the sampling unit was a classroom of ninth-grade male students. In each selected school, all classes of ninth-grade males were stratified by ability grouping (high-achieving class or low-achieving class). For the schools where males and females were separated, one male class was randomly selected from the high-achieving classes and one from the low-achieving classes. However, the number of sampled classes was doubled in the schools having coed classes only. The potential number of students in the selected classes was 875; 828 (94.6%) students attended the class during the period of investigation. All 828 students in attendance answered the questionnaire, and 797 questionnaires were found to be valid, indicating a response rate of 96.3 percent.

Instrumentation

The survey was conducted in December 1988 and January 1989. The data were collected by using a group self-administered questionnaire. The questionnaire was administered to all students in attendance in the sampled classes on the day of the survey. Subjects were assured that their responses would be kept anonymous. The study instrument comprised three parts. The independent variables consisted of social learning and social bonding variables, with the dependent variable being cigarette smoking status.

Cigarette smoking status was measured by one 5-point item ranging from 1 to 5, with 1 indicating never smoking, 2 indicating an experimental smoker, 3 indicating an ex-smoker, 4 indicating an occasional smoker, and 5 indicating a regular smoker. The social learning variables were measured by a 37-item scale derived from one developed by Akers et al. (1979), Krohn et al. (1985), and Becker and Lauer (1984) and revised by the investigator to fit Chinese cultural characteristics. The social bonding variables were measured by an 36-item scale adapted from the questionnaire developed by Akers et al. (1979), Krohn et al. (1983), and Becker and Lauer (1984). A pilot study was conducted by the investigator before data collection in order to check the readability and possible problems of the instrument and also to judge the time-length of the questionnaire.

III. RESULTS

Cigarette Smoking Status

Among the 797 student respondents, 49.8 percent had never smoked cigarettes, and 27.9 percent were experimental smokers (Table 1). However, 22.2 percent of the respondents reported being smokers, including ex-smokers (5.1%), occasional smokers (10.5%), and regular smokers (6.6%). The smoking status variable was further verified by the smoking frequency reported by the students. Smoking frequency was significantly and positively correlated with smoking status ($r = .91$, $p < .001$). Support was therefore given to the hypothesis that the smoking status variable had high concurrent validity and was an appropriate assessment of cigarette smoking.

Social Learning Predictors of Smoking Status

A descriptive analysis was performed to examine the frequency distribution of the social learning variables (Table 2). In terms of imitation, the student respondents reported having 2.47 smoking role models. The student's family members, mass media, role models on television or movies, peers, and teachers provided important smoking role models for the students. For the component of definitions favorable or unfavorable to smoking, the results indicated that the respondents had unfavorable definitions and disapproved of adolescent smoking. Regarding the differential association component, the outcomes revealed that the student group as a whole was associated with antismoking norms and a predominantly nonsmoking peer group. The six scales of differential social reinforcement component consistently demonstrated that the student respondents believed that they would get negative social reactions from smoking. Similarly, the two variables of the differential social/nonsocial reinforcement component linked smoking to negative consequences.

Reliability and Validity

The reliability of the social learning and social bonding scales has been tested. Krohn et al.'s (1985) study of adolescent cigarette smoking used the factor

Table 1. Smoking Prevalence Among Student Respondents

Variables	*Response*	*n*	%	*Skewness*[a]
Smoking Status	1. Never Smoke	397	49.8	1.2
	2. Experimentally Smoke	222	27.9	
	3. Ex-Smoker	41	5.1	
	4. Occasionally Smoke	84	10.5	
	5. Regularly Smoke	53	6.6	
Smoking Frequency	1. Never Smoke	397	49.8	1.8
	2. Only Once or Twice	217	27.2	
	3. 1 Cigarette per month	45	5.6	
	4. 1 Cigarette per week	50	6.3	
	5. 1-5 Cigarettes per day	38	4.8	
	6. 6-10 Cigarettes per day	23	2.9	
	7. 11-20 Cigarettes per day	13	1.6	
	8. More than 20 Cigarettes per day	7	.9	
	9. Unknown	7	.9	

Notes: $N = 797$.

[a] Smoking status and smoking frequency had skewness values of 1.2 and 1.8, respectively, which were below the criterion of normality $\pm$ 2.58 (Tabachnick & Fidell, 1983). Therefore, the assumption of normality was met for both variables.

analysis method to yield six social learning factors for their initiation model. The reliability for those social learning factors was moderate, with Cronbach's alpha of .73 for both the parental definition scale and the friends' definition scale, .60 for the parental imitation scale, and .66 for the friends definition scale, .60 for the parental imitation scale, and .66 for the friends' imitation scale. Within the same study project, Skinner, Massey, Krohn, and Lauer (1985) used the factor analysis method to create nine social bonding factors. The reliability of those social bonding factors ranged from medium to high, with Cronbach's alpha ranging from .64 to .88 for the attachment scales, from .62 to .76 for the commitment to conventional activities and institutions scales, and from .55 to .85 for the belief scales, respectively. In this study, Cronbach's Alpha coefficient was recomputed to estimate the internal consistency of each scale. The reliability tests showed that both the social learning and social bonding scales had a medium to high level of reliability, with Cronbach's Alpha coefficients ranging from .65 to .91 and .57 to .92, respectively (see Table 2).

The social learning variables and social bonding variables have been found to be valid in explaining adolescent cigarette smoking. In their 3-year panel study of adolescent cigarette smoking in a community in the American Midwest, Krohn et al.'s (1985) utilized the path analysis method to test the causal model of the theory. Their study demonstrated that the 12 social learning variables could explain 41 percent of the variance in smoking maintenance

Table 2. Descriptive Data and Reliability Coefficients for Social Learning Variables

		Scale (Mean)				*Reliability*
Variables (Number of items)	*N*[a]	Low-High	*Mean*	*S.D.*	*Skewness*[b]	*Alpha(N)*[c]
Imitation						
SL1: Index of Imitation (1)	791	0-6	2.47	1.74	0.30	—
Definitions Favorable or Unfavorable to Smoking						
SL3: Law Abiding/Violating Definitions (2)	794	1-6	5.17	.92	−1.40	.65(791)
SL2: Techniques of Neutralization (3)	795	1-6	2.55	1.17	.57	.75(794)
SL4: Positive/Negative Definition (1)	788	1-6	2.31	1.36	.68	—
Differential Association						
SL6: Significant Peers' Norm Qualities (3)	781	1-6	2.42	1.12	.59	.77(483)
SL5: Significant Adults' Norm Qualities (3)	796	1-6	2.08	.94	1.07	.70(697)
SL7: Differential Peer Association (6)	784	1-4	1.56	.64	1.50	.85(451)
Differential Social Reinforcement						
SL8: Priase for Not Smoking (8)	791	1-6	5.12	.90	−1.50	.89(287)
SL13: Interference with School Activities (3)	785	1-6	4.78	1.11	−.61	.91(784)
SL11: Informal Deterrence (1)	794	1-6	4.10	1.52	−.70	—
SL13: Formal Deterrence (1)	791	1-6	3.97	1.44	−.60	—
SL9: Friends' Rewarding or Punishing Reactions (1)	777	1-5	2.33	.70	.99	—
SL10: Parent's Rewarding or Punishing Reactions (1)	792	1-5	1.71	.50	−.12	—
Differential Social/Nonsocial Reinforcement						
SL14: Social/Nonsocial Rewards-Costs of Smoking (2)	796	(−12)	−5.02	4.46	.13	—
SL15: Overall Reinforcement Balance (1)	795	1-3	1.42	.53	.68	—

Notes: [a] The number of cases involved in the calculation of the mean of each subscale.

[b] The skewness values for all the social learning variables were below the criterion of normality (±2.58), with a range of −1.50 to 1.50. Therefore, the social learning variables were nonproblematic for parametric data analyses.

[c] The number of cases involved in the calculation of the Cronbach's Alpha of each subscale represented the number of respondents having complete data for all questions in the subscale.

among adolescents, but the variables could only explain 3 percent of the variance in smoking initiation. In another analysis of the same research project, Krohn et al. (1983) indicated that the social bonding model, as measured by 10 social bonding variables, could explain 33 percent of the variance in cigarette smoking among adolescents.

A test of translation validity was performed to examine the accuracy of the translation of the instrument from an English version to a Chinese edition. First, the investigator translated the English version of the instrument to a Chinese edition. Then another bilingual individual translated the Chinese edition of the instrument back to an English version. The discrepancy between the original English form and the final English form was examined. The translation validity coefficient was calculated to be .82. This result demonstrated that the Chinese version of the instrument had a moderately satisfying translation validity.

A multiple regression analysis was completed to examine the overall relationship between the social learning model variables and smoking status (Table 3). The social learning model variables were significant predictors of cigarette smoking status ($R = .81$, $p < .001$). The total social learning model variables could account for 64.4 percent of the variation of smoking status, indicating a fairly strong relationship. Altogether, the multiple regression analysis indicated that four of the five major social learning components were significant predictors of smoking status. Definitions favorable or unfavorable to smoking was the most predictive social learning component, followed by differential association, differential social reinforcement, and differential social/nonsocial reinforcement. The component imitation was not significantly related to smoking status.

To determine the specific social learning variables that could best predict smoking status, individual social learning variables were entered separately into a stepwise regression equation (Table 4). The outcome revealed that six social learning variables were entered in the stepwise regression equation, which together explained 64.0 percent of the variance in smoking status among the students. The positive/negative definition variable was the strongest predictor of smoking status, singularly accounting for 83.0 percent of the total explained variance (.536/.640). The second most powerful social learning predictor was differential peer association, which could additionally account for 10.9 percent of the total explained variation of smoking status (.070/.640). Interference with school activities, the third most powerful predictor of smoking status, could uniquely contribute an additional 3.1 percent to the total explained variance of smoking status (.020/.640). Three other variables, namely overall reinforcement balance, adult norm qualities, and techniques of neutralization, while significant, could only add a minimal amount to the explained variance.

Table 3. Multiple Regression Analysis of Smoking Status by Social Learning Variables

Social Learning Variables	*B Value*	*Beta*	*Significance*
Imitation			
SL1: Index of Imitation	.03	.04	
Definitions Favorable or Unfavorable to Smoking			
SL2: Techniques of Neutralization	.08	.08	*
SL3: Law Abiding/ Violating Definitions	−.06	−.04	
SL4: Positive/Negative Definition	.42	.46	***
Differential Association			
SL5: Significant Adults' Norm Qualities	−.12	−.09	***
SL6: Significant Peers' Norm Qualities	−.07	−.06	
SL7: Differential Peer Association	.49	.25	***
Differential Social Reinforcement			
SL8: Praise for Not Smoking	−.06	−.04	
SL9: Friends' Rewarding or Punishing Reaction	.05	.03	
SL10: Parents' Rewarding or Punishing Reaction	−.03	.01	
SL11: Informal Deterrence	.02	.02	
SL12: Formal Deterrence	−.03	−.03	
SL13: Interference with School Activities	−.13	−.12	***
Differential Social/Nonsocial Reinforcement			
SL14: Social/Nonsocial Rewards-Costs of Smoking	.01	.05	
SL15: Overall Reinforcement Balance	.19	.08	**

Notes: $N = 712$. Multiple $R = .81$. Adjusted $R^2 = .6436$.
F ratio = 86.60 ($p = .0000$).
* $p < .05$.
** $p < .01$.
*** $p < .001$.

Overall, the directionality of correlation values indicated that the students who were smokers were more likely to have the following six characteristics: (a) They tended to approve adolescent smoking, (b) associate with smoking friends, (c) think that smoking would not interfere with their school activities, (d) believe that they would get mainly positive results from cigarette smoking, (e) perceive that their significant adults would approve of adolescent cigarette smoking, and (f) justify adolescent cigarette smoking.

Social Bonding Predictors of Smoking Status

A descriptive analysis was done to offer information about the social bonding variables (Table 5). In terms of the attachment to conventional others component, the student group tended to report a moderately high degree of

Table 4. Stepwise Regression of Smoking Status by Social Learning Variables

Social Learning Variables	*Adj.* R^2	*Adj.* R^2 *Change*	F *(R^2 Change)*
SL4: Positive/Negative Definition	.536	.536	823.79***
SL7: Differential Peer Association	.606	.070	125.89***
SL13: Interference with School Activities	.626	.020	38.27***
SL15: Overall Reinforcement Balance	.631	.005	12.23***
SL5: Adult Norm Qualities	.636	.005	9.91**
SL2: Techniques of Neutralization	.640	.004	8.74**

Notes: $N = 712$
** $p < .01$.
*** $p < .001$.

Table 5. Descriptive Data and Reliability Coefficients for Social Bonding Variables

Social Bonding Variables *Variables (Number of items)*	N[a]	*Scale (Mean)* *Low-High*	*Mean*	*S.D.*	*Skewness*[b]	*Reliability* *Alpha(N)*[c]
Attachment to Conventional Others						
SB: Peer Attachment	796	1-5	3.41	.83	−.28	.90(793)
SB1: Maternal Attachment (7)	797	1-5	3.36	.90	−.47	.89(794)
SB2: Paternal Attachment (7)	797	1-5	3.11	1.03	−.23	.92(789)
Commitment to Conventional Activities						
SB6: Commitment to School Activities (3)	797	1-6	4.70	.73	−.57	.57(794)
SB5: Educational Aspirations (1)	794	1-5	3.61	1.09	−.28	—
SB7: Religiosity(1)	794	1-4	2.32	.88	−.06	—
SB4: School Grades & Academic Endeavors[d] (2)	797	0-4	2.00	.86	−.21	.65(786)
Beliefs in Conventional Norms						
SB9: Legal Norms (2)	794	1-6	5.17	.92	−1.40	.65(791)
SB8: Parental Norms (1)	791	1-6	4.91	.99	−1.01	—
SB10: Belief about Cigarette Smoking (1)	793	1-6	4.74	1.37	−1.30	—
SB11: Belief about Drinking Alcohol (1)	793	1-6	4.17	1.48	−.42	—

Notes: [a] The number of cases involved in the calculation of the mean of each subscale.
[b] The skewness values for all social bonding variables were below the criterion of normality (±2.58), with a range of −.06 to −1.40. Therefore, parametric data analyses of social bonding variables were completed.
[c] The number of cases involved in the calculation of Cronbach's Alpha coefficient of each subscale was based on the people who answered all the questions in the subscale.
[d] The variable school grades and academic endeavors was computed by the following formula: [z score (average school grades) + z score (average time spent studying every weekday)]/2.

attachment to their parents and peers. For the commitment to conventional activities component, the student group as a whole tended to report a high degree of commitment to conventional activities (e.g., school activities, educational aspirations, and school grades and academic endeavors), with religiosity being the only exception. With regard to the beliefs in conventional norms component, the student group tended to adhere to both legal norms and parental norms and also thought cigarette smoking to be wrong. However, the students only slightly agreed that drinking alcohol was wrong.

A multiple regression analysis was done to examine the overall predictability of the social bonding model variables on smoking status (Table 6). The total social bonding model variables were significantly related to smoking status ($R = .63$, $p < .001$). The social bonding model variables explained 39 percent of the variance of smoking status among the student respondents, which demonstrated a strong relationship. Additional inspection of the standardized regression coefficients showed that two of the three major social bonding components, namely commitment to conventional activities and beliefs in conventional norms, were significantly associated with the smoking status of the students.

To identify the specific social bonding variables that offer the most predictive ability to smoking status, individual social bonding variables were entered separately into a stepwise regression equation (Table 7). The results indicated that four social bonding variables were entered in the stepwise regression equation, collectively explaining 39.2 percent of the variance of the smoking status of the students. Belief about cigarette smoking was the strongest social bonding predictor of smoking status, which could account for more than 64.0 percent of the total explained variation (.253/.392). The school grades and academic endeavors variable was the second strongest social bonding predictor of smoking status, which singularly accounted for 26.8 percent of the total explained variance (.105/.392). Legal norms contributed an additional 7.6 percent to the total explained variance (.030/.392). Educational aspiration, while significant, only added 1.0 percent to the total explained variance (.004/.392). The directionality of the correlation demonstrated that, compared to the students who did not smoke cigarettes, the students who smoked tended to have the following four characteristics: (a) thought cigarette smoking was not wrong, (b) received low grades and spent less time studying and doing homework, (c) did not adhere to general laws and smoking laws, and (d) had a low level of educational expectations.

Comparison of the Explanatory Power of Two Models in Predicting Smoking Status

Two procedures were performed in order to compare the explanatory power of the two models in predicting cigarette smoking status among male students.

Table 6. Multiple Regression Analysis of Smoking Status by Social Bonding Variables

Social Bonding Variables	*B Value*	*Beta*	*Significance*
Attachment to Conventional Others			
SB1: Maternal Attachment	.02	.01	
SB2: Paternal Attachment	−.06	−.04	
SB3: Peer Attachment	.04	.02	
Commitment to Conventional Activities			
SB4: School Grades & Academic Endeavors	−.37	−.25	***
SB5: Educational Aspirations	−.10	−.09	*
SB6: Commitment to School Activities	.01	.01	
SB7: Religiosity	−.03	−.02	
Beliefs in Conventional Norms			
SB8: Parental Norms	.02	.01	
SB9: Legal Norms	−.29	−.21	***
SB10: Belief about Cigarette Smoking	−.31	−.34	***
SB11: Belief about Drinking Alcohol	.04	.04	

Notes: $N = 781$. Multiple $R = .63$. Adjusted $R^2 = .3900$.
F ratio = 46.34($p = .0000$).
* $p < .05$
*** $p < .001$.

Table 7. Stepwise Regression Analysis of Smoking by Social Bonding Variables

Social Bonding Variables	*Adj.* R^2	*Adj.* R^2 *Change*	$F(R^2$ *Change)*
SB: Belief about Cigarette Smoking	.253	.253	265.52***
SB4: School Grades and Academic Endeavors	.358	.105	127.48***
SB9: Legal Norms	.388	.030	39.78***
SB5: Educational Aspirations	.392	.004	6.07*

Notes: $N = 781$.
* $p < .05$.
*** $p < .001$.

In the first procedure, two methods of setwise hierarchical regression analysis were used (Table 8). Using the first method, the set of social learning variables was initially entered into the regression equation. The social learning model variables uniquely explained 64.3 percent of the variation of smoking status ($p < .001$). Then, the set of social bonding variables was entered into the equation, contributing an additional .7 percent to the explained variance of smoking status ($p < .05$). Using the second method, the set of social bonding model variables was initially entered, which accounted for 40.5 percent of the variance of smoking status ($p < .001$). The results indicated that both models

Table 8. Setwise Hierarchical Regression Analysis of Smoking Status by Social Learning and Social Bonding Variables

Sets	*Adj. R^2*	*Adj. R^2 Change*	*F (R^2 Change)*
Method 1			
Step 1: Social Learning Variables	.643***	.643	84.86***
Step 2: Social Bonding Variables	.650***	.007	2.30*
Method 2			
Step 1: Social Bonding Variables	.405***	.405	44.13***
Step 2: Social Learning Variables	.650***	.245	35.36***

Notes: $N = 699$.
* $p < .05$.
*** $p < .001$.

Table 9. Stepwise Regression Analysis of Smoking Status by All Social Learning and Social Bonding Variables

Predictors	*Adj. R^2*	*Adj. R^2 Change*	*F (R^2 Change)*
Social Learning Variables			
SL4: Positive/Negative Definition[a]	.533	.533	798.46***
SL7: Differential Peer Association[a]	.602	.069	121.70***
SL13: Interference with School Activities[a]	.622	.020	38.06***
SL15: Overall Reinforcement	.628	.006	12.72***
SL5: Adult Norm Qualities	.634	.006	10.84***
SL2: Techniques of Neutralization	.638	.004	10.19**
Social Bonding Variables			
SB4: School Grade and Academic Endeavors	.643	.005	9.30**
SB7: Religiosity	.645	.002	4.48*

Notes: $N = 699$
[a] Three social learning variables contributed substantially to the variance of smoking status.
* $p < .05$.
** $p < .01$.
*** $p < .001$.

contributed uniquely and significantly to the variance of smoking status. However, the social learning model explained more variation of smoking status than did the social bonding model. Together, both models could account for 65.0 percent of the variance of smoking status.

In the second procedure, to decide the specific social learning and social bonding variables that offered the most predictive ability to smoking status, individual variables of both models were entered separately into a stepwise regression equation (Table 9). The result revealed that six social learning variables and two social bonding variables contributed significantly to the variation of smoking status at the .05 level. These eight variables together explained 64.5 percent of the variance of smoking status. Nevertheless, only three social learning variables, named positive/negative definition, differential peer association, and interference with school activities, contributed substantially to the variance of smoking status. It was concluded that none of the social bonding variables could explain a substantial amount of the variance of smoking status after the social learning variables were held constant. This finding was congruent with the previous hierarchical regression analysis in concluding that Akers' Social Learning Model contributed more in predicting adolescent smoking than did Hirschi's Social Bonding Model.

IV. DISCUSSION

The present study showed that the prevalence of smoking among ninth-grade male students in Taipei was high. Among the 797 male student respondents, over 50 percent had tried cigarettes. This result approximates those found in a study of a similar youth group (Chen, 1985). However, the smoking rate found in the present study is higher than those reported by S.C. Huang (1982) and C.C. Chen (1987). Both studies of junior high school students in Taipei found that about one third of the ninth-grade male students had ever smoked cigarettes.

In terms of the amount of cigarettes smoked by the current smokers, the present research found that the smoking frequency among the students was higher than that found in the earlier studies. The present study revealed that 8.8 percent of the students smoked less than one cigarette per day while only 5.0 percent to 6.0 percent of the students in S.C. Chen's (1985) and S.C. Huang's (1982) studies did so. In addition, 9.3 percent of the students in the present study smoked more than one cigarette every day, compared to only 3.0 percent to 4.0 percent in the previous studies. The difference in smoking frequency between the present study and past research could be attributed to the fact that the earlier studies were with a younger population (seventh- to ninth-grade male students). However, it is possible that the high smoking frequency rates in the present study reflect a trend toward increased frequency. In order to explore the smoking trend among teenagers, a longitudinal study should be performed.

The present study demonstrated that Akers' Social Learning theory provided a useful theoretical framework in predicting adolescents' smoking behavior. The findings are congruent with previous research (Krohn et al, 1985). More specifically, the present study demonstrated that definition favorable or unfavorable to smoking was the most predictive social learning component of smoking status, followed by differential association, differential social reinforcement, and differential social/nonsocial reinforcement, with imitation being the only component failing to make a contribution. Nevertheless, the outcomes differ from Akers et al.'s (1979) conclusions that (a) differential association was the most powerful social learning component in predicting drug use and (b) social/nonsocial reinforcement was more predictive of drug use than was purely social reinforcement. In other words, the present research shows that the components definitions favorable or unfavorable to smoking and social reinforcement play a more important role in predicting smoking status.

Additionally, the findings that the Social Bonding Model is a valid theoretical framework in explaining adolescent smoking and the components beliefs in conventional norms and commitment to conventional activities had the strongest constraining effect on adolescent smoking are supported by past research (Krohn et al., 1983).

Both Byram's (1984) research of adolescent drinking behavior and Akers and Cochran's (1985) study of adolescent marijuana use indicated that the social learning model was more powerful in predicting drug use than was the social bonding model. This study tends to support previous research. This study indicates that both models contributed uniquely and significantly to the variation of smoking status; however, the Social Learning Model was more powerful in predicting smoking status than was the Social Bonding Model. The finding may be explained in two ways. First, the social bonding model variables (attachment, commitment, and beliefs) are usually general in nature, while the social learning model variables (imitation, definitions, association, and reinforcement) appear to be specific to smoking. Thus, the outcome that the social learning variables could predict smoking better than could the social bonding variables seems to be reasonable. Second, the conceptual overlap between the social learning and social bonding theories, as mentioned by Akers and Cochran (1985), may contribute to the limited unique contribution of the social bonding variables after the social learning variables are held constant.

Among all the social learning and social bonding variables, three social learning variables offered a substantial level of explanation. Positive/negative definition contributed the most, followed by differential peer association and interference with school activities. These findings imply that both individual factors (positive/negative definition and interference with school activities) and external factors (peer association) are determinants of teenage smoking behavior, but the former are far more influential. Similarly, J.W. Chen (1988) asserted that adolescent smoking was related more to internal factors (e.g., smoking intention, attitudes toward smoking, and educational goals) than to external factors (e.g., perceived smoking prevalence among close friends). The phenomenon can be explained by the selective characteristics of the learning process. Although external factors, such as smoking peers, offer the important smoking models which one can comply and identify with, smoking behavior will not occur until one truly accepts and internalizes the external influence and sets up his own definitions about smoking. Just as Akers et al. (1979) mentioned, the definitions (internal factors) are learned through imitation of and social reinforcement from the people with whom one is associated (external factors). Once learned, the definitions serve as discriminative stimuli for the behavior. Accordingly, to effectively help prevent teenagers from starting to smoke, the antismoking program needs to emphasize both the individual and external factors related to smoking.

The seven most predictive social learning and social bonding variables are further discussed below. The finding that positive/negative definition was the strongest predictor of smoking is congruent with the previous studies that reported positive attitudes toward smoking to be linked to adolescent smoking (Chassin, Presson, Sherman, Corty, & Olshavsky, 1984; Pederson, Baskerville, & Lefcoe, 1981; Rooney & Wright, 1982). In addition, the result that techniques of neutralization were significantly correlated with smoking status supports Sykes and Matza's (1957) position that the definitions toward smoking and justifying delinquent behavior were associated with deviant behavior. However, cause-effects between the definitions of smoking behavior cannot be drawn from the study due to its cross-sectional characteristics. A longitudinal study is suggested in order to explore the relationship between teenage smoking and the development of definitions/views toward smoking over time.

Next, the outcome that differential peer association was the second most powerful social learning predictor of smoking status supports previous studies' conclusions that smokers tended to have smoking friends while nonsmokers usually having nonsmoking friends (Gordon, 1986; Huang, 1982; Levitt & Edwards, 1970; Rooney & Wright, 1982). Just as Ellis, Indyke, and Debevoise (1980) mentioned, "Peer pressure—the powerful influence exerted by friends in the same age group to conform to group behavior—is a major factor in initiating smoking behavior, particularly among younger adolescents" (p. 6). One possible explanation for this finding is that identity through conformity to a particular group is an important human need, especially for adolescents. According to Erikson, the crisis of identify versus confusion occurs in adolescence, and the central problem of this period is establishing a sense of identity (Gage & Berliner, 1988). This result implies that school educational process needs to help students recognize the influence of the peer group on their behavior and assist them to make informed decisions regarding smoking. However, of particular surprise was that peer norm qualities, a variable similar to differential peer association, did not make a unique contribution after other variables were held constant. This finding conflicts with previous studies reporting that close friends' cigarette smoking did not make a unique contribution after other variables were held constant (Rooney & Wright, 1982). Taken together, the outcome indicates that the association with smoking peers is a more important determinant of adolescents' smoking behavior than is their perception of smoking norms for their peers.

Furthermore, interference with school activities, one variable of the social reinforcement component, uniquely contributed to the variance of smoking status. In contrast, the other five variables of the same component (praise for not smoking, friends' and parents' rewarding and punishment, and formal and informal deterrence), while mostly independently significant, were not significant predictors of smoking status after other social learning and social bonding variables were entered. The outcome implies that the internal social reinforcement (interference with school activities) is a more important factor in predicting smoking than are the external social reinforcement factors (e.g., rewarding and punishing reactions of others).

Additionally, overall reinforcement balance was predictive of smoking status. This significant finding was consistent with Hunter, Baugh, Webber, Sklov, and Berenson's (1982) study that reported current smokers as having stronger beliefs about the rewards of smoking than did nonsmokers. Besides that, the finding that adult norm qualities variable was also a significant social learning predictor of smoking status is congruent with S.C. Chen's (1985) and Nolte, Smith, and O'Rourke's (1983) findings that nonsmoking students were more likely to perceive that their significant adults would disapprove of their smoking than were the smokers. The implication is that to effectively facilitate nonsmoking behavior among adolescents, the school should foster family involvement and enhance parental nonsmoking norms.

The finding that the school grades and academic endeavors variable was a predictor of smoking status is congruent with studies in the literature that report school grades and time spent on doing homework to be negatively related to tobacco uses (Chen, 1988; Rooney & Wright, 1982; Young & Rogers, 1986). Just as Newman (1970) mentioned, cigarette smoking may be a compensatory action by teenagers who do not succeed academically, especially for those anticipating failing the examination. If this inference is real, helping the students with low academic performance to establish a positive self-concept and to find ways to obtain achievement may be a possible method to address the teenage smoking problem. Additionally, the present study indicated that commitment to school activities was not uniquely predictive of teenage smoking. The finding is similar to an earlier study (McCaul, Glasgow, O'Neill, Freeborn & Rump, 1982) reporting no significant difference in the number of school activities between smokers and nonsmokers. As a whole, the result reflects that the commitment to school academic work is a stronger predictor of youth smoking than is the commitment to the overall school activities. Compared to nonsmokers, the student smokers may be less involved in school academic work, but not participate differentially in general school activities.

Moreover, the outcome that the social learning component imitation, while independently related to smoking status, was not uniquely associated with smoking status after other variables were entered, is supported by other, researchers. Akers et al. (1979), in their study of alcohol and marijuana use, also reported imitation to be the weakest explanatory social learning component of drug use. The limited nature of the index of imitation (number of smoking models) may explain the insignificant result. Compared to other social learning variables, imitation is more stationary, rather than socially interactive, in nature. Therefore, it is anticipated that merely observing smoking models would not be a powerful predictor of smoking behavior.

Finally, the social bonding component attachment to conventional others was not found to be uniquely linked to smoking status. The outcome supports Krohn et al.'s (1983) conclusion that parental attachment, compared to other social bonding variables, had a relatively small effect on adolescent smoking. However, the present outcome is incongruent with Krohn et al.'s findings that parental attachment was negatively related to adolescent smoking. The difference between the present study and Krohn et al.,'s research may be due to the cultural differences between the American family and the Chinese family. Generally, Chinese parents are not as child-centered, or as verbal with their children, as are American parents. Hence, the parental attachment scale designed by Akers et al. (1979) that focuses on understanding, praising, listening, being close, and talking over plans may not be a valid measurement of the bond between Chinese parents and children. A scale measuring parental supervision and child-raising attitudes may be a more appropriate measurement of the bond that ties Chinese children to their parents.

V. RECOMMENDATIONS

The present study has provided a basic understanding about the social learning and social bonding factors contributing to smoking behavior in a Chinese youth population. Several recommendations are made for future endeavors and study. First, because a substantial proportion of the ninth-grade male students smoked cigarettes, the antismoking program needs to focus on prevention in the early grades and encourage students' decisions not to smoke in all later grades. The program should also include smoking cessation programs that are attractive to adolescents in order to support and facilitate nonsmoking behaviors. Teachers and school administrators should positively encourage the student smokers to actively seek assistance. Second, because the students' definitions of smoking are the prime determinants of their smoking behavior, the educational program needs to address the normative meaning of smoking. For example, the program may involve value clarification techniques to help students clarify their own values, beliefs, and attitudes, and to help them establish unfavorable definitions toward smoking. More studies should also be completed to explore the process of the development of negative views of smoking in order to facilitate nonsmoking behavior among adolescents.

Third, because social reinforcement would influence students' decisions concerning smoking, the antismoking program should promote a school environment that discourages smoking and fosters positive social reinforcement for nonsmoking behavior. Fourth, since low academic performance is associated with adolescent smoking, the program needs to actively identify the high-risk group and help prevent them from initiating smoking. The school needs to carefully diagnose the problems existing in the educational process and develop strategies to assist the students with achievement deficiencies in achieving a higher level of academic performance, increasing achievement, and developing positive self-concepts.

In addition, research methods other than the self-administered questionnaires are suggested in order to provide a triangulation check and comprehensive evaluation of adolescent smoking. Finally, future studies may include psychosocial factors, personality characteristics, individual factors, and social environmental factors to improve the predictability of adolescent smoking behavior and enhance practical implementation. More studies, such as longitudinal and cross-section studies, could verify the applicability of the theories. However, researchers should carefully consider the cultural differences between Chinese and American societies in order to make necessary adjustments in applying the theories in a Chinese population.

ACKNOWLEDGMENTS

We wish to express our sincere appreciation to Dr. Ronald Akers and Dr. Samuel Becker for their kind permission to use and modify their research instruments. Our sincere acknowledgment also goes to all school administrators and students in the 12 participating public junior high schools for their assistance with data collection.

REFERENCES

Akers, R.L., & J.K. Cochran (1985). Adolescent marijuana use: A test of three theories of deviant behavior. *Deviant Behavior* 6, 323-346.

Akers, R.L., M.D. Krohn, L.L. Kaduce, & M. Radosevich. (1979). Social learning and deviant behavior: A specific test of a general theory. *American Sociological Review* 44, 636-655.

Becker, S.L., & R.M. Lauer. (1984). *Questionnaire: Survey of youth smoking and behavior.* (Available from S.L. Becker, Department of Communication Studies, University of Iowa, Iowa City, Iowa 52242).

Byram, O.W. (1984). *A Study of adolescent drinking behavior with emphasis on four explanatory models.* Doctoral dissertation, Mississippi State University, 1983. *Dissertation Abstracts International*, 45, 952A.

Burgess, R.L. & R.L. Akers. (1966). A differential association reinforcement theory of criminal behavior. *Social Problems* 14, 128-147.

Chassin, L., C.C. Presson, S.J. Sherman, E. Corty, & R.W. Olshavsky. (1984). Predicting the onset of cigarette smoking in adolescents: A longitudinal study. *Journal of Applied Social Psychology* 14, 224-243.

Chen, C.C. (1987). *A study of the reactions to second-hand smoking and the related factors among junior high school students.* Unpublished master's thesis, National Taiwan Normal University, Taipei, ROC.

Chen J.W. (1988). *Adolescents' knowledge, behavior patterns, and attitudes related to cigarette smoking in the Republic of China.* Unpublished doctoral dissertation, Indiana University, Bloomington.

Chen, S.C. (1985). *A study of smoking intentions of junior high school students in Taipei.* Unpublished master's thesis, National Taiwan Normal University, Taipei, ROC.

Chen, T.T.L. (1988). *The impact of American tobacco trade on Taiwan: A case study.* Paper presented at Interagency Committee on Smoking and Health, National Advisory Committee's meeting of "Tobacco and Health Internationally."

Ellis, B.H., D. Indyke, & N.M. Debevoise. (Eds.) (1980). *Smoking programs for youth.* (NIH Publication No. 80-2156). Bethesda, MD: National Cancer Institute.

Gage, N.L. & Berliner, D.C. (1988). *Educational Psychology* (4th ed.). Boston, MA: Houghton Mifflin.

Gordon, N.P. (1986). Never smokers, triers and current smokers: Three distinct target groups for school-based antismoking programs. *Health Education Quarterly* 13, 163-180.

Huang, S.C. (1982). *A study of reasons for cigarette smoking and smoking role models of junior high school students.* Unpublished master's thesis, National Taiwan Normal University, Taipei, ROC.

Huang, S.S. (1981). *A study of the influence of recognitive smoking cessation strategy on the smoking behavior of junior high school students.* Unpublished master's thesis, National Taiwan Normal University, Taipei, ROC.

Hunter, S.M., J.G. Baugh, L.S. Webber, M.C. Sklov, & G.S. Berenson. (1982). Social learning effects on trial and adoption of cigarette smoking in children: The Bogalusa heart study. *Preventive Medicine* 11, 29-42.

Krohn, M.D., Skinner, W.F., Massey, J.L., & Akers, R.L. (1985). Social learning theory and adolscent cigarette smoking: A longitudinal study. *Social Problems*, 32 455-471.

Krohn, M.D., J.L. Massey, W.F. Skinner, & R.M. Lauer. (1983). Social bonding theory and adolescent cigarette smoking: A longitudinal analysis. *Journal of Health and Social Behavior* 24, 337-349.

Levitt, E.E., & J.A. Edwards. (1970). A multivariate study of correlative factors in youth cigarette smoking. *Developmental Psychology* 2, 5-11.

McCaul, K.D., R. Glasgow, H.K. O'Neill, V. Freeborn, & B.S. Rump. (1982). Predicting adolescent smoking. *Journal of School Health* 52, 342.

Newman, I.M. (1970). Adolescent cigarette smoking as compensatory behavior. *Journal of School Health* 40, 316-321.

Nolte, A.E., Smith, B.J., & O'Rouke, T. (1983). The relative importance of parental attitudes and behavior and behavior upon youth smoking behavior. *Journal of School Health*, 53, 264-271.

Pederson, L.L., J.C. Baskervile, & N. Lefcoe. (1981). Multivariate prediction of cigarette smoking among children in grades, six, seven and eight. *Journal of Drug Education* 11, 191-203.

Rooney, J.F., & T.L. Wright. (1982). An extension of Jessor and Jessor's problem behavior theory from marijuana to cigarette use. *The International Journal of the Addictions* 17, 1273-1287.

Skinner, W.F., J.L. Massey, M.D. Krohn, & R.M. Lauer. (1985). Social influences and constraints on the initiation and cessation of adolescent tobacco use. *Journal of Behavioral Medicine* 8, 353-377.

Sutherland, E.H. & Cressey, D.R. (1960). *Principles of Criminology* (6th ed.). Chicago, IL: J.B. Lippincott.

Sykes, G.M., & D. Matza. (1957). Techniques of neutralization: A theory of delinquency. *American Sociological Review* 22, 664-670.

Tabachnick, B.G., & L.S. Fidell. (1983). *Using multivariate statistics.* New York: Harper & Row.

Union Press. (1987). Foreign tobacco import increased twenty-two times. *Union Press*, November 5, p. 3.

Young, T.L., & K.D. Rogers (1986). School performance characteristics preceding onset of smoking in high school students. *American Journal of Diseases of Children* 140, 257-259.

BEHAVIORAL AND HEALTH EFFECTS OF THE ANTISMOKING CAMPAIGN IN THE UNITED STATES

Kenneth E. Warner

I. INTRODUCTION

The history of cigarette smoking in the United States consists of two equally remarkable phases. From the turn of the century through 1963, cigarette consumption rose virtually monotonically, growing from 54 per year per adult in 1900 to more than 4300 in 1963. Since 1963, per capita consumption has fallen to fewer than 3000, to levels last seen in the early 1940s; per capita consumption has fallen annually, without exception, every year since 1973 (see Figure 1).

The first phase might well be labeled the "love affair." Glorified in movies, endorsed by athletes, sent to war with our soldiers, and modeled by prominent politicians and intellectuals, cigarette smoking became a virtual social necessity, initially among males and then, later, among females too. In the late 1940s and early 1950s, almost three-quarters of American men born between 1911 to 1930 were smokers (U.S. Department of Health and Human Services, 1989).

Research in Human Capital and Development, Volume 7, pages 135-148.

ISBN: 1-55938-132-9

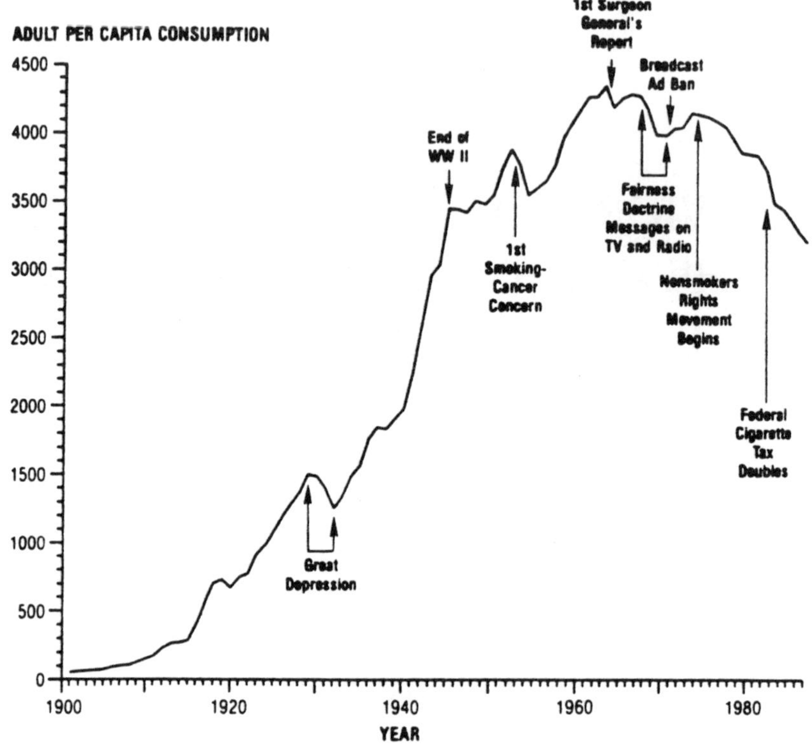

Source: U.S. Dkepartment of Health and Human Services (1989).

Figure 1. Adult Per Capita Cigarette Consumption and Major Smoking-and-Health Events

The love affair with the cigarette was jolted in the early 1950s by prominent articles in the popular press describing the findings of epidemiologic studies strongly linking smoking to lung cancer (Doll & Hill, 1954; Wynder & Graham, 1950). Cigarette consumption dropped sharply in 1953 and 1954, rebounding thereafter as the public was "reassured" by the development of filter-tipped cigarettes, a product sold with the theme—often implicit, sometimes explicit—that filters "removed" the hazardous elements from cigarette smoke. (The filter-tip share of the market rose from 1 percent in 1952 to become the dominant product by 1960.)

The event marking the beginning of the end of America's love affair with the cigarette was publication in January 1964 of the first Surgeon General's report on smoking and health (U.S. Public Health Service, 1964), a landmark government report that initiated what has come to be known in the United

States as "the antismoking campaign." While there has never been a coordinated campaign against smoking in the United States, publication of the report marked the beginning of a sustained period of diverse antismoking education, publicity, and policy development activities by a wide variety of governmental agencies, at the federal, state, and local level, medical and voluntary health agencies, and private for-profit concerns.

Collectively, these activities have contributed to an extraordinary change in the social acceptability of smoking and in patterns of smoking behavior (U.S. Department of Health and Human Services, 1989). Whereas 40 years ago, failure to smoke verged on social deviance (at least among men), today government officials and health professionals confidently plan for a near-future "smoke-free society." This paper reviews findings from the author's research on the effects of the antismoking campaign on smoking behavior and the associated health benefits.

II. CAMPAIGN-INDUCED CHANGES IN SMOKING BEHAVIOR

Introduction

While Figure 1 exhibits a clear change in smoking trends, the behavioral measure—adult per capita consumption (total cigarette consumption divided by the population over 17 years of age)—masks important changes in the composition of the smoking population, the mix of smoking prevalence and daily consumption (the combination of which determines aggregate consumption), the nature of the product, and so on. There are numerous obvious and subtle measures of behavior change that, owing to space limitations, will not receive attention here. These include the rapid shift from unfiltered to filtered cigarettes, referred to above, a similar shift two decades later from "full-flavored" cigarettes to "low tar and nicotine" brands, and the transition from a male-dominated market to today's parity in smoking by the sexes. For discussion of these developments, the interested reader should consult the 1989 Surgeon General's report on smoking and health (U.S. Department of Health and Human Services, 1989).

The author's research on behavioral effects of the campaign has focused on two dimensions of smoking behavior. The following section describes an analysis of how per capita consumption has changed relative to the pattern it would have followed in the absence of the antismoking campaign. The second section considers how age-sex cohort-specific smoking prevalence rates have been affected by the campaign. Details on methods and findings are presented elsewhere (Warner, 1989).

Campaign Effects on Per Capita Consumption

As observed in Figure 1, the decrease in adult per capita cigarette consumption since 1964 has been substantial. Nevertheless, that decrease *understates* the effect of the antismoking campaign on per capita consumption. The reason is that the diffusion of smoking throughout the public, reflected in the escalating consumption prior to 1964, likely would have persisted in the absence of publicity linking smoking to disease. The prevalence of smoking among men had leveled off at 53 percent by the 1930s (a rate sustained through the mid-1950s). By contrast, the prevalence of smoking among women was increasing rapidly, from an estimated 18 percent in 1935, to 25 percent in 1955, to 34 percent in 1965. Had women's prevalence eventually caught up with that of men, and had daily consumption rates been comparable, annual per capita consumption would have reached approximately 6000 cigarettes.

To assess the likely pattern of per capita consumption in the absence of the antismoking campaign, I fitted data on per capita consumption and a series of independent variables, for the years 1947-1987, through use of ordinary least squares regression analysis. Independent variables included standard economic variables, such as cigarette price, a measure of lagged consumption (reflecting the addictiveness of smoking), and measures of antismoking "events," including publication of the first Surgeon General's report, growth of the nonsmokers' rights movement, and so forth. Estimated regression coefficients for the antismoking variables indicated the specific association between each "event" and per capita consumption.

The aggregate impact of the antismoking campaign in any given year was estimated by adding the values of all the relevant antismoking variables, multiplied by their regression coefficients, to the year's actual per capita consumption. (This includes an antismoking effect carried forward into future years through the lagged dependent variable, the "addiction" measure.) Comparison of actual per capita consumption with the resulting estimates of consumption in the absence of the antismoking events (and hence "campaign") provided the study's measure of the aggregate impact of the campaign.

The analysis concluded that individual antismoking "events" were associated with statistically significant decreases in per capita consumption ranging from 3.5 to 7.5 percent in the year of the event. The aggregate impact of the campaign, during each year from 1964 through 1987, is depicted in Figure 2. (The dotted and dashed lines reflect alternative treatment of cigarette price trends. See Warner, 1989 for an explanation.) All told, the analysis indicated that in 1987 per capita consumption would have been 79 to 89 percent greater than the level actually experienced had the campaign never materialized. This is a much more substantial impact than the typical interpretation comparing the level of consumption in 1963, the year prior to initiation of the campaign, with the level in 1987. That difference amounts to 35 percent (still a substantial impact).

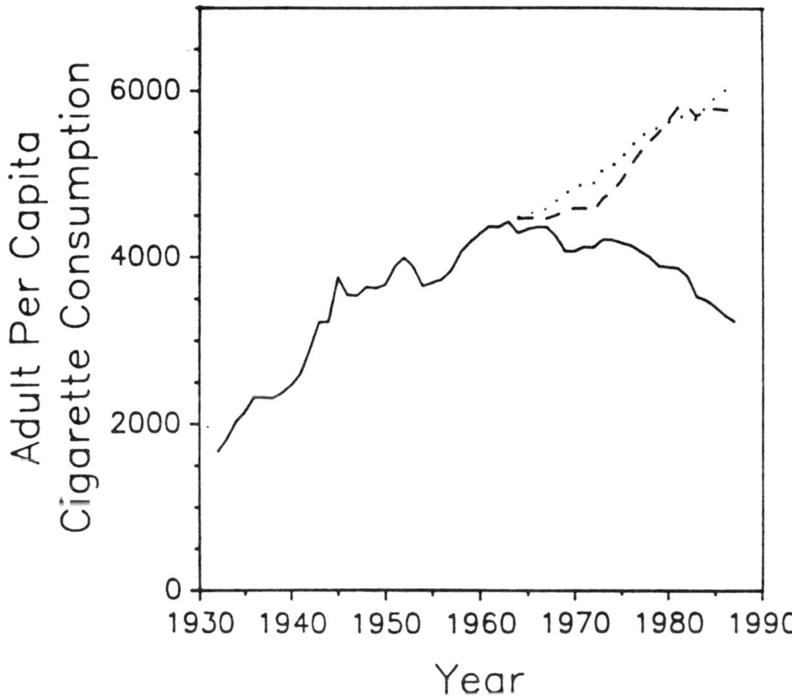

Source: Warner (1989).

Figure 2. Comparison of actual per capita cigarette consumption (solid line) with estimated consumption in the absence of the antismoking campaign (dashed line = actual cigarette prices; dotted line = real price held constant)

Campaign Effects on Cohort-Specific Smoking Prevalence

The most common measure of smoking behavior is prevalence. Every age-sex birth cohort has a unique pattern of growth in prevalence and then, for those that are old enough, decline. Decreasing prevalence results from many smokers quitting while few are starting, and from the differential mortality experience of smokers and nonsmokers.

While each cohort's prevalence pattern is unique, there are distinct similarities in rates of growth, ages of peak prevalence, and time and rate of decline. This is particularly true for men. Drawing on the "traditional" patterns of prevalence growth and decline, and factoring in diffusion trends, a colleague

Table 1. Smoking Prevalence for Males (%) 1964 through 1985, Reported and Expected in the Absence of the Antismoking Campaign

Birth Cohorts	*Year (19–)* 64	65	66	67	68	69	70	71	72	73	74	75	76	77	78	79	80	81	82	83	84	85	*Expected minus reported 1985*
1901-10																							
Reported	45	45	45	43	42	39	39	36	35	34	31	30	28	27	26	20	18	18	19	19	17	16	9
Expected	46	46	46	45	44	42	42	40	39	38	37	37	36	36	35	34	32	31	29	28	26	25	
1911-20																							
Reported	61	60	59	59	58	54	53	51	50	48	46	46	43	40	39	32	30	29	28	26	24	22	23
Expected	62	61	60	60	59	57	56	56	55	55	54	54	53	52	51	50	49	48	47	46	45	45	
1921-30																							
Reported	63	62	62	61	60	56	55	53	52	51	48	47	47	45	44	42	41	39	36	34	33	32	21
Expected	66	66	66	65	65	64	64	64	63	63	63	62	62	61	61	59	58	57	56	55	54	53	
1931-40																							
Reported	59	59	58	57	56	53	53	51	50	49	47	46	45	44	44	42	44	43	42	40	38	35	19
Expected	62	63	63	64	64	64	64	63	63	63	62	62	62	61	61	59	58	57	56	55	55	54	
1941-50																							
Reported	42	46	50	54	58	58	58	57	56	55	54	53	51	49	47	44	44	43	41	40	39	38	22
Expected	43	48	53	57	61	61	62	62	63	63	64	64	64	64	64	63	63	62	62	62	61	60	
1951-60																							
Reported	1	2	4	7	10	14	18	23	27	31	36	38	40	40	39	40	42	41	40	40	39	38	28
Expected	2	3	5	8	11	16	21	26	32	39	44	50	54	58	61	62	64	65	65	66	66	66	

Source: Warner (1989).

and I compared actual reported prevalence patterns in 10-year age-sex birth cohorts with those that might have been expected in the absence of the antismoking campaign. The method is described in two papers (Warner, 1989; Warner & Murt, 1982). The findings of this analysis are presented in Tables 1 and 2 and illustrated in Figures 3 and 4.

In each of the figures, the actual cohort prevalence experience over time is plotted as the solid line. The dashed line represents the prevalence trend we would have anticipated in the absence of the campaign. The two figures illustrate two different phenomena. In Figure 3, representing an older male cohort (born 1921-1930), actual prevalence peaked in the early 1950s (when the men were in their 20s) and began to decline thereafter, as would be expected (because few people start smoking after the age of 21, while many quit (U.S. Department of Health and Human Services, 1989)). According to our analysis, the antismoking campaign accelerated a declining prevalence trend; the effect of the campaign is measured by the gap between the dashed and solid lines. The precise numbers are found in Table 1.

Figure 3 depicts the smoking prevalence of a cohort of younger women, born 1941-1950. This cohort's reporting of its actual prevalence experience suggests that prevalence peaked in the early 1970s (when the women were in their 20s and early 30s) and declined thereafter. Had the cohort's smoking history not been influenced by the antismoking campaign, we estimated that prevalence would have continued to rise throughout the 1970s and remain near peak levels through the mid-1980s (the end point of this analysis).

As the data in Tables 1 and 2 indicate, by 1985 all six of the age-sex birth cohorts studied were experiencing smoking prevalence rates well below those that would have been anticipated in the absence of the antismoking campaign. Numerically, the smallest percentage point differences were found in the oldest cohorts of each sex, but this primarily reflected the very low smoking prevalence of these cohorts in the 1980s. (In 1985, these individuals were 75 to 84 years old. Their peak prevalence never rose as high as that of later cohorts, and at this relatively advanced age, smoking had killed a significant percentage of the smokers. This affects the accuracy of retrospective reporting of smoking behavior as a measure of the cohort's true historic experience [Harris, 1983].)

The largest gaps between reported prevalence and that expected in the absence of the campaign were found in the youngest cohorts. According to our estimates, in 1985 fully two-thirds of men born 1951-1960 would have been smokers had the campaign never materialized. In fact, only 38 percent were smoking that year. Among women, we would have expected 54 percent to be smokers, without the campaign; with the campaign, only a third reported themselves to be smokers.

Combining the reported and estimated prevalence figures with the size of the corresponding cohorts (and adjusting the latter for differences due to differential death rates of smokers and nonsmokers), I estimated that there

Table 2. Smoking Prevalence for Females (%) 1964-1985, Reported and Expected in the Absence of the Antismoking Campaign

Birth Cohorts	*Year (19–)*																						*Expected minus reported 1985*
	64	*65*	*66*	*67*	*68*	*69*	*70*	*71*	*72*	*73*	*74*	*75*	*76*	*77*	*78*	*79*	*80*	*81*	*82*	*83*	*84*	*85*	
1901-10																							
Reported	22	21	21	20	20	19	18	17	17	16	15	15	13	13	13	13	15	13	10	8	8	8	6
Expected	22	21	21	20	20	19	19	19	19	18	18	18	17	17	17	17	16	16	15	15	14	14	
1911-20																							
Reported	36	36	36	36	35	33	33	31	31	30	29	28	27	26	26	25	26	24	22	20	19	18	13
Expected	37	37	37	37	36	36	36	35	35	35	35	35	34	34	34	34	33	33	32	32	31	31	
1921-30																							
Reported	43	43	43	42	42	40	40	39	39	39	38	38	38	37	36	31	31	30	30	39	28	27	17
Expected	44	45	46	47	48	48	48	49	49	49	48	48	48	47	47	47	47	46	46	45	44	44	
1931-40																							
Reported	44	44	44	44	44	43	43	43	42	42	42	42	41	40	39	39	35	34	34	34	33	32	17
Expected	45	46	46	47	47	48	48	48	49	49	50	50	50	51	51	51	51	51	50	50	49	49	
1941-50																							
Reported	25	30	34	38	40	40	41	41	41	41	41	40	39	38	37	35	34	34	33	33	32	32	20
Expected	27	32	36	40	42	44	46	47	48	49	50	50	51	51	52	52	52	52	52	52	52	52	
1951-60																							
Reported	1	1	2	3	6	10	13	17	22	27	31	35	38	38	37	34	32	33	34	34	33	32	22
Expected	1	2	3	5	8	12	15	20	25	31	36	40	45	47	49	50	50	51	52	53	54	54	

Source: Warner (1989).

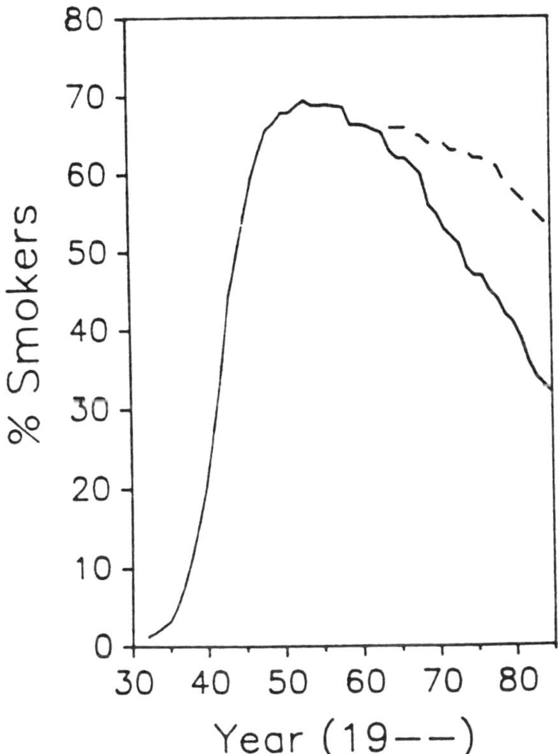

Source: Warner (1989).

Figure 3. Actual Smoking Prevalence History (solid line) and Estimated Prevalence for 1964-85 in the Absence of the Antismoking Campaign (dashed line), 1921-30 Male Cohort

would have been 91 million smokers in the United States in 1985 had the antismoking campaign never occurred. In fact, there were an estimated 56 million smokers that year.

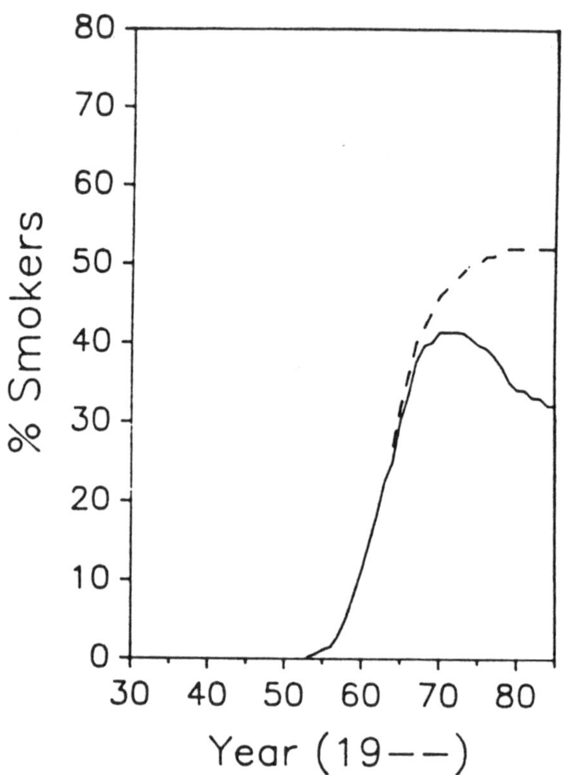

Source: Warner (1989).

Figure 4. Actual Smoking Prevalence History (solid line) and Estimated Prevalence for 1964-85 in the Absence of the Antismoking Campaign (dashed line), 1941-50 Female Cohort

III. DEATHS POSTPONED BY CAMPAIGN-INDUCED DECREASES IN PREVALENCE

The cohort smoking prevalence analysis constituted the base for estimation of the number of premature smoking-related deaths that were postponed or avoided as a result of the antismoking campaign. This study also estimated

Table 3. Death Postponed by Campaign-related Smoking Cessation and Noninitiation, 1964-85 (in thousands)

Birth year	*Males*	*Females*	*Total*
1901-10	103.6	16.7	120.3
1911-20	182.0	46.0	228.0
1921-30	182.7	59.6	242.3
1931-40	83.2	22.7	105.9
1941-50	44.0	15.5	59.5
1951-60	29.0	4.2	33.2
Total	624.5	164.7	789.2

Source: Warner (1989).

the increase in life expectancy experienced by those who benefitted from campaign-produced decisions to quit smoking or not to start.

The number of deaths postponed was estimated by applying epidemiologic data on age- and sex-specific mortality rates of smokers, quitters, and never smokers to the cohort-specific changes in smoking prevalence just described. The reduced mortality rates of quitters (compared with continuing smokers) were multiplied by the estimated number of campaign-induced quitters and non-initiators in each cohort and in each year from 1964 through 1985. To estimate the number of life-years saved associated with each death postponed, life expectancy gained was calculated by comparing the former smoker's life expectancy with that of a continuing smoker, using life table analysis (see Warner, 1989 for details).

The results of the deaths postponed analysis are presented in Table 3. The bottom line, found in the lower right-hand corner of the table, is that 789,200 premature smoking-produced deaths were avoided or postponed between 1964 and 1985 as a result of the American public's behavioral responses to the antismoking campaign. A large majority of the health benefit was derived by men, because many more men were smokers, men's smoking prevalence exhibited more substantial change in response to the campaign, and men's smoking-related death rates were greater than those of women. For both men and women combined, according to the life table analysis, the average life expectancy gained associated with each premature death postponed or avoided was 20.6 years.

Much of the postponement of death associated with campaign-related nonsmoking through 1985 would not be realized by 1985. Quitting in the 1980s, for example, is likely to avoid many more deaths in the 1990s than in the years immediately following cessation, reflecting the gradual decline in former smokers' relative risk of death. By "aging" the population of quitters and noninitiators alive in 1985 and applying to them the differential mortality rates of former smokers, I estimated the avoidance or postponement of death

Table 4. Death Postponed 1986-2000 by Campaign-related Smoking Cessation and Noninitiation through 1985 (in thousands)

Birth year	*Males*	*Females*	*Total*
1901-10	18.8	5.9	24.7
1911-20	194.6	83.8	278.4
1921-30	429.5	162.6	592.1
1931-40	315.3	128.6	443.9
1941-50	290.5	109.8	400.3
1951-60	241.7	76.3	318.0
Total	1490.4	567.0	2057.4

Source: Warner (1989).

between 1986 and the year 2000 as a result of quitting or noninitiation through 1985. The results of this analysis are presented in Table 4. These figures demonstrate that the principal health benefit of the antismoking campaign lies in the future. Between 1986 and 2000, over 2 million additional smoking-related deaths will be avoided or postponed as a consequence of campaign responses occurring *before* 1986. (These results, as well as those of the analysis pertaining to 1964-1985 were subjected to sensitivity analyses. For results, see Warner, 1989.)

IV. CONCLUSION

The findings from these studies indicate that the antismoking campaign in the United States has achieved truly remarkable changes in behavior, and impressive health gains associated with them. The estimated mortality avoidance represents one of the most substantial public health success stories of the century. At the same time, the massive toll of continuing smoking means that this success represents only a small portion of smoking's disease burden. As seen in Figure 5, between 1964 and 1985 Americans born between 1901 and 1960 experienced an estimated 5.7 million smoking-related deaths. In the absence of the antismoking campaign, 6.5 million cumulative deaths would have been expected. The estimated 789,200 deaths postponed or avoided represented just 12 percent of the anticipated mortality toll.

For several reasons, the results presented in this paper should be interpreted in terms of their qualitative meaning. Assumptions made in each analysis (particularly the cohort prevalence analysis) create uncertainties about the precise magnitudes of the various estimates. Sensitivity analyses help to clarify the potential importance of such uncertainty (Warner, 1989).

Use of the then-available data also affects the results. For example, the American Cancer Society has recently completed collection and tabulation of data from a six-year prospective study of 1.2 million people that is providing

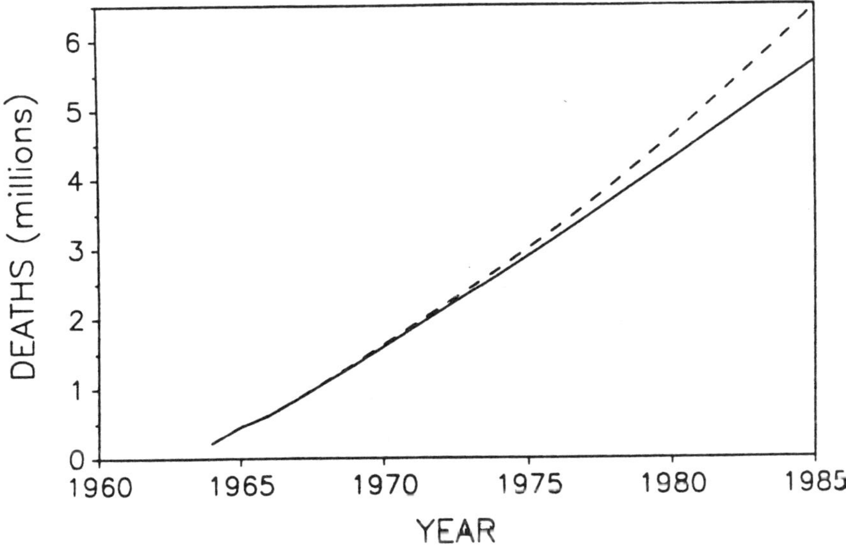

Source: Unpublished data from study reported by Warner (1989).

Figure 5. Comparison of Estimated Cumulative Smoking-Related Deaths (solid line) with Estimate of the Number That Would Have Occurred without the Antismoking Campaign (dashed line), 1964-85.

more contemporary estimates of the health effects of smoking. An important finding of this new ACS study is that the deleterious effects of smoking by women are virtually identical to those experienced by men: the relative risks of various smoking-related diseases in women are seen, in the new study, to equal those of men documented two to three decades earlier (U.S. Department of Health and Human Services, 1989). Given that the diffusion of smoking among women lagged behind that of men by a comparable period, this finding confirms the expectation of similar health effects for similar smoking behaviors in men and women. Application of these newer relative risks to the mortality analysis discussed earlier would produce greater estimates of life savings among women. (Similarly, the new ACS study is finding that relative risks of disease and death have risen substantially among men too, reflecting the much earlier initiation and greater intensity of smoking by men dying in the 1980s from smoking-related causes. As such, the men's mortality savings are undoubtedly underestimated here as well.)

Regardless of the quantitative precision of the estimates presented in this paper, the essential qualitative message of these analyses is an important one: a sustained, if disorganized national campaign to educate the public about the hazards of smoking, combined with social and policy measures to discourage smoking, has had a substantial impact on smoking in America. As a consequence, a perhaps unparalled avoidance of premature death has been achieved. That both behavior change and health benefit have to be pointed out demonstrates the enormous burden of the legacy of a half century of unfettered growth in smoking.

Smoking kills approximately 400,000 Americans each year, accounting for more than one death of every six (U.S. Department of Health and Human Services, 1989). According to recent estimates by the World Health Organization, smoking annually kills 3 million people worldwide. WHO projects that, absent significant changes in current trends in smoking, fully 500 million people now alive—one tenth of the world's population—will die as a result of cigarette smoking (Peto & Lopez, 1991). The lessons of America's antismoking campaign offer intellectual insights to the interested behavioral scientist. Nevertheless, given their pragmatic importance, it is to be hoped that their principal students will be health policy makers around the world.

REFERENCES

Doll, R., & Hill, A.B. (1954). The mortality of doctors in relation to their smoking habits. A preliminary report. *British Medical Journal* 1(4877), 1451-55.

Harris, J.E. (1983). Cigarette smoking among successive birth cohorts of men and women in the United States during 1900-80. *Journal of the National Cancer Institute* 71, 473-9.

Peto, R. & A. Lopez. (1991). Worldwide mortality from current smoking patterns. In B. Durston & K. Jamrozik, (eds.), *Tobacco and Health 1990: The Global War Proceedings of the 7th World Conference on Tobacco and Health.* Perth, Western Australia, (April 1-5). Perth, WA: Health Department of Western Australia.

U.S. Department of Health and Human Services. (1989). Reducing the Health Consequences of Smoking: 25 Years of Progress. A Report of the Surgeon General. U.S. Department of Health and Human Services, Public Health Service, Centers for Disease Control, Office on Smoking and Health. Department of Health and Human Services, Pub. No. (CDC) 89-8411. Washington, DC: Government Printing Office.

U.S. Public Health Service. (1964). Smoking and Health. Report of the Advisory Committee to the Surgeon General of the Public Health Service. U.S. Dept. of Health, Education, and Welfare, Public Health Service, Center for Disease Control. PHS Pub. No. 1103. Washington, DC: Government Printing Office.

Warner, K.E. (1989). Effects of the antismoking campaign: An update. *American Journal Public Health* 79, 144-51.

Warner, K.E., & H.A. Murt. (1982). Impact of the antismoking campaign on smoking prevalence: A cohort analysis. *Journal of Public Health Policy* 3, 374-89.

Wynder, E.L., & E.A. Graham. (1950). Tobacco smoking as a possible etiologic factor in bronchiogenic carcinoma: A study of 684 proved cases. *Journal American Medical Association* 143, 329-96.

A COST-BENEFIT ANALYSIS OF SMOKING IN CANADA

Bernard C.K. Choi

I. INTRODUCTION

Health effects of smoking, such as lung cancer, bladder cancer, and cardiovascular diseases, have been well studied (IARC, 1986). However, there has been very little research into the economic effects of smoking (Thompson & Forbes, 1982). This cost-benefit analysis of smoking in Canada was part of a much bigger project conducted by the Metropolitan Toronto District Health Council in Toronto, Canada to look at smoking reduction strategies for Metropolitan Toronto.

The objective of this study was to examine societal costs and benefits associated with smoking in Canada, and in three regions within Canada. The three regions included a province, namely Ontario, a municipality, namely Metropolitan Toronto, and a city, namely the City of Toronto.

The word "societal" in the objective of this study must be emphasized. The model that was used to look at costs and benefits was based on the society as a whole, and not on the individual. In some cases, the costs and benefits to the society may not be the same as the costs and benefits to an individual.

Research in Human Capital and Development, Volume 7, pages 149-175.

ISBN: 1-55938-132-9

By using the attributable risk model, Collishaw and Myers (1984) were able to show that for Canada as a whole, the cost of smoking in 1979 totalled 5.2 billion Canadian dollars, over 2 billion dollars more than the consumer expenditure for tobacco products in the same year. The research question that followed was: would this economic impact be the same for various regions within Canada? This study attempted to provide an answer. Preliminary results of this study have been published elsewhere (Choi & Nethercott, 1988). This paper describes the final results, with all cost and benefit estimates adjusted to 1990 Canadian dollars.

II. MATERIALS AND METHODS

The model that was followed was the one proposed by Collishaw and Myers (1984).

In this study, costs were those losses attributable to smoking, including: foregone future income due to premature death, partial income loss due to disability, cost of hospitalization, cost of physician visits, and property and forest fire losses.

For benefits, there were three major categories that were considered: dollars spent by consumers on tobacco paid to retailers, wholesalers, manufacturers, leaf processors, and farmers; federal government tax on tobacco products; and provincial government tax on tobacco products.

Smokers were defined in this study as all current smokers of cigarettes, pipes or cigars and all former smokers who smoked for 10 or more years and quit smoking less than 5 years ago. This is the same definition as the one that was used in the Canada Health Survey (Statistics Canada, 1985). Former smokers who quit are also included as smokers because the effects of smoking do not disappear immediately when they stop smoking.

The concept of attributable risk, first proposed by MacMahon and Cole (1971), has been used extensively in the mathematical model. Attributable risk (AR) is that proportion of excess disease, death, or use of health services which can be attributed to smoking, and is estimated by the following equation.

$$AR = \frac{f(RR-1)}{1+f(RR-1)} \qquad (1)$$

where f represents the fraction of exposure, or the proportion of the population who are smokers, and RR represents the relative risk.

The first part of the mathematical model looked at lost income due to premature deaths caused by smoking. Smoking causes premature death. At the time of death, all of the future income which could have been generated if there were no death, would be lost. For each age group and for males and females separately the relative risk of mortality and fraction of exposure with respect to smoking were estimated. From these, the age and sex specific attributable risks were calculated. Each attributable risk represented the proportion of excess deaths caused by smoking, and when multiplied with the total number of deaths in a year in that age-sex category, gave the number of deaths attributable to smoking. When this number was multiplied with the present value of future income, it gave the foregone income due to premature death which was attributable to smoking. This was then added up across all age-sex strata to obtain the total foregone income for the society in a year.

For disability, the calculation was basically the same, with relative risk of disability and fraction of exposure being used to estimate the attributable risk of disability. However, weighting factors were used to adjust the daily income for the fact that a day of disability does not necessarily mean that all activities are gone for that day. For each day of disability, part of the daily income was lost due to lower level of productivity. This calculation gave the partial income loss due to disability attributable to smoking.

With regards cost of hospitalization, patients who die in the hospitals, and those who are still alive at the time when they leave the hospitals, were treated differently in the model.

For hospitalization costs ending in death, relative risk of mortality and fraction of exposure were used to calculate attributable risk of death due to smoking. From total number of days of hospitalization ending in death, the number of days of hospitalization attributable to smoking were calculated. And from the cost per day of hospitalization, the cost of hospitalization attributable to smoking was calculated.

For those patients who require hospitalization but who were alive at the end of the hospitalization period, the calculation was different. Instead of relative risk of mortality, the relative risk of hospitalization was used. With fraction of exposure, the attributable risk of hospitalization was calculated. From the total number of days of hospitalization, which ended with the patient leaving alive, the number of days of hospitalization attributable to smoking was calculated. And from the cost per day of hospitalization, the cost of hospitalization attributable to smoking was calculated.

The two costs of hospitalization, for those ending in death, and ending with the patient leaving alive, were then combined to give the total cost of hospitalization.

For physician visits, relative risk of physician visits, fraction of exposure, attributable risk, total number of visits in a year, number of visits attributable to smoking, and average cost per visit, were used to come up with the cost of physician visits attributable to smoking.

For fires, both property fires and forest fires that were started by smoking materials with respect to property losses, forestry losses, forest fire fighting costs, and forest fire protection costs, were considered.

For the societal benefits, the consumer expenditure for tobacco products paid to retailers, wholesalers, manufacturers, leaf processors, farmers, federal government, and provincial government were considered.

Data for this study were obtained from various sources: relative risk estimates were taken from the original paper by Collishaw and Myers (1984); fractions of exposure for various age and sex groups were obtained from the Canada Health Survey (Statistics Canada, 1983) and the City of Toronto Health Survey (MacPherson, 1984); total number of deaths, days of disability, days of hospitalization, and physician visits, were obtained from the Ontario Ministry of Health (1980a, 1984a, 1985) reports, Canada Health Survey (Statistics Canada, 1983), and the City of Toronto Health Survey (MacPherson, 1984); income data, cost of hospitalization, and cost of visits were obtained from Statistics Canada (1981, 1985) reports, and Ontario Ministry of Health (1980b, 1984b, 1985) reports; weighting factors for disability days were taken from Collinshaw and Myers (1984); information on property and forest fire losses was obtained from the Ontario Ministry of the Solicitor General (Office of the Fire Marshall, 1979, 1983), City of Toronto Fire Department (1985), and the Ontario Ministry of Natural Resources (1985); and information on the benefits or consumer expenditure for tobacco products was obtained from the Canadian Tobacco Manufacturers' Council (1985), and Peat, Marwick and Partners (1983) report.

III. RESULTS

The mathematical model was applied to estimate costs and benefits of smoking in Ontario in 1979, Metropolitan Toronto in 1983 and the City of Toronto in 1983. Results are shown in the following tables.

Table 1 shows the costs and benefits of smoking in the 3 study regions, in millions of dollars. Details of the derivations are shown in the Appendices.

In Ontario in 1979, the foregone income due to mortality was 1017 million dollars, partial income loss due to disability 61 million dollars, direct costs of hospitalization 239 million dollars, direct costs of physician visits 22 million dollars, and fire damage 13 million dollars. The total was 1352 million, in 1979 Canadian dollars. When adjusted to 1990 dollars based on inflation (Consumer Price Index or CPI), the total becomes 2530 million dollars.

On the other hand, for consumer expenditure, the industry share was 490 million dollars, federal tax 296 million dollars, provincial tax 219 million dollars. The total was 1005 million dollars which, when adjusted to 1990 dollars, becomes 1881 million dollars.

Therefore, the excess of costs over benefits, in terms of 1990 Canadian dollars, was estimated to be 649 million dollars.

Table 1. Costs and Benefits of Smoking in 3 Regions in Canada, in Millions of Dollars

	Ontario 1979	*Metro Toronto 1983*	*City of Toronto 1983*
Costs			
1. Foregone income due to mortality	1017	333	100
2. Partial income loss due to disability	61	8	2
3. Direct costs of hospitalization	239	92	42
4. Direct costs of physician visits	22	11	3
5. Fire damage	13	2	1
Totals of costs	1352	446	148
(Totals-adjusted to 1990 dollars)	2530	605	201
Benefits			
1. Industry share	490	186	54
2. Federal tax	296	110	32
3. Preovincial tax	219	121	35
Totals of benefits	1005	417	121
(Totals-adjusted to 1990 dollars)	1881	567	164
Excess of costs over benefits in 1990 dollars	649	38	37

Similar trends of excess of costs over benefits were observed using Metropolitan Toronto 1983 data, and the City of Toronto 1983 data. For Metropolitan Toronto, the estimated cost was 605 million dollars and the benefit 567 million dollars. The excess was 38 million dollars. For the City of Toronto, the estimated cost was 201 million dollars, and the benefits 164 million dollars. The excess was 37 million dollars.

Results for the 3 regions within Canada are therefore consistent with those obtained by Collishaw and Myers (1984) for Canada. At the national level, at the provincial level, at the municipal level, and at the city level, costs of smoking in all cases exceed the benefits.

Because the sizes of the population of these three regions are not the same, the figures are not directly comparable to one another. To allow comparison, the figures have to be standardized according to population size.

Table 2 shows the per capita costs and benefits, adjusted to 1990 dollars. This table has also included the Canadian 1979 data, calculated from Collishaw and Myers (1984) results.

It can be seen that the per capita costs of foregone income due to mortality attributable to smoking are very similar in Canada ($265 per person per year), Ontario ($224), Metropolitan Toronto ($212), and the City of Toronto ($228).

For partial income loss due to disability, the figures are: Canada $49 per person per year, Ontario $14, Metro Toronto $5, and City of Toronto $5. The discrepancy among these figures is mainly due to the fact that total days of

Table 2. Per Capita Costs and Benefits of Smoking in Canada, in 1990 Dollars

	*Canada**	*Ontario*	*Metro Toronto*	*City of Toronto*
Costs				
1. Foregone income due to mortality	265	224	212	228
2. Partial income loss due to disability	49	14	5	5
3. Direct costs of hospitalization	87	53	58	97
4. Direct costs of physician visits	1	5	7	7
5. Fire damage	7	3	1	1
Totals of costs	409	299	283	338
Benefits				
1. Industry share	116	107	118	124
2. Federal tax	69	65	69	73
3. Provincial tax	52	48	78	80
Totals of benefits	237	220	265	277
Excess of costs over benefits in 1990 dollars	172	79	18	61

Note: * Calculated from results of Collishaw and Myers (1984).

disability for Canada and Ontario were estimated from the Canada Health Survey (Statistics Canada, 1983), and those for Metropolitan Toronto and the City of Toronto were from the City of Toronto Health Survey (MacPherson, 1984).

Direct costs of hospitalization range from $53 to $97 per person per year, and direct costs of physician visits range from $1 to $7.

Fire damage due to careless smoking in Canada is $7 per person per year, Ontario $3, Metro Toronto $1 and the City of Toronto $1. The costs for Canada and Ontario are high because of forest fires. In Metro Toronto and the City of Toronto there are no forest fires.

Therefore, the total estimated costs of smoking, at 1990 price levels, are $409 per person for Canada, $299 for Ontario, $283 for Metro Toronto, and $338 for the City of Toronto. These figures are alarming. For example, on the average, it is estimated that each year $409 is paid by each person residing in Canada to cover the costs due to losses attributable to smoking in the society.

In terms of the benefits, the industry share ranges from $107 to $124 per person per year, federal tax ranges from $65 to $73, and the provincial tax ranges from $48 to $80.

Total societal benefit for Canada is $237 per person per year, Ontario $220, Metropolitan Toronto $265, and the City of Toronto $277.

The excess of costs over benefits for Canada is $172 per person per year, Ontario $79, Metropolitan Toronto $18, and the City of Toronto $61.

Table 3 shows that by eliminating smoking in the society for one year, Canada could save 4102 million dollars, Ontario 649 million dollars, Metro

Table 3. Extra Burden on the Society that Can be Removed by Eliminating Smoking in the Society for One Year

	*Canada**	*Ontario*	*Metro Toronto*	*City of Toronto*
Total (and per capita) excess of costs over benefits in 1990 Canadian Dollars	$4102 million ($172/ person)	$649 million ($79/ person)	$38 million ($18/ person)	$37 million ($61/ person)
Number of (and percentage of all) deaths	27458 (17%)	7996 (13%)	1953 (13%)	641 (12%)
Number of (and percentage of all) days of disability	45.6 million days (5%)	5.0 million days (5%)	0.5 million days (4%)	0.1 million days (4%)
Number of (and percentage of all) days of hospitalization	767 thousand days (14%)	80 thousand days (13%)	27 thousand days (12%)	13 thousand days (12%)
Number of (and percentage of all) physician visits	1.7 million visits (3%)	0.8 million visits (3%)	0.3 million visits (2%)	0.1 million visits (2%)

Note: * From results of Collishaw and Myers (1984).

Toronto 38 million dollars, and the City of Toronto 37 million dollars. It can be translated into a savings of from $18 to $172 per person per year, at 1990 price levels.

In addition, by eliminating smoking for just one year, we would be able to avoid about 27 thousand unnecessary deaths in Canada, 8 thousand in Ontario, 2 thousand in Metro Toronto, and 600 in the City of Toronto, which represent from 12 percent to 17 percent of all deaths. We would also be able to eliminate about 4 to 5 percent of disability days, 12 to 14 percent of hospitalization days, and 2 to 3 percent of physician visits.

IV. CONCLUSIONS

A few conclusions can be drawn from this study:

1. There was a consistent excess of smoking-related expenses over revenues generated in Canada, Ontario, Metro Toronto, and the City of Toronto.
2. The potential impact that could be made through elimination or reduction of smoking in the society is staggering.
3. It is both necessary and timely to take steps to reduce the proportion of smokers in the society—if only for purely economic reasons.

4. Cost-benefit analysis can provide important information for healthy public policy making.

In this study, there are a number of limitations which are potential sources of underestimation. There are now more heavy smokers than when the major studies of the relative risks of smoking were conducted. No consideration has been given to second-hand smoke. The real costs of treating smoking related disease may exceed the average cost of hospitalization. No data were available on the cost of pharmaceuticals, property fire fighting, extra ventilation, maintenance, depreciation, productive time lost, and extra fire and life insurance related to smoking. No estimation has been made of the cost in terms of decrements in the quality of life due to disability. No consideration has been given to the costs associated with teratogenic effects of smoking, such as low birth weights. In future cost-benefit analysis, these must be taken into consideration, when appropriate data are available.

APPENDICES FOLLOW

Table A1. Derivation of Present Value of Foregone Income by Reason of Mortality Attributable to Tobacco Use, by Age and Sex, Ontario, 1979

Sex	*Age*	[a] *Percentage exposed to tobacco's risk*	[b] *Relative risk of mortality*	*Attributable fraction*	[c] *Total number of deaths*	*Number of deaths attributable to tobacco use*	[d] *Present value of future income in millions of dollars*	*Total foregone income by reason of mortality attributable tobacco use in millions of dollars*
Males	15-24	.4703	.00	.000	1127	0	.362	.000
	25-34	.4867	1.52	.202	798	161	.387	62.373
	35-44	.4869	1.82	.285	1130	322	.334	107.691
	45-54	.5065	2.20	.378	3056	1155	.247	285.351
	55-64	.4492	1.86	.279	5930	1652	.147	242.912
	65+	.3038	1.58	.150	20955	3139	.071	222.884
Subtotal					32996	6431.		921.212
Females	15-24	.4534	.00	.000	378	0	.184	.000
	25-34	.3748	.00	.000	390	0	.184	.000
	35-44	.4073	1.12	.047	647	30	.158	4.764
	45-54	.3772	1.31	.105	1621	170	.122	20.704
	55-64	.3368	1.27	.083	3347	279	.080	22.319
	65+	.1831	1.31	.054	20221	1086	.044	47.789
Subtotal					26604	1565		95.576
Total					59600	7796		1016.787

Notes: [a] Fraction exposed to tobacco's risk is derived from unpublished results of the Canada Health Survey (Statistics Canada, 1983). Population exposed to tobacco's risk includes all current daily and occasional smokers of cigarettes, pipes or cigars and all former cigarette smokers who smoked for ten or more years and quit less than five years ago.

[b] These relative risks are taken from Collishaw and Myers (1984).

[c] Total number of deaths of residents of Ontario in 1979 is taken from Report of the Registrar General for 1979/1980, Table 22 (Ontario Ministry of Health, 1980a).

[d] These estimates are drived from 1979 income data (Statistics Canada, 1981) for Ontario, using the method described in Collishaw and Myers (1984).

Table A2. Dollars Estimates of Cost Reductions in the Quality of Life Due to Disability Attributable to Tobacco Use, by Age and Sex, Ontario, 1979

Sex	*Age*	[a]*Percentage exposed to tobacco's risk*	[e]*Relative risk of disability*	*Attributable fraction*	[f]*Total days of disability (millions)*	*Days of disability attributable to tobacco use (millions)*	[g]*Average daily income $*	[h]*Weighting factor*	*Total cost of disability attributable to tobacco use (millions of dollars)*
Males	15-24	.4703	.93	−.034	7.38	−.25	20.00	.41	−2.059
	25-34	.4867	.94	−.030	6.25	−.19	49.00	.40	−3.684
	35-44	.4869	.98	−.010	5.19	−.05	58.00	.40	−1.184
	45-54	.5065	1.30	.132	4.40	.58	55.00	.43	13.739
	55-64	.4492	1.18	.075	10.61	.79	49.00	.43	16.723
	65+	.3038	1.05	.015	7.86	.12	25.00	.43	1.264
Subtotal					41.68	1.00			24.799
Females	15-24	.4534	1.26	.105	8.50	.90	15.00	.41	5.511
	25-34	.3748	1.32	.107	14.08	1.51	25.00	.40	15.081
	35-44	.4073	1.24	.089	8.70	.77	26.00	.40	8.057
	45-54	.3772	1.27	.092	8.62	.80	25.00	.40	7.968
	55-64	.3368	.97	−.010	10.41	−.11	21.00	.40	−.892
	65+	.1831	1.06	.011	12.28	.13	15.00	.41	.820
Subtotal					62.58	4.00			36.545
Total					104.27	5.00			61.343

Notes: [a] Fraction exposed to tobacco's risk is derived from unpublished results of the Canada Health Survey (Statistics Canada, 1983). Population exposed to tobacco's risk includes all current daily and occasional smokers of cigarettes, pipes or cigars and all former cigarette smokers who smoked for ten or more years and quit less than five years ago.

[e] These relative risks are taken from Collishaw and Myers (1984).

[f] Canada Health Survey (Statistics Canada, 1983). Unpublished results.

[g] These data are drived from Statistics Canada (1981) income distribution data for Ontario, 1979.

[h] These weights are taken from Collishaw and Myers (1984).

Table A3. Direct Costs of Hospitalization Attributable to Tobacco Use for Persons Deceased at Time of Separation, by Age and Sex, Ontario, 1979

Sex	Age	[a] *Percentage exposed to tobacco's risk*	[b] *Relative risk of mortality*	*Attributable fraction*	[i] *Total number of days of hospitalization (thousands)*	*Number of days of hospitalization attributable to tobacco use (thousands)*	[j] *Cost per day of hospitalization*	*Cost of hospitalization attributable to tobacco use for those deceased on separation (millions of dollars)*
Males	15-24	.4703	.00	.000	2.92	.00	152.00	.000
	25-34	.4867	1.52	.202	3.01	.61	152.00	.092
	35-44	.4869	1.82	.285	6.74	1.92	152.00	.292
	45-54	.5065	2.20	.378	23.57	8.91	152.00	1.354
	55-64	.4492	1.86	.279	56.19	15.66	152.00	2.380
	65+	.3038	1.58	.150	218.75	32.77	152.00	4.981
Subtotal					311.18	59.87		9.100
Females	15-24	.4534	.00	.000	2.56	.00	152.00	.000
	25-34	.3748	.00	.000	3.00	.00	152.00	.000
	35-44	.4073	1.12	.047	6.81	.32	152.00	.048
	45-54	.3772	1.31	.105	22.83	2.39	152.00	.363
	55-64	.3368	1.27	.083	46.70	3.89	152.00	.592
	65+	.1831	1.31	.054	225.14	12.09	152.00	1.838
Subtotal					307.04	18.69		2.841
Total					618.21	78.56		11.941

Notes: [a] Fraction exposed to tobacco's risk is derived from unpublished results of the Canada Health Survey (Statistics Canada, 1983). Population exposed to tobacco's risk includes all current daily and occasional smokers of cigarettes, pipes or cigars and all former cigarette smokers who smoked for ten or more years and quit less than five years ago.

[b] These relative risks are taken from Collishaw and Myers (1984).

[i] Ontario Ministry of Health, Corporate and Community Services Information Resources and Services Branch, unpublished tabulations (1985).

[j] Taken from Ontario Ministry of Health (1980b).

Table A4. Direct Costs of Hospitalization Attributable to Tobacco Use for Persons Alive at Time of Separation, by Age and Sex, Ontario, 1979

Sex	Age	[a] *Percentage exposed to tobacco's risk*	*Relative risk of hospitalization*	*Attributable fraction*	[i] *Total number of days of hospitalization (millions)*	*Number of days attributable to tobacco use (millions)*	*Cost per day of hospitalization*	*Cost of hospitalization attributable to tobacco use for those alive on separation (millions of dollars)*
Males	15-24	.4703	2.20	.361	.39	.14	152.00	21.276
	25-34	.4867	.91	−.046	.36	−.02	152.00	−2.507
	35-44	.4869	1.30	.127	.37	.05	152.00	7.149
	45-54	.5065	1.50	.202	.61	.12	152.00	18.736
	55-64	.4492	2.00	.310	.83	.26	152.00	39.199
	65+	.3038	2.00	.233	1.62	.38	152.00	57.200
Subtotal					4.17	.93		141.053
Females	15-24	.4534	1.50	.185	.73	.13	152.00	20.506
	25-34	.3748	1.20	.070	.99	.07	152.00	10.483
	35-44	.4073	1.30	.109	.55	.06	152.00	9.152
	45-54	.3772	3.70	.505	.64	.32	152.00	49.314
	55-64	.3368	1.20	.063	.77	.05	152.00	7.415
	65+	.1831	.83	−.032	2.13	−.07	152.00	−10.397
Subtotal					5.82	.57		86.474
Total					9.99	1.50		227.527

Notes: [a] Fraction exposed to tobacco's risk is derived from unpublished results of the Canada Health Survey (Statistics Canada, 1983). Population exposed to tobacco's risk includes all current daily and occasional smokers of cigarettes, pipes or cigars and all former cigarette smokers who smoked for ten or more years and quit less than five years ago.

[k] These relative risks are taken from Collishaw and Myers (1984).

[i] Ontario Ministry of Health, Corporate and Community Services, Information Resources and Services Branch, unpublished tabulations (1985).

[j] Taken from Ontario Ministry of Health (1980b).

Table A5. Direct Costs of Physician Visits Attributable to Tobacco Use, by Age and Sex, Ontario, 1979

Sex	Age	[a] Percentage exposed to tobacco's risk	[m] Relative risk of physician visit	Attributable fraction	[n] Total number of visits (millions)	Visits attributable to tobacco use (millions)	[o] Average cost per visit	Directs costs of physician visits attributable to tobacco use (millions of dollars)
Males	15-24	.4703	1.07	.032	2.02	.06	26.68	1.714
	25-34	.4867	1.02	.010	1.51	.01	37.36	.543
	35-44	.4869	.96	−.020	1.36	−.03	35.58	−.964
	45-54	.5065	.94	−.031	1.51	−.05	36.56	−1.725
	55-64	.4492	1.15	.063	1.60	.10	37.16	3.742
	65+	.3038	1.03	.009	1.93	.02	41.65	.726
Subtotal					9.92	.12		4.036
Females	15-24	.4534	1.16	.068	2.86	.19	34.08	6.595
	25-34	.3748	.99	−.004	3.44	−.01	37.09	−.479
	35-44	.4073	.99	−.004	1.86	−.01	42.08	−.320
	45-54	.3772	1.38	.125	2.61	.33	27.98	9.145
	55-64	.3368	1.26	.081	2.24	.18	30.11	5.438
	65+	.1831	.87	−.024	2.46	−.06	43.24	−2.598
Subtotal					15.47	.62		17.780
Total					25.39	.74		21.817

Notes: [a] Fraction exposed to tobacco's risk is derived from unpublished results of the Canada Health Survey (Statistics Canada, 1983). Population exposed to tobacco's risk includes all current daily and occasional smokers of cigarettes, pipes or cigars and all former cigarette smokers who smoked for ten or more years and quit less than five years ago.

[m] These relative risks are taken from Collishaw and Myers (1984).

[n] Canadian Health Survey (Statistics Canada, 1983).

[o] Calculated from unpublished tabulations of Ontario Ministry of Health, (1985).

Table A6. Cost of Fires Attributable to Tobacco Use, Ontario, 1979, in Millions of Dollars

	Property loss	*Forestry loss*	*Fire fighting costs*	*Fire protection costs*
Property fires[p]	10.1	—	—	—
Forest fires[q]	—	0.2	0.8	1.7
Total	10.1	0.2	0.8	1.7

Notes: [p] Taken from Office of the Fire Marshal (1979). Estimates of property fire fighting costs are unavailable.
[q] Total forest fire figures are obtained from the Ontario Ministry of Natural Resources (1985). Using the method of Collishaw and Myers (1979), it is estimated that 10% of the total costs are attributable to tobacco use.

Table A7. Distribution of Expenditure on Tobacco in Ontario, 1979

	Millions of dollars[r]
Retailers	123
Wholesalers	51
Manufacturers, Leaf processors, Farmers	316
Federal Tax	296
Provincial Tax	219
Total	1005

Note: [r] Cigarette sales figures in Canada and Ontario are provided by the Canadian Tobacco Manufacturers' Council (1985).

Table A8. Dollar Estimates of the Consequences of Tobacco Use, Ontario, 1979

	Consequences (millions of dollars)		*Consumer expenditure (millions of dollars)*
Foregone income due to mortality	1017	Industry share	490
Disability	61	Federal tax	296
Direct costs of hospitalization	239	Provincial tax	219
Direct costs of physician services	22		
Fire damange	13		
Totals-1979 dollars	1352		1005

Table B1. Derivation of Present Value of Foregone Income by Reason of Mortality Attributable to Tobacco Use, by Age and Sex, Metro Toronto, 1983

Sex	*Age*	[a] *Percentage exposed to tobacco's risk*	[b] *Relative risk of mortality*	*Attributable fraction*	[c] *Total number of deaths*	*Number of deaths attributable to tobacco use*	[d] *Present value of future income in millions of dollars*	*Total foregone income by reason of mortality attributable tobacco use in millions of dollars*
Males	15-24	.4703	.00	.000	139	0	.495	.000
	25-34	.4867	1.52	.202	170	34	.542	18.609
	35-44	.4869	1.82	.285	235	67	.469	31.448
	45-54	.5065	2.20	.378	599	226	.347	78.575
	55-64	.4492	1.86	.279	1530	426	.207	88.255
	65+	.3038	1.58	.150	5152	772	.099	76.409
Subtotal					7825	1526.		293.297
Females	15-24	.4534	.00	.000	62	0	.282	.000
	25-34	.3748	.00	.000	79	0	.282	.000
	35-44	.4073	1.12	.047	186	9	.242	2.097
	45-54	.3772	1.31	.105	421	44	.187	8.242
	55-64	.3368	1.27	.083	883	74	.123	9.053
	65+	.1831	1.31	.054	5602	301	.068	20.461
Subtotal					7233	427.		39.854
Total					15058	1953.		333.150

Notes: [a] Fraction exposed to tobacco's risk for Metropolitan Toronto, 1983 is assumed to be the same as that for Ontario, 1979.

[b] These relative risks are taken from Collishaw and Myers (1984).

[c] Total number of deaths of residents of Metropolitan Toronto in 1983 is taken from Report of the Registrar General for 1983/1984, Table 25 (Ontario Ministry of Health, 1984a).

[d] Figures for Metropolitan Toronto are assumed to be the same as those for Ontario, which are estimated from 1983 income data (Statistics Canada, 1985) for Ontario, using the method described in Collishaw and Myers (1984).

Table B2. Dollars Estimates of Cost Reductions in the Quality of Life Due to Disability Attributable to Tobacco Use, by Age and Sex, Metro Toronto, 1983

Sex	*Age*	[a] *Percentage exposed to tobacco's risk*	[c] *Relative risk of disability*	*Attributable fraction*	[f] *Total days of disability (millions)*	*Days of disability attributable to tobacco use (millions)*	[g] *Average daily income $*	[h] *Weighting factor*	*Total cost of disability attributable to tobacco use (millions of dollars)*
Males	15-24	.4703	.93	−.034	.80	−.03	29.00	.41	−.323
	25-34	.4867	.94	−.030	2.00	−.06	69.00	.40	−1.657
	35-44	.4869	.98	−.010	.71	−.01	82.00	.40	−.230
	45-54	.5065	1.30	.132	.51	.07	77.00	.43	2.237
	55-64	.4492	1.18	.075	1.05	.08	69.00	.43	2.329
	65+	.3038	1.05	.015	.33	.00	34.00	.43	.071
Subtotal					5.39	.06			2.428
Females	15-24	.4534	1.26	.105	1.77	.19	24.00	.41	1.834
	25-34	.3748	1.32	.107	1.29	.14	38.00	.40	2.102
	35-44	.4073	1.24	.089	.84	.08	39.00	.40	1.171
	45-54	.3772	1.27	.092	.35	.03	38.00	.40	.492
	55-64	.3368	.97	−.010	.65	−.01	31.00	.40	−.082
	65+	.1831	1.06	.011	.78	.01	24.00	.41	.084
Subtotal					5.69	.43			5.600
Total					11.08	.49			8.028

Notes: [a] Fraction exposed to tobacco's risk for Metropolitan Toronto, 1983 is assumed to be the same as that for Ontario, 1979.

[c] These relative risks are taken from Collishaw and Myers (1984).

[f] Calculated from unpublished results of the City of Toronto Community Health Survey, 1983, by making a projection to Metro Toronto using appropriate age and sex specific population structures.

[g] Figures for Metropolitan Toronto are assumed to be the same as those for Ontario, which are estimated from 1983 income data (Statistics Canada, 1985) for Ontario using the method described in Collishaw and Myers (1984).

[h] These weights are taken from Collinshaw and Myers (1984).

Table B3. Direct costs of Hospitalization Attributable to Tobacco Use for Persons Deceased at Time of Separation, by Age and Sex, Metro Toronto, 1983

Sex	*Age*	[a]*Percentage exposed to tobacco's risk*	[b]*Relative risk of mortality*	*Attributable fraction*	[i]*Total number of days of hospitalization (thousands)*	*Number of days of hospitalization attributable to tobacco use (thousands)*	[j]*Cost per day of hospitalization*	*Cost of hospitalization attributable to tobacco use for those deceased on separation (millions of dollars)*
Males	15-24	.4703	.00	.000	.71	.00	252.00	.000
	25-34	.4867	1.52	.202	.84	.17	252.00	.043
	35-44	.4869	1.82	.285	1.86	.53	252.00	.134
	45-54	.5065	2.20	.378	5.29	2.00	252.00	.504
	55-64	.4492	1.86	.279	17.60	4.90	252.00	1.236
	65+	.3038	1.58	.150	82.45	12.35	252.00	3.113
Subtotal					108.74	19.95		5.028
Females	15-24	.4534	.00	.000	.88	.00	252.00	.000
	25-34	.3748	.00	.000	.74	.00	252.00	.000
	35-44	.4073	1.12	.047	2.67	.12	252.00	.031
	45-54	.3772	1.31	.105	6.27	.66	252.00	.165
	55-64	.3368	1.27	.083	13.27	1.11	252.00	.279
	65+	.1831	1.31	.054	91.66	4.92	252.00	1.241
Subtotal					115.49	6.81		1.716
Total					224.23	26.76		6.744

Notes: [a] Fraction exposed to tobacco's risk for Metropolitan Toronto, 1983 is assumed to be the same as that for Ontario, 1979.
[b] These relative risks are taken from Collishaw and Myers (1984).
[i] Ontario Ministry of Health, Corporate and Community Services, Information Resources and Services Branch, unpublished tabulations (1985).
[j] Estimated from Ontario Ministry of Health (1984b).

Table B4. Direct Costs of Hospitalization Attributable to Tobacco Use for Persons Alive at Time of Separation, by Age and Sex, Metro Toronto, 1983

Sex	*Age*	[a]*Percentage exposed to tobacco's risk*	*Relative risk of hospitalization*	*Attributable fraction*	[i]*Total number of days of hospitalization (millions)*	*Number of days attributable to tobacco use (millions)*	[j]*Cost per day of hospitalization*	*Cost of hospitalization attributable to tobacco use for those alive on separation (millions of dollars)*
Males	15-24	.4703	2.20	.361	.07	.03	252.00	6.637
	25-34	.4867	.91	−.046	.08	.00	252.00	−.947
	35-44	.4869	1.30	.127	.08	.01	252.00	2.505
	45-54	.5065	1.50	.202	.12	.03	252.00	6.314
	55-64	.4492	2.00	.310	.22	.07	252.00	16.794
	65+	.3038	2.00	.233	.43	.10	252.00	25.014
Subtotal					1.00	.22		56.318
Females	15-24	.4534	1.50	.185	.15	.03	252.00	6.753
	25-34	.3748	1.20	.070	.23	.02	252.00	4.094
	35-44	.4073	1.30	.109	.13	.01	252.00	3.677
	45-54	.3772	3.70	.505	.13	.07	252.00	17.038
	55-64	.3368	1.20	.063	.20	.01	252.00	3.165
	65+	.1831	.83	−.032	.67	−.02	252.00	−5.432
Subtotal					1.52	.12		29.295
Total					2.51	.34		85.612

Notes: [a] Fraction exposed to tobacco's risk for Metropolitan Toronto, 1983 is assumed to be the same as that for Ontario, 1979.

[k] These relative risks are taken from Collinshaw and Myers (1984).

[i] Ontario Ministry of Health, Corporate and Community Services, Information Resources and Services Branch, unpublished tabulations (1985).

[j] Estimated from Ontario Ministry of Health (1984b).

Table B5. Direct Costs of Physician Visits Attributable to Tobacco Use, by Age and Sex, Metro Toronto, 1983

Sex	*Age*	[a]*Percentage exposed to tobacco's risk*	[m]*Relative risk of physician visit*	*Attributable fraction*	[n]*Total number of visits (millions)*	*Visits attributable to tobacco use (millions)*	[o]*Average cost per visit*	*Directs costs of physician visits attributable to tobacco use (millions of dollars)*
Males	15-24	.4703	1.07	.032	.92	.03	35.32	1.037
	25-34	.4867	1.02	.010	1.02	.01	49.46	.486
	35-44	.4869	.96	−.020	.56	−.01	47.10	−.523
	45-54	.5065	.94	−.031	.57	−.02	48.39	−.863
	55-64	.4492	1.15	.063	.85	.05	49.19	2.639
	65+	.3038	1.03	.009	.82	.01	55.14	.406
Subtotal					4.73	.07		3.181
Females	15-24	.4534	1.16	.068	1.71	.12	45.12	5.219
	25-34	.3748	.99	−.004	2.55	−.01	49.10	−.471
	35-44	.4073	.99	−.004	1.10	.00	55.71	−.250
	45-54	.3772	1.38	.125	.55	.07	37.04	2.555
	55-64	.3368	1.26	.081	.74	.06	39.86	2.367
	65+	.1831	.87	−.024	1.02	−.02	57.24	−1.423
Subtotal					7.66	.21		7.997
Total					12.40	.28		11.178

Notes: [a] Fraction exposed to tobacco's risk for Metropolitan Toronto, 1983 is assumed to be the same as taht for Ontario, 1979.

[m] These relative risks are taken from Collishaw and Myers (1984).

[n] Calculated from unpublished results of the City of Toronto Community Health Survey, 1983, by making a projection to Metro Toronto using appropriate age and sex specific population structures.

[o] Calculated from unpublished tabulations of Ontario Ministry of Health (1985).

Table B6. Cost of Fires Attributable to Tobacco Use, Metro Toronto, 1983, in Millions of Dollars

	Property loss	*Forestry loss*	*Fire fighting costs*	*Total*
Property fires[p]	1.7	—	—	1.7
Forest fires[q]	—	—	—	—
Total	1.7	—	—	1.7

Notes: [p] Calculated from Office of the Fire Marshal (1983), assuming that 7 percent (percentage for Ontario property fires in 1983) of total property fire losses were caused by smoker's material. Estimates of property fire fighting costs are unavailable.

[q] Forest fire figures are not a significant problem in Metropolitan Toronto.

Table B7. Distribution of Expenditure on Tobacco in Metro Toronto, 1983

	Millions of dollars[r]
Retailers	63
Wholesalers	9
Manufacturers, Leaf processors, Farmers	114
Federal Tax	110
Provincial Tax	121
Total	417

Note: [r] Calculated from Peat, Marwick and Partners (1983), and projected to Metropolitan Toronto by using appropriate population structures.

Table B8. Dollar Estimates of the Consequences of Tobacco Use, Metro Toronto, 1983

	Consequences (millions of dollars)		*Consumer expenditure (millions of dollars)*
Foregone income due to mortality	333	Industry share	186
Disability	8	Federal tax	110
Direct costs of hospitalization	92	Provincial tax	121
Direct costs of physician services	11		
Fire damange	2		
Totals-1983 dollars	446		417

Table C1. Derivation of Present Value of Foregone Income by Reason of Mortality Attributable to Tobacco Use, by Age and Sex, City of Toronto, 1983

Sex	*Age*	[a]*Percentage exposed to tobacco's risk*	[b]*Relative risk of mortality*	*Attributable fraction*	[c]*Total number of deaths*	*Number of deaths attributable to tobacco use*	[d]*Present value of future income in millions of dollars*	*Total foregone income by reason of mortality attributable tobacco use in millions of dollars*
Males	15-24	.4703	.00	.000	37	0	.495	.000
	25-34	.4867	1.52	.202	53	11	.542	5.802
	35-44	.4869	1.82	.285	68	19	.469	9.100
	45-54	.5065	2.20	.378	154	58	.347	20.201
	55-64	.4492	1.86	.279	407	113	.207	23.477
	65+	.3038	1.58	.150	1995	299	.099	29.588
Subtotal					2714	501		88.168
Females	15-24	.4534	.00	.000	17	0	.282	.000
	25-34	.3748	.00	.000	24	0	.282	.000
	35-44	.4073	1.12	.047	51	2	.242	.575
	45-54	.3772	1.31	.105	105	11	.187	2.056
	55-64	.3368	1.27	.083	229	19	123	2.348
	65+	.1831	1.31	.054	2002	108	.068	7.312
Subtotal					2428	140		12.291
Total					5142	641		100.458

Notes: [a] Fraction exposed to tobacco's risk for City of Toronto, 1983 is assumed to be the same as that for Ontario, 1979.

[b] These relative risks are taken from Collishaw and Myers (1984).

[c] Calculated from number of deaths of residents of Metropolitan Toronto in 1983 (Ontario Ministry of Health, 1984a), by making a projection to the City of Toronto using appropriate age and sex specific population structures.

[d] Figures for City of Toronto are assumed to be the same as those for Ontario, which are estimated from 1983 income data (Statistics Canada, 1985) for Ontario, using the method described in Collishaw and Myers (1984).

Table C2. Dollars Estimates of Cost Reductions in the Quality of Life Due to Disability Attributable to Tobacco Use, by Age and Sex, City of Toronto, 1983

Sex	*Age*	[a]*Percentage exposed to tobacco's risk*	[e]*Relative risk of disability*	*Attributable fraction*	[f]*Total days of disability (millions)*	*Days of disability attributable to tobacco use (millions)*	[g]*Average daily income $*	[h]*Weighting factor*	*Total cost of disability attributable to tobacco use (millions of dollars)*
Males	15-24	.4703	.93	−.034	.21	−.01	29.00	.41	−.087
	25-34	.4867	.94	−.030	.62	−.02	69.00	.40	−.518
	35-44	.4869	.98	−.010	.21	.00	82.00	.40	−.067
	45-54	.5065	1.30	.132	.13	.02	77.00	.43	.577
	55-64	.4492	1.18	.075	.28	.02	69.00	.43	.619
	65+	.3038	1.05	.015	.13	.00	34.00	.43	.028
Subtotal					1.58	.01			.552
Females	15-24	.4534	1.26	.105	.48	.05	24.00	.41	.501
	25-34	.3748	1.32	.107	.39	.04	38.00	.40	.642
	35-44	.4073	1.24	.089	.23	.02	39.00	.40	.324
	45-54	.3772	1.27	.092	.09	.01	38.00	.40	.122
	55-64	.3368	.97	−.010	.17	.00	31.00	.40	−.021
	65+	.1831	1.06	.011	.28	.00	24.00	.41	.030
Subtotal					1.65	.12			1.599
Total					3.23	.14			2.151

Notes: [a] Fraction exposed to tobacco's risk for City of Toronto, 1983 is assumed to be the same as that for Ontario, 1979.

[e] These relative risks are taken from Collishaw and Myers (1984).

[f] These data are calculated from unpublished results of the City of Toronto Community Health Survey, 1983, by making a projection to the City of Toronto using appropriate age and sex specific population structures.

[g] Figures for City of Toronto are assumed to be the same as those for Ontario, which are estimated from 1983 income data (Statistics Canada, 1985) for Ontario, using the method described in Collishaw and Myers (1984).

[h] These weights are taken from Collishaw and Myers (1984).

Table C3. Direct costs of Hospitalization Attributable to Tobacco Use for Persons Deceased at Time of Separation, by Age and Sex, City of Toronto, 1983

Sex	*Age*	[a]*Percentage exposed to tobacco's risk*	[b]*Relative risk of mortality*	*Attributable Fraction*	[i]*Total number of days of hospitalization (thousands)*	*Number of days of hospitalization attributable to tobacco use (thousands)*	[j]*Cost per day of hospitalization*	*Cost of hospitalization attributable to tobacco use for those deceased on separation (millions of dollars)*
Males	15-24	.4703	.00	.000	.46	.00	252.00	.000
	25-34	.4867	1.52	.202	.26	.05	252.00	.013
	35-44	.4869	1.82	.285	1.08	.31	252.00	.078
	45-54	.5065	2.20	.378	2.13	.80	252.00	.203
	55-64	.4492	1.86	.279	9.32	2.60	252.00	.654
	65+	.3038	1.58	.150	39.30	5.89	252.00	1.484
Subtotal					52.54	9.65		2.431
Females	15-24	.4534	.00	.000	.63	.00	252.00	.000
	25-34	.3748	.00	.000	.25	.00	252.00	.000
	35-44	.4073	1.12	.047	1.49	.07	252.00	.018
	45-54	.3772	1.31	.105	2.83	.30	252.00	.075
	55-64	.3368	1.27	.083	5.64	.47	252.00	.118
	65+	.1831	1.31	.054	39.89	2.14	252.00	.540
Subtotal					50.73	2.98		.751
Total					103.28	12.63		3.182

Notes: [a] Fraction exposed to tobacco's risk for City of Toronto, 1983 is assumed to be the same as that for Ontario, 1979.
[b] These relative risks are taken from Collishaw and Myers (1984).
[i] Ontario Ministry of Health, Corporate and Community Services, Information Resources and Services Branch, unpublished tabulations (1985).
[j] Estimated from Ontario Ministry of Health (1984b).

Table C4. Direct Costs of Hospitalization Attributable to Tobacco Use for Persons Alive at Time of Separation, by Age and Sex, City of Toronto, 1983

Sex	*Age*	[a]*Percentage exposed to tobacco's risk*	[b]*Relative risk of hospitalization*	*Attributable fraction*	[i]*Total number of days of hospitalization (millions)*	*Number of days attributable to tobacco use (millions)*	[j]*Cost per day of hospitalization*	*Cost of hospitalization attributable to tobacco use for those alive on separation (millions of dollars)*
Males	15-24	.4703	2.20	.361	.03	.01	252.00	2.909
	25-34	.4867	.91	−.046	.05	.00	252.00	−.519
	35-44	.4869	1.30	.127	.04	.01	252.00	1.317
	45-54	.5065	1.50	.202	.06	.01	252.00	2.954
	55-64	.4492	2.00	.310	.10	.03	252.00	7.655
	65+	.3038	2.00	.233	.21	.05	252.00	12.214
Subtotal					.48	.11		26.528
Females	15-24	.4534	1.50	.185	.06	.01	252.00	2.887
	25-34	.3748	1.20	.070	.10	.01	252.00	1.828
	35-44	.4073	1.30	.109	.06	.01	252.00	1.564
	45-54	.3772	3.70	.501	.06	.03	252.00	7.073
	55-64	.3368	1.20	.063	.09	.01	252.00	1.400
	65+	.1831	.83	−.032	.32	−.01	252.00	−2.623
Subtotal					.69	.05		12.129
Total					1.17	.15		38.657

Notes: [a] Fraction exposed to tobacco's risk for City of Toronto, 1983 is assumed to be the same as that for Ontario, 1979.

[k] These relative risks are taken from Collishaw and Myers (1984).

[i] Ontario Ministry of Health, Corporate and Community Services, Information Resources and Services Branch, unpublished tabulations (1985).

[j] Estimated from Ontario Ministry of Health (1984b).

Table C5. Direct Costs of Physician Visits Attributable to Tobacco Use, by Age and Sex, City of Toronto, 1983

Sex	Age	*[a] Percentage exposed to tobacco's risk*	*[m] Relative risk of physician visit*	*Attributable fraction*	*[n] Total number of visits (millions)*	*Visits attributable to tobacco use (millions)*	*[o] Average cost per visit*	*Directs costs of physician visits attributable to tobacco use (millions of dollars)*
Males	15-24	.4703	1.07	.032	.25	.01	35.32	.278
	25-34	.4867	1.02	.010	.32	.00	49.46	.152
	35-44	.4869	.96	−.020	.16	.00	47.10	−.152
	45-54	.5065	.94	−.031	.15	.00	48.39	−.222
	55-64	.4492	1.15	.063	.23	.01	49.19	.702
	65+	.3038	1.03	.009	.32	.00	55.14	.157
Subtotal					1.42	.02		.915
Females	15-24	.4534	1.16	.068	.47	.03	45.12	1.427
	25-34	.3748	.99	−.004	.78	.00	49.10	−.144
	35-44	.4073	.99	−.004	.30	.00	55.71	−.069
	45-54	.3772	1.38	.125	.14	.02	37.04	.635
	55-64	.3368	1.26	.081	.19	.02	39.86	.614
	65+	.1831	.87	−.024	.36	−.01	57.24	−.509
Subtotal					2.24	.05		1.954
Total					3.66	.07		2.869

Notes: [a] Fraction exposed to tobacco's risk for City of Toronto, 1983 is assumed to be the same as that for Ontario, 1979.

[m] These relative risks are taken from Collishaw and Myers (1984).

[n] These data are calculated from unpublished results of the City of Toronto Community Health Survey, 1983, by making a projection to the City of Toronto using appropriate age and sex specific population structures.

[o] Average cost per visit in the City of Toronto 1983 is assumed to be the same as that in Metropolitan Toronto, 1983.

Table C6. Cost of Fires Attributable to Tobacco Use, City of Toronto, 1983, in Millions of Dollars

	Property loss	*Forestry loss*	*Fire fighting costs*	*Total*
Property fires[p]	0.5	—	0.3	0.8
Forest fires[q]	—	—	—	—
Total	0.5	—	0.3	0.8

Notes: [p] Calculated from unpublished tabulations of City of Toronto Fire Department (1985), assuming that 7 percent (percentage for Ontario property fires in 1983) of total property fire losses were caused by smoker's material.

[q] Forest fire figures are not a problem in the City of Toronto.

Table C7. Distribution of Expenditure on Tobacco in City of Toronto, 1983

	Millions of dollars[r]
Retailers	18
Wholesalers	3
Manufacturers, Leaf processors, Farmers	33
Federal Tax	32
Provincial Tax	35
Total	121

Note: [r] Estimated from Peat, Marwick and Partners (1983), and projected to the City of Toronto by using appropriate population structures.

Table C8. Dollar Estimates of the Consequences of Tobacco Use, City of Toronto, 1983

	Consequences (millions of dollars)		*Consumer expenditure (millions of dollars)*
Foregone income due to mortality	100	Industry share	54
Disability	2	Federal tax	32
Direct costs of hospitalization	42	Provincial tax	35
Direct costs of physician services	3		
Fire damange	1		
Totals-1983 dollars	148		121

ACKNOWLEDGMENTS

This work was supported in part by a grant from the Metropolitan Toronto District Health Council and a computer grant from the Cancer Research Society.

REFERENCES

Canadian Tobacco Manufacturers' Council. (1985). Unpublished Tabulations.

Choi, B.C.K., & Nethercott, J.R. (1988). The economist impact of smoking in Canada. *International Journal of Health Planning and Management* 3, 197-205.

City of Toronto Fire Department. (1985). Unpublished Tabulations.

Collishaw, N.E., & Myers, G. (1984). Dollar estimates of the consequences of tobacco use in Canada, 1979. *Canadian Journal of Public Health* 75, 192-199.

IARC. (1986). *Evaluation of the carcinogenic risk of chemicals to humans: Tobacco smoking.* (IARC publication no. 38), pp. 282-292. International Agency for Research on Cancer, Lyon.

MacMahon, B., & Cole, R. (1971). Attributable risk percent in case-control studies. *British Journal of Preventive and Social Medicine* 25, 242-244.

MacPherson, A.S. (1984). *The city of Toronto community health survey: A description of the health status of Toronto residents, 1983.* City of Toronto Department of Public Health.

Office of the Fire Marshall. (1979). Fire losses in Ontario, 1979. Ontario Ministry of the Solicitor for General.

Office of the Fire Marshall. (1983). Fire losses in Ontario, 1983. Ontario Ministry of the Solicitor General.

Ontario Ministry of Health. (1980a). Report of the Registrar General for 1979/1980.

Ontario Ministry of Health. (1980b). Hospital Statistics for 1979/1980.

Ontario Ministry of Health (1984a). Report of the Registrar General for 1983/1984.

Ontario Ministry of Health. (1984b). Hospital Statistics for 1983/1984.

Ontario Ministry of Health. (1985). Unpublished Tabulations. Information Resources & Services Branch.

Ontario Ministry of Natural Resources. (1985). Unpublished Tabulations. Aviation and Fire Management Centre.

Peat, Marwick and Partners. (1983). *Economic impact of the tobacco industry in 1982: Ontario.* Canadian Tobacco Manufacturers' Council, Montreal.

Statistics Canada. (1981). *Income distribution by size in Canada 1979.* Statistics Canada Catalogue 13-207, Ottawa.

Statistics Canada. (1983). *Canada's health survey.* Unpublished tabulations. Department of National Health and Welfare, Research and Analysis Section, Ottawa.

Statistics Canada. (1985). *Income distribution by size in Canada 1983.* Statistics Canada Catalogue 13-207, Ottawa.

Thompson, M.E. & Forbes, W.F. (1982). Costs and "benefits" of cigarette smoking in Canada. *Canadian Medical Association Journal*, 127, 831-832.

DRINKING HABITS AND PREVALENCE OF HYPERTENSION AMONG JAPANESE WORKERS OF DIFFERENT WORKING CONDITIONS

Masao Ishizaki, Yuichi Yamada, Teruhiko Kido,
Ryumon Honda, Ikiko Tsuritani, and Eriko Ikai

I. INTRODUCTION

It is well-known that the economy of Japan has developed very rapidly during the last 30 years. According to reports from the Japanese Ministry of Health and Welfare, the number of patients visiting medical facilities for the treatment of hypertension has continued to increase in Japan during the same period. The number of hypertensive patients was about 3.9 per 1,000 population in 1960, but has increased to about 30.7 at the present time (Ministry of Health and Welfare, Japan 1991). Thus, the rapid economic growth in Japan may have an association with the rapid increase in the number of hypertensive patients.

Research in Human Capital and Development, Volume 7, pages 177-187.

ISBN: 1-55938-132-9

Recently, excessive alcohol consumption has been recognized as a cause of hypertension. The consumption of alcoholic beverages among Japanese people has also increased rapidly during the last 30 years. The volume of pure alcohol consumed in 1987 in Japan was 754,000 kl, which was about twice the amount consumed 20 years previously (Japanese Public Health Association, 1991). Ueshima, Ohsaki, Tatara, and Asakura (1984), therefore, proposed that increased alcohol consumption may play an important role in the increase in the number of hypertensive patients found in Japan.

Considerably wide variations in the prevalence of hypertension and in drinking habits among the workers of different working conditions, such as scales of companies and kinds of occupations, are often recognized. The present study, therefore, was designed to clarify whether the differences in the prevalence of hypertension in different worker populations are associated with different drinking habits, that is, different alcohol consumption.

II. MATERIALS AND METHODS

The study subjects comprised 107,692 workers (62,336 men and 45,356 women) who received annual health check-ups during the one-year period extending from January, 1988 to December, 1988 at a medical facility in Ishikawa Prefecture, Japan. They were asked about their drinking habits (non-drinker, drink more than once a month, drink more than once a week, daily drinker), smoking habits (non-smoker, ex-smoker, smoker) by means of a self-report questionnaire at the time of the health check-up.

The data of blood pressure (BP) and body mass index (BMI) were also obtained from the health check-ups. BP above 140/90 mmHg was defined as hypertension, and BMI above 25.0 kg/m^2 in males and above 24.0 kg/m^2 in females was defined as obesity. 20,119 of the 62,336 male subjects (32.3%) and 12,888 of the 45,356 female subjects (28.4%) were examined at the health check-up for serum gamma-glutamyl transpeptidase (γ-GTP) activity and serum total-cholesterol (T- chol) concentration. γ-GTP above 50 U/L and T-chol above 230 mg/dl were defined as abnormal elevations.

The age-adjusted ratios of the frequencies of hypertensive and obese workers, those of daily drinkers, smokers, and those of workers with high γ-GTP and high T-chol were obtained among the worker-groups divided by different scales of companies (1 to 4 employees, 5 to 29 employees, 30 to 99 employees, 100 to 299 employees, 300 to 999 employees, more than 1000 employees), and among the worker-groups divided by different kinds of occupations (manager, engineer, clerk, laborer, salesman, driver, and farmer).

III. RESULTS

Among the 62,336 male workers, 18,807 (30.2%) were non-drinkers, and 28,282 (45.4%) were daily drinkers. 38,076 (61.1%) were smokers. Hypertension was found in 19,627 (31.0%), and obesity was found in 11,553 (18.5%). Among the 20,119 male workers whose blood was examined, 827 (4.1%) showed elevated serum γ-GTP activity and 3,193 (15.9%) showed elevated serum T-chol concentrations.

On the other hand, 35,316 (77.9%) of the 45,356 female workers were non-drinkers, and only 1,908 (4.2%) were daily drinkers. 4,167 (9.2%) were smokers. Hypertension was found in 7,106 (15.7%), and obesity was found in 9,474 (20.9%) of the female workers. Only 19 (0.1%) of the 12,888 women whose blood was examined showed elevated serum, γ-GTP activity. 2,029 (15.7%) showed elevated serum T-chol concentrations.

The frequencies of hypertension, obesity, daily drinkers, smokers, and workers with elevated serum γ-GTP and T-chol levels among the worker-groups of different scales of companies, after adjustment for differences in the age distributions, are illustrated in Figure 1A (men) and in Figure 1B (women). The frequencies among the worker-groups of different kinds of occupations are illustrated in Figure 2A (men) and in Figure 2B (women).

As shown in Figure 1A, the frequencies of hypertension and obesity were generally high in the male workers belonging to the smaller scale companies, although workers in the biggest scale companies where the number of employees was above 1000 showed relatively higher frequencies. Daily drinkers and smokers were also more frequent in the smaller scale companies. On the other hand, workers with high serum γ-GTP levels were found more frequently in the larger scale companies. There were no associations between the frequencies of high serum T-chol and the scale of company.

In the female workers (Figure 1B), the frequencies of hypertension were higher in the workers of middle scale companies with 30 to 299 employees. Daily drinkers and smokers were also more frequent in the workers of middle-scale companies. Workers with elevated serum γ-GTP levels were found most frequently in the workers of companies with 300-999 employees.

Among the male occupational groups (Figure 2A), drivers, farmers and managers showed hypertension more frequently. Obesity was found more frequently in managers and drivers. Daily alcohol consumers and smokers were found more frequently in farmers, drivers, salesmen and managers, although there were fewer smokers among the managers. Elevated serum γ-GTP levels were more frequent in managers, engineers and clerks, but elevated serum T-chol levels did not show marked differences among the occupational groups.

As shown in Figure 2B for female workers, hypertension was somewhat more frequent in laborers, saleswomen and farmers. Obesity was found more

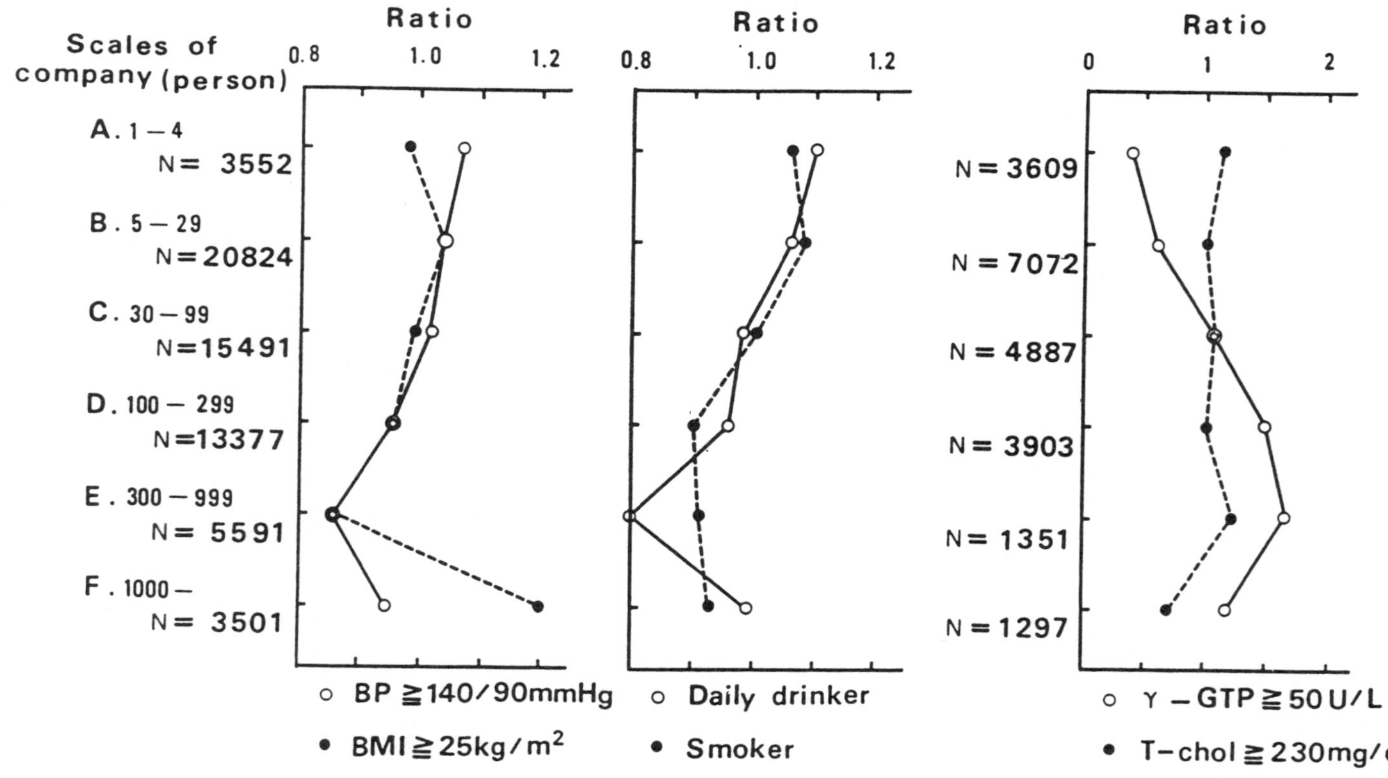

Figure 1A. Age-adjusted Ratios of Hypertension, Obesity, Daily Drinkers, Smokers, and Workers with Elevated Serum γ-GTP and T-chol Levels Among Male Worker-Groups of Different Scales of Companies.

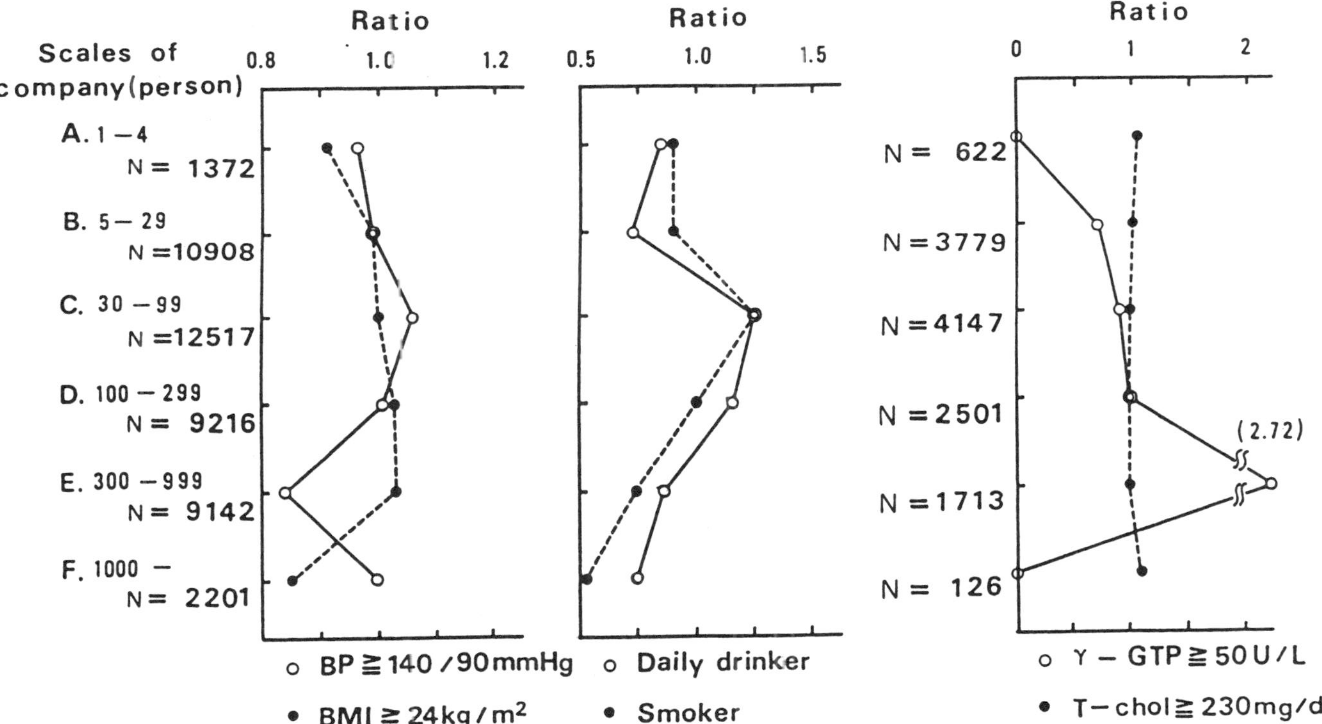

Figure 1B. Age-adjusted Ratios of Hypertension, Obesity, Daily Drinkers, Smokers, and Workers with Elevated Serum γ-GTP and T-chol Levels Among Female Worker-Groups of Different Scales of Companies.

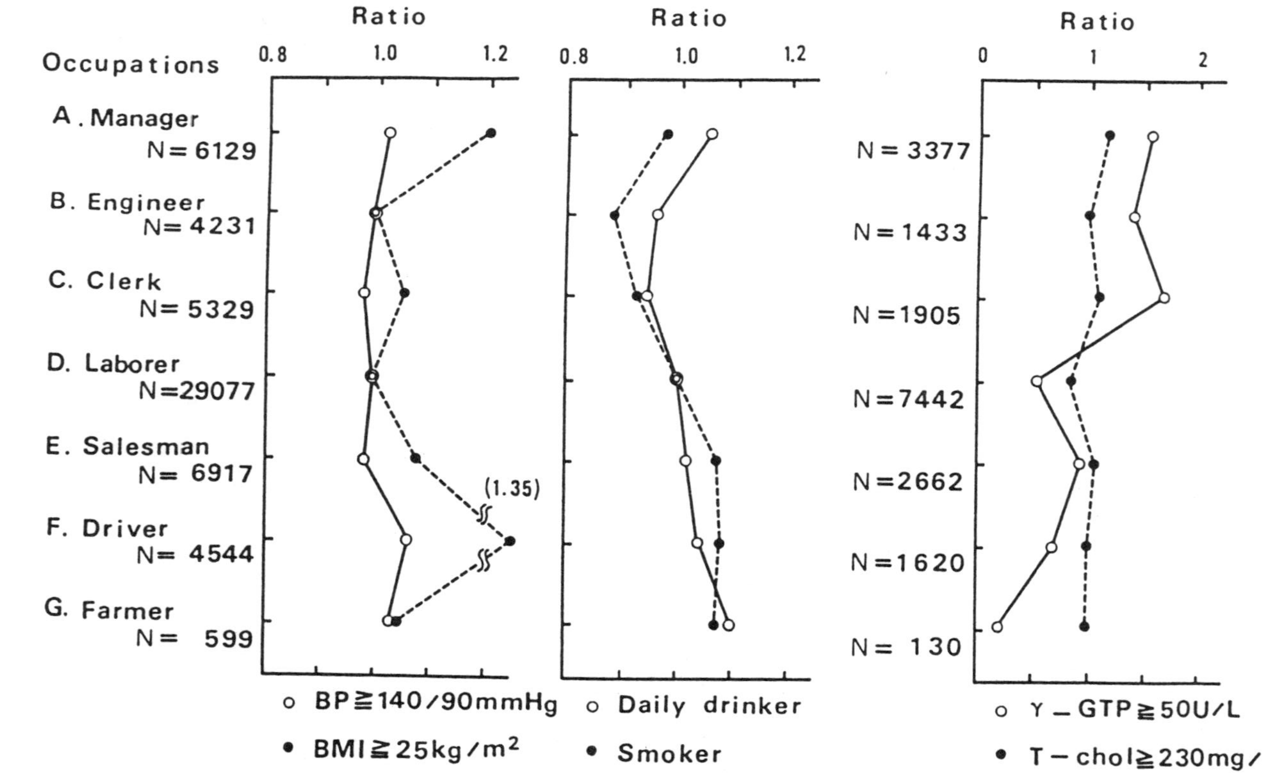

Figure 2A. Age-adjusted Ratios of Hypertension, Obesity, Daily Drinkers, Smokers, and Workers with Elevated Serum γ-GTP and T-chol Levels Among Male Worker-Groups of Different Kinds of Occupations.

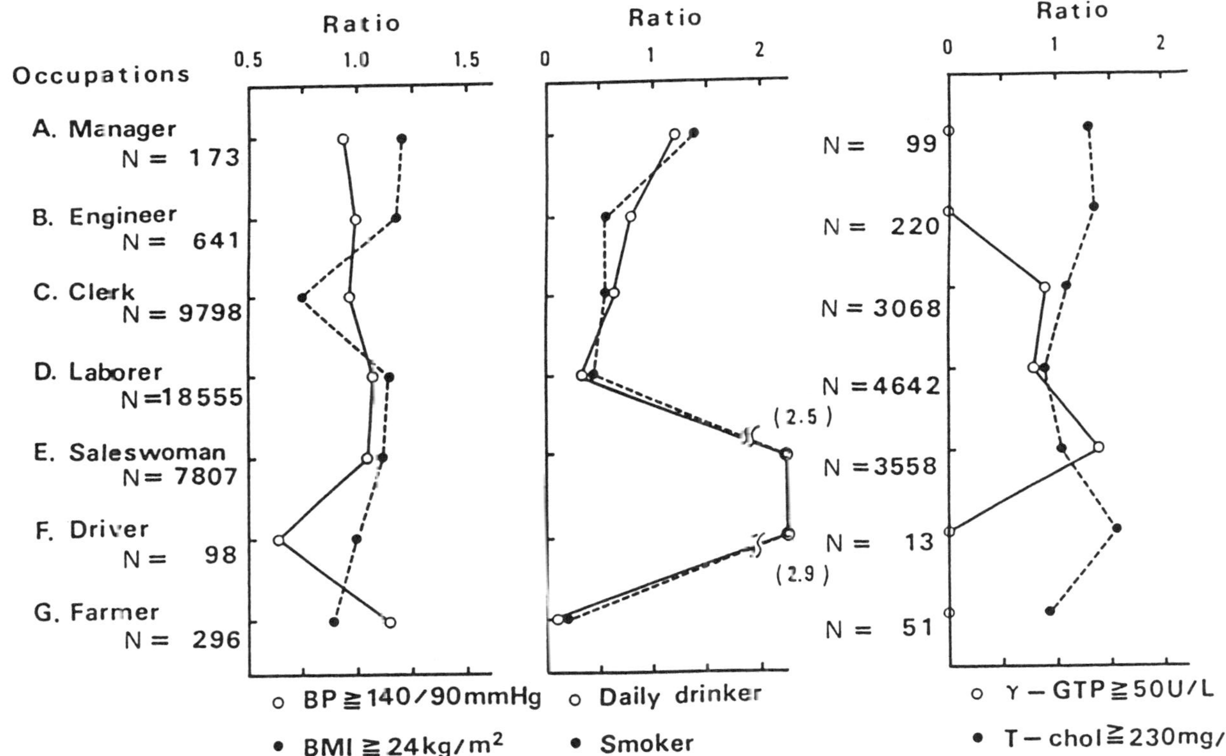

Figure 2B. Age-adjusted Ratios of Hypertension, Obesity, Daily Drinkers, Smokers, and Workers with Elevated Serum γ-GTP and T-chol Levels Among Female Worker-Groups of Different Kinds of Occupations.

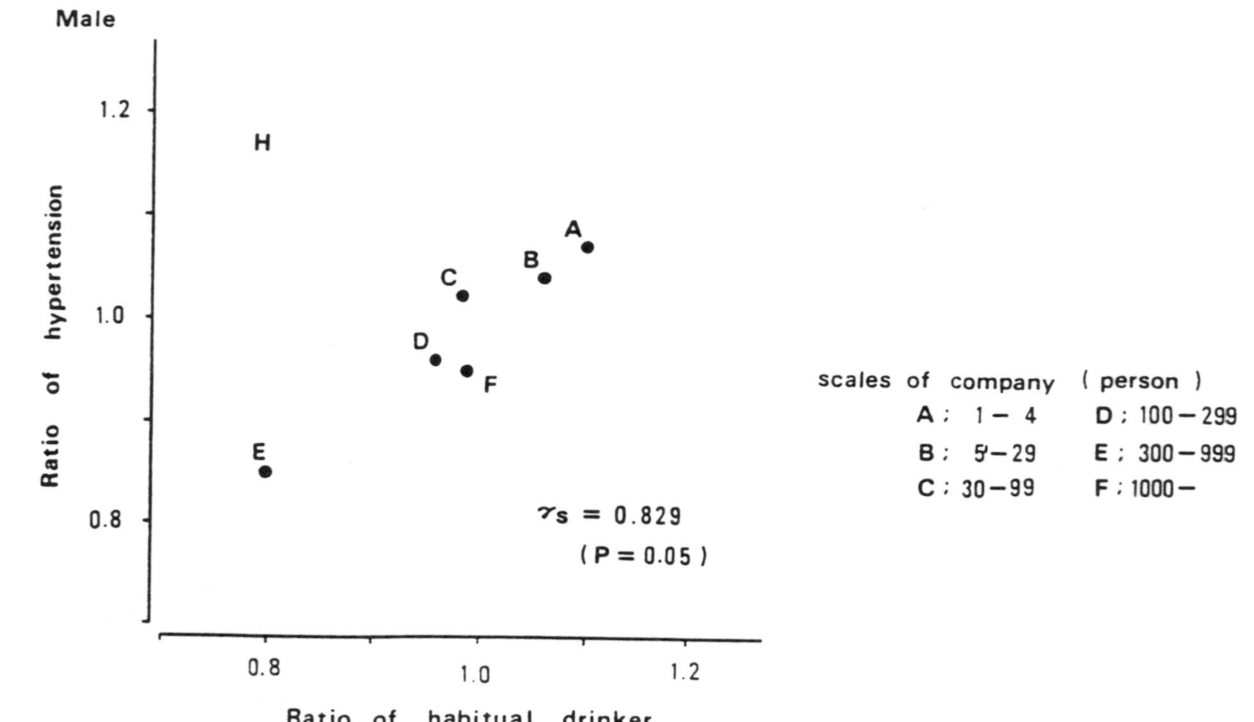

Figure 3. Spearman's Rank Correlation Coefficient Obtained Between the Frequencies of Hypertension and those of Daily Drinkers Among the Six Male Worker-Groups of Different Company Scales.

frequently in managers, engineers, laborers and saleswomen. Daily drinkers and smokers were more frequent in saleswomen, drivers and managers.

As shown in Figure 3, Spearman's rank correlation coefficient obtained between the frequencies of hypertension and those of daily drinkers among the six male worker-groups of different company scales was 0.829 ($p = 0.05$), and in Figure 4 that among the seven different occupational groups was 0.750 ($p < 0.05$). In female workers, however, these were not significant. No other significant associations were found between the frequencies of hypertension and those of obesity, smokers, and those of workers with high γ-GTP, and those with high serum T-chol.

IV. DISCUSSION

Modernization of Japanese society, accompanied by rapid economic growth, has brought about profound changes in the lifestyle of the Japanese people. With regard to the development of hypertension, excessive salt intake is known to be one of the major causes. Salt intake per capita among Japanese, however, has decreased during the last 30 years (Ministry of Health and Welfare, Japan, 1991), probably due to westernization of dietary habits. Obesity due to excessive intake of food energy may cause hypertension. Energy intake per capita increased rapidly during the first 10 years of this period, although it has decreased slowly during the last 10 years (Ministry of Health and Welfare, Japan, 1991). Thus, these nutritional factors cannot explain the recent increase in the number of hypertensive patients in Japan.

In the results of the present study, a higher prevalence of hypertension was found in male workers who belong to smaller scale companies, in drivers, farmers and managers. These findings suggest that hypertension is more prevalent in the workers with poorer working conditions, or in those with heavier psychological loads. Higher alcohol consumption among the workers may be one factor involved in the development of hypertension. Indeed, the present study showed an association between the frequency of hypertension and the frequency of daily drinkers among male workers with different working conditions, such as different scales of companies and different kinds of occupations. No significant association was found between alcohol consumption and the prevalence of hypertension among the female workers in the present study. Few Japanese women are daily drinkers, which may explain the lack of an association.

It is said that hypertension is observed more often in lower socioeconomic and lower educational groups (Schlussel, Schnall, Zimbler, Warren, & Pickering, 1990), and these groups are known to consume more alcohol (Lang, Degoulet, Aime, DeVries, Jacquinet-Salord, & Fouriaud, 1987).

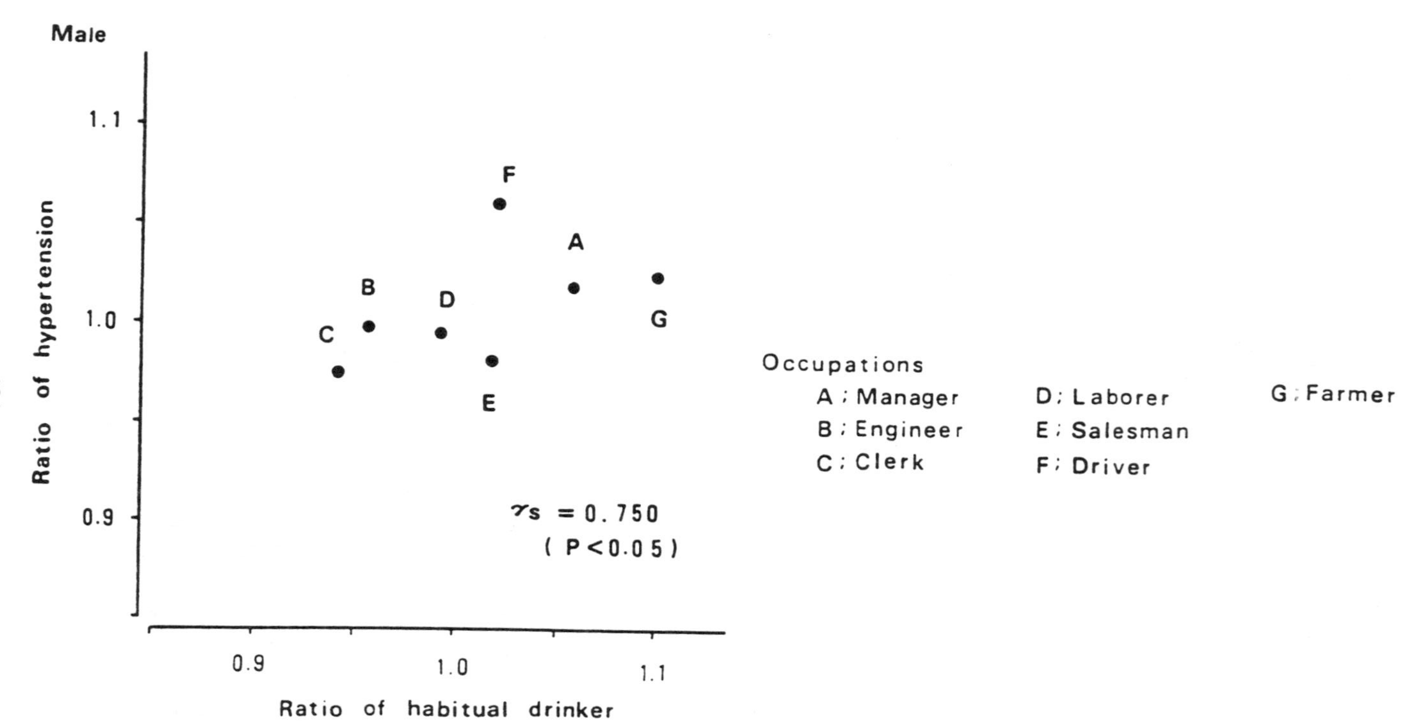

Figure 4. Spearman's Rank Correlation Coefficient Obtained Between the Frequencies of Hypertension and those of Daily Drinkers Among the Seven Different Occupational Groups.

It is also known that Japanese male workers in managerial posts, who feel more psychological stress, tend to drink more alcohol for relaxation. One study has indicated that Japanese managers are absent or ill due to hangover on average 30 days per year, in contrast to 10 days for unskilled workers (Hishimura & Saito, 1985). Therefore, alcohol consumption may play a role in producing differences in the prevalence of hypertension among Japanese male workers of different working conditions.

However, whether alcohol consumption is the major cause of these differences is still open to question because the frequencies of hypertensive workers did not correlate with those of workers with elevated serum γ-GTP levels in the present worker-groups of different working conditions. In our previous studies on workers in a factory (Yamada, Ishizaki, Kido, Honda, Tsuritani, Nogawa, & Yamaya, 1989a, 1989b) in which working conditions were similar, levels of serum γ-GTP, a biological marker for alcohol consumption, were shown to correlate with blood pressure or the prevalence of hypertension more closely than alcohol consumption itself. Other confounding factors should also be considered.

REFERENCES

Hishimura, M., & Saito, M. (1985). Problem between occupation and alcohol. *Handbook of Alcohol Clinic*, 321-324.

Japanese Public Health Association. (1991). Circumstance of alcohol consumption in Japanese. *Public Health Information*, 21 (6):5. (in Japanese).

Lang, T., Degoulct, P., Aime, F., DeVries, C., Jacquinet-Salord, M.C., & Fouriaud, C. (1987). Relationship between alcohol consumption and hypertension prevalence and control in a French population. *Journal of Chronic Disease*, 40:713.

Ministry of Health and Welfare, Japan. (1991). Present condition of national nutrition. *Journal of Health and Welfare Statistics Association*. 38 (9):92-93, 446. (in Japanese).

Schlussel, Y.R., Schnoll, P.L., Zimber, M., Warren, K., & Pickerg, T.G. (1990). The effect of work environments on blood pressure: Evidence from seven New York organizations. *Journal of Hypertension*, 8:679.

Ueshima, H., Ohsaka T., Tatara K., & Asakura S. (1984). Alcohol consumption, blood pressure and stroke mortality in Japan. *Journal of Hypertension*, 2(3):191.

Yamada, Y., Ishizaki, M., Kido, T., Honda, R., Tsuritani, I., Nogawa, K., & Yamaya, H. (1989a). The effect of small volume alcohol consumption on blood pressure: With special reference to the relationship between serum gamma-GTP activity and blood pressure. *Japanese Journal of Public Health*, 36:375.

Yamada, Y., Ishizaki, M., Kido, T., Honda, R., Tsuritani, I., Nogawa, K., & Yamaya, H. (1989b). Relationship between serum gamma-glutamyl transpeptidase activity, blood pressure and alcohol consumption. *Journal of Human Hypertension*, 3:409.

IT CAN'T BE A DRUG, MISS, IT'S NOT ILLEGAL: STUDENT PERCEPTIONS OF DRUG EDUCATION IN VICTORIAN POST PRIMARY SCHOOLS

Monica Slattery and Jan Garrard

I. INTRODUCTION

'Smoking is a health habit,' or so believe 30 percent of New South Wales secondary school students. These 30 percent of students understood 'hazard' to mean 'habit' and as such would read the cigarette packet message (prior to 1987) as promotion rather than warning (Long, 1975).

Curiously, only 26 percent of the males and 86 percent of the females who described themselves as 'chain smokers' in a recent Australian study, had in fact smoked recently (Hill, Willcox, Gardner, & Houston, 1986). The explanation, it seems, lay in the students' understanding of the term 'chain smoker';

> It has subsequently come to our attention that the term (chain smoker) is taken by some children to refer to a person who smokes only when a lighted cigarette is being handed from person to person (i.e., in a chain of people) (Hill et al., 1986, p. 59).

Research in Human Capital and Development, Volume 7, pages 189-207.

ISBN: 1-55938-132-9

These two instances are associated with one of the fundamental principles in education; that is, that learners/people construct their own views of reality (Driver, Guesne, & Tiberghien, 1985; Gunstone & Northfield, 1986; West & Pines, 1985). This 'constructivist' view of learning sees learning as a process of interaction between existing beliefs and attitudes and new information. Existing beliefs can negate new information that does not match. New learning takes place in the context of existing conceptions and hence, is most effective when it is based on the learner's existing beliefs. Stated succinctly, this view is,

> The most important single factor influencing learning is what the learner already knows. Ascertain this and teach him (her) accordingly (Ausubel, 1968, p. vi).

The National Drug Education Committee seems to hold this view of learning when they advocate that:

> Drug education should proceed from what people already know, and should recognise that the level of existing knowledge will vary with the age and general education level of the target group (Commonwealth Department of Health, 1987).

The fundamental questions then become not only the standard curriculum questions of what do we teach and how do we teach it, but also what do the learners already know and believe and what do they want or need to know? (Rowling, 1987).

Studies of student drug use provide some of what learners already know; that is, their experiential knowledge. A recent Victorian study indicated that analgesics, other medicines, alcohol, and tobacco were the most commonly used drugs. Among the illegal drugs, marijuana was the most common with usage increasing with the age of the student:

1. 3.4 percent of year 7 students reported using marijuana;
2. 16 percent of year 9 students; and
3. 26.7 percent of year 11 students.

Other illicit drug usage rates were low with less than 7 percent of students ever having used narcotics, stimulants or hallucinogens (Ministry of Education and Health Commission Victoria, 1986).

Licit drugs usage rates indicate that a percentage of the class have experiential knowledge of substances such as analgesics, tobacco or alcohol. Alcohol consumption levels for years 7, 9, and 11 students show that the 'drinkers' form a significant sub-group. The figures given below refer to students who report having consumed at least five drinks in a row in the last fortnight.

1.	Year 7	males	11.3 percent
		females	8.8
2.	Year 9	males	25.8 percent
		females	18.3
3.	Year 11	males	43.4 percent
		females	30.0

(Ministry of Education and Health Commission Victoria, 1986)

Other studies show a reduction in student drug use (with the exception of marijuana where the usage rate has stopped increasing) (Baker, Homel, Flaherty, & Trebilco, 1987), but still identify a group who will have experiential knowledge of drugs both licit and illicit.

Other information about student knowledge and beliefs about drugs is contained in 'death prediction statistics' studies wherein students associate specific drugs with the number of deaths they cause. These studies indicate that the misconception of narcotics as the drug type that causes the most drug-related deaths is widespread. One study found that 48 percent of males and 52 percent of females held this view (Baker et al., 1987). The accurate perception of tobacco as the major cause of drug-related deaths has been found to be held by between 11 percent (Chapman & Homel, 1987) and 20 percent (Baker et al., 1987) of students. Neither the criteria nor the source that students use for these predictions are elucidated.

Studies of factors that influence students knowledge, behavior and beliefs about drugs have found the following factors significant; families' and friends' attitudes and behaviors (Ahlgren, Norem, Hockhauser, & Garvin, 1982; Nolte, Smith, & O'Rourke, 1987); teachers' behavior (Bewley, Johnson, & Banks, 1979); school policy (Crow, 1984; Murray, Swan, & Clarke, 1984); packaging (Wilson, Wakefield, Easterman, & Baker, 1987); availability, legal restrictions on sale, pricing (Wallack, & Corbett, 1987); advertising (Bjartveit, Lochsen, & Aaro, 1981; Chapman, & Fitzgerald, 1982; Fisher, Blaze-Temple, Cross, & Howat, 1987); and the media (Bell, 1985).

This study set out to increase the understanding of what students know and believe about drugs and to explore the origins of their knowledge and beliefs.

II. THE RESEARCH PROJECT

The study of students was a subset of a wider study of drug education programs in Victorian Schools (Garrard & Northfield, 1987); a study replicated since then in other schools.

The research methodology included a survey questionnaire which was sent to 561 Victorian Post Primary Schools, case studies of 18 schools (16 post primary and 2 primary) and small group-structured interviews with students at 14 of those 18 schools.

The students ranged in age from 10/11 year olds at year 5 to 16/17 year olds at year 11. These small group discussions were designed to explore:

(a) students' responses to their drug education programs, and
(b) students' beliefs and attitudes about drugs.

This latter topic is the subject of the present paper. Other information is available from the report (Garrard & Northfield, 1987).

Discussions with Students

Audio tape-recorded interviews were conducted with one or more groups of approximately five students at each of the 14 schools.

The discussion topics included:

1. Students' beliefs and attitudes about a series of 17 substances which included a wide range of legal and illegal drugs. These 17 substances were presented to the students as picture cards which they were asked to:
   (a) sort into groups and explain the groupings;
   (b) place on a continuum of most to least dangerous for an individual to use;
   (c) place on a continuum of most dangerous to least dangerous in terms of causing problems for the community; and
   (d) place on a continuum of most to least dangerous in terms of long-term effects.
2. Students' understanding of the terms 'drug,' 'drug problem,' and 'addiction.'
3. Sources of students' beliefs about drugs.
4. Students' predictions of which drugs are the major causes of drug related deaths in Australia.

III. BRIEF SUMMARY OF FINDINGS AND DISCUSSION

The numerical data in this study were derived from the pooling of results from individual case studies and should be seen as pointing to possible trends and raising issues rather than allowing firm conclusions to be drawn. The students are not a random sample as they were all recipients of a drugs education course prior to the study.

The Card-Sort Task

'Substance groupings'

Most students grouped the substances into four categories as follows:

1. 'hard drugs' commonly consisting of crack, heroin, cocaine, marijuana, LSD, and occasionally glue, pep pills, sedatives, or cigarettes;
2. 'medical drugs' commonly consisting of analgesics, OTCs, sedatives and occasionally pep pills;
3. 'minor drugs' commonly consisting of beer, wine coolers and vitamin pills, coffee and occasionally including cigarettes;
4. 'not drugs' commonly consisting of salad roll, milk, and occasionally including vitamin pills, coffee, wine coolers and cigarettes.

Some students grouped the substances according to method of use (drinking, sniffing, smoking, swallowing); while others used availability and cost as the criteria (cost most, available in everyday houses, buy at chemist only).

'Most to least dangerous for an individual to use'

Each substance was scored from 1-17 according to its position on the students' spectrum of least dangerous (1) to most dangerous (17) for an individual to use. The mean scores and standard deviations for each substance over all the student groups is presented below in Table 1.

These results show clearly that most student groups believed crack to be the most dangerous drug and the other four illicit drugs (heroin, cocaine, LSD, and marijuana) followed. The drug which causes the most drug related deaths in Australia (tobacco) was rated as the eighth most dangerous drug.

All student groups perceived wine coolers to be less dangerous than beer even though the alcoholic content of the substances was visible and one of the coolers had a higher alcoholic content than beer (Island Cooler 6.0 percent, Foster's Lager 4.9 percent).

The data show that the student groups were in agreement about the two 'most dangerous' drugs, crack and heroin, and the 'non-drugs,' the salad roll and milk, but there was less agreement about the danger of the drugs between these two types.

A verbal analysis of the tape-recorded discussions that accompanied this ranking task provided information about how students responded to the substances. These findings are used where relevant in this paper. Some of the salient findings not used elsewhere, are that there was wide variability in student beliefs and behaviors about analgesics, vitamins and coffee; students had very little to say about pep pills, heroin, milk, salad roll, OTCs, and sedatives (knew

Table 1. Mean Scores and Standard Deviations; Most to Least Dangerous for the Individual User
n = 20 student groups

Substance	*Mean*	*Standard Deviation*
Crack	16.6	0.9
Heroin	15.9	0.6
Cocaine	14.7	1.5
LSD	14.2	0.5
Marijuana	11.9	2.9
Sedatives	9.8	2.7
Pep Pills	9.2	2.6
Cigarettes	9.0	2.9
Beer	8.9	2.4
Glue	8.2	3.8
Wine Coolers	7.8	2.9
Over the Counter	7.7	2.0
Analgesics	6.4	2.1
Vitamin Tablets	5.3	2.6
Coffee	4.3	1.8
Salad Roll	1.7	0.6
Milk	1.6	0.6

little/spoke little is not clear); students knew very little about LSD; students were clear that marijuana was a drug, but expressed different views as to its dangerousness; students believed that glue was a drug and made negative comments about it with the only debate being whether you would die before you became addicted to it.

Criteria Used to Rank the Substances

The verbal analysis revealed that students mostly used two pharmacological properties as criteria to judge the dangerousness of a substance for individual use:

1. the speed of addiction, and
2. the amount needed to cause death.

Most to Least Dangerous for Community Problems

Beer was perceived as the drug that causes the most problems for the wider community. Many students meant 'alcohol' not 'beer' when they placed the card and linked beer to spirits and fortified wines. The criteria used were the road toll and domestic violence as well as, to a lesser extent, physiological effects. There was little mention of the percentage of the population that used the drug as a criterion for its placement in the ranking.

Table 2. Mean Scores and Standard Deviations; Most to Least Dangerous for Community Problems
n = 10 student groups

Substance	*Mean*	*Standard Deviation*
Beer	14.3	3.8
Crack	12.5	4.7
Wine Coolers	11.8	4.8
Pep Pills	11.4	2.6
Cocaine	11.3	3.6
Heroin	11.3	3.4
Cigarettes	11.0	5.5
Marijuana	10.5	2.6
Sedatives	10.5	2.8
LSD	9.9	4.1
Glue	8.5	3.7
Over the Counter	8.3	2.7
Analgesics	7.2	3.0
Vitamin Pills	5.2	2.6
Coffee	4.4	3.5
Milk	1.7	0.7
Salad Roll	1.5	0.5

Crack remained high in the ratings while cigarettes moved up one place and still hovered around the mid-point. The standard deviations for the substances except the roll and the milk, were generally higher than in Table 1 and the standard deviation for the cigarette ranking (SD 5.5) is the highest of all. This indicates that there is higher variability among student groups on the issue of community issues about drug use. It is unclear why pep pills became so dangerous.

The discussion about 'beer' and 'alcohol' revealed that most students did not understand 'alcoholic volume' nor the relationship between potency and quantity when applied to drinking. Students commented that alcoholics drank fortified wines or spirits not beer or wine cooler. There was marked ambivalence amongst students whether alcohol was in fact a drug.

Most to Least Dangerous Substances in Terms of Long Term Effects

Beer and cigarettes were considered to be the most dangerous drugs in terms of long-term effects. Once again, wine coolers were rated lower than beer.

It is interesting to note that while alcohol and tobacco were rated as more dangerous in the contexts of community problems and long-term effects than in the context of individual use (interpreted as short-term by students), students' ratings of analgesics were always low and varied little between Tables 1, 2, and 3.

Table 3. Means and Standard Deviations; Most to Least Dangerous in Terms of Long Term Effect
n = 8 student groups

Substance	*Mean*	*Standard Deviation*
Beer	14.2	2.8
Cigarettes	13.8	3.6
Heroin	13.3	2.6
Crack	12.9	4.0
Wine Coolers	11.8	5.2
Cocaine	11.6	3.1
Marijuana	10.8	2.5
LSD	10.6	2.1
Sedatives	9.9	5.0
Pep Pills	7.9	4.3
Glue	7.8	4.0
Over the Counters	7.3	2.6
Coffee	6.8	4.4
Analgesics	6.5	3.0
Vitamin Pills	3.6	0.7
Milk	2.5	2.7
Salad Roll	2.3	2.4

Weekly analgesic use among post primary students in New South Wales has nearly doubled between 1971 and 1983, and analgesics are the most widely used drugs by years 7 and 9 students in Victorian post primary schools (overtaken by alcohol and tobacco among year 11 students) (Commonwealth Department of Health, 1986; Ministry of Education and Health Department, Victoria, 1986).

Within the present study, a survey of drug education programs in Victorian post primary schools showed that school drug education programs included analgesics less frequently than alcohol and tobacco.

Once again, as in Table 2, Table 3 is characterized by greater variability in drug rankings among different student groups (as indicated by high standard deviations in the ratings for most drugs) than was the case in Table 1. Some students linked milk and the salad roll to heart disease and obesity.

Word Meanings

'Drug'

Commonly, students defined 'drug' by giving an example of a 'hard' drug or describing highly addictive or lethal properties. Some students offered more formal-type definitions and (without being asked) attributed these to school learning; however, these students gave 'hard drug' examples when asked. While such dual understandings of concepts can be functional, they can also hinder learning (Gleitman, Armstrong, & Gleitman, 1983). The student can use each understanding exclusively in its particular context and hence *not* see their own 'out of school' behavior as drug taking.

That the 'exemplary' or prototypical definitions persisted indicates the strength of these pre-existing beliefs as these students had all participated in drug education courses where 97 percent of the courses included alcohol and 59 percent included prescribed tablets. Studies of cognitive dissonance indicate that the individual either negates the dissonant element in his/her cognitions or devalues its importance. Students did devalue school as a *source* of data about drugs (see sources of students' beliefs) and, it seems, devalued the data.

One group of students who gave an exemplar definition were pushed by the interviewer to provide a 'formal-type' definition:

Interviewer: What's a drug?
Student: Depends what kind of drug it is—like medical drug, that can help you. Like coke and all that—you can die from them.
Interviewer: So if you have drugs—some of which you can die from and some of which help you—what's a drug?
[Long pause]
Interviewer: I'll give you an example. There are foods that you don't like and there are foods that you do like—what's food?
Student: Energy.
Student: It keep you going.
Student: Just energy.
Interviewer: You see under the category food there are ones that you like and ones that you don't like, but you have a definition for food. So there's drugs, ones that are good for you and ones that are bad for you—what's a drug?
Student: Something that you rely on.
Student: Something that makes you feel good—like when you have Big Mac you feel good.

Drug Problem

The 'drug problem' was variously seen in terms of:

1. specific drugs (i.e., the drug problem is crack, heroin, cocaine, etc.);
2. the properties and effects of drug use (i.e., the drug problem is addiction, dying, getting hooked, etc.);
3. the people who take drugs (i.e., the drug problem is junkies, pushers, drug addicts, etc.);
4. how people handle drugs (i.e., the drug problem is misuse of drugs, going a bit overboard, etc.);
5. organizations associated with drug use/abuse (e.g., the National Campaign, Operation Noah, etc.); and
6. there is no drug problem.

Table 4. The Meaning of 'Drug Problem' 20 Student Groups

Category of response	*Percentage of responses*
Specific drugs	41
Properties of drugs and effects of drug use	29
People who take drugs	11
How people handle drugs	9
Organizations	4
No drug problem	2

Table 4 indicates that the most students see the drug problem in terms of specific (usually illicit) drugs, and their properties and effects. Very few students perceived the drug problem as a 'people' problem or a social problem.

'Addiction'

Addiction was also defined by some in terms of illicit drugs. For example, 'Oh well, physical addiction—wouldn't that be heroin'.

However, most students had some concept of dependence apart from a specific drug of dependence. One student interview explored 'addictive' as follows:

Student: Addictive is when you can't live without it.
Interviewer: So, you could be addicted to air?
Student 1: Yes.
Student 2: No.
Student 3: Um.
Student 1: Well, you'd die if you couldn't breathe.
Interviewer: So you're addicted to anything you can't live without.
Student 2: No. Addictive is if you think you can't live without it, but you really can.
Interviewer: People sometimes say they will die if their girlfriend or boyfriend goes away. Does that make friends addictive?
Student 2: No. It is body things you think you can't live without.

Some students were unaware that tobacco can result in physical dependence and expressed the belief that it is easy to give up cigarettes. In fact, psychological addiction was seen as easy to overcome.

Some of Students' Beliefs About Drugs

Two measures of students' sources of beliefs about drugs were used: a direct measure and an indirect measure.

The direct measure consisted of asking students directly where they thought they got most of their ideas about drugs from. The indirect measure consisted of an analysis of all indirect references to sources of beliefs made by students during the entire discussion.

Table 5 indicates that the various media (but mainly television) are the main sources of students' beliefs about drugs. Parents were frequently mentioned by students, but most often in a negative context (e.g., 'the kid knows more than the parent'). Similarly school as a source of drug knowledge was cited more frequently in a negative than a positive sense (e.g., 'the teachers don't know much more than what we do').

Friends, acquaintances, and 'other kids' were frequently mentioned. Personal experience was an underrated source of drug knowledge when students responded to the direct question. However, personal experience was an important factor according to the indirect measure (e.g., 'I've tried smoking. It was pretty disgusting . . . that was the last time I ever tried it').

The indirect measure of students' beliefs produced some different results from the direct measure. for example, the percentage of responses attributed to the personal experience category of responses was 3 percent from the direct measure and 22 percent from the indirect measure. This difference in the measures is congruent with other studies that have used these methods (Garrard, 1987). However, it raises an issue about student learning. In the constructivist model many studies have shown the persistence of existing beliefs and that these beliefs can negate new information that is discrepant. Students indirectly or spontaneously cited experience as a source and studies of student drug use confirm these statistics, yet the students were not aware of or did not admit this source when asked. This may mean in their thinking about drug-related issues they see their outside of school lives as separate from school learning and this may reduce the impact of school learning on their lives.

Media as Educator

Table 5 indicates that the Media are a very potent and salient source of student beliefs about drugs. Some of the things the media taught students is that crack is cheap, fast acting, available and made from household products and that Wine Cooler is made from fruit juice and sugar, is good for you and available in six packs. As many students believe advertisements (Fisher et al., 1987) and presumably even more believe documentaries, biographies and feature stories, it is understandable that the media have been accused of being drug peddlers because of the role they play in: (1) actually creating a ready market for the drug they are ostensibly warning people about; and (2) providing the type of explicit information (e.g., where to buy, how to prepare, how to ingest) which actually enables access to and use of the particular drug (Wallace, 1987).

Table 5. Sources of Students' Beliefs About Drugs; Percentages of Responses in Seven Categories 20 Student Groups

	Percentage of Responses	
Source of beliefs	*Direct Measure*	*Indirect Measure*
Media (total)	35	30
-electronic	19	21
-print	8	4
-general	8	5
Friends	17	21
Parents (total)	19	21
-positive	5	
-negative	14	
School (total)	12	4
-positive	8	
-negative	4	
Community	4	2
Personal experience	3	22
Health professionals	1	1

Media and Illicit Drugs

Media exposés of illicit drug use are contrary to nearly all of the principles of drug education formulated by the National Drug Education Committee and stated in the National Drug Education Guidelines (Commonwealth Department of Health,1987). Thus they: (1) use scare tactics and rely on fear arousal; (2) are 'one-off' sessions rather than long-term consistent programs; (3) focus on providing information about specific drugs; (4) use addict and ex-addict testimonials; and (5) focus on illicit drugs.

'Educational' approaches such as exposés have been shown to be counter-productive in that they can actually lead to increased rather than decreased drug use (Jones, 1981).

The argument that media drug programs such as '48 Hours on Crack Street' are designed, not to 'educate people,' but to raise community awareness about drug problems is questionable on several grounds.

First, the importance of raising community awareness about a non-existent (in Australia) drug is highly questionable. As mentioned earlier, this very activity of awareness raising can in itself lead to the problem it is purportedly trying to prevent. Secondly, the 'hidden curriculum' in media drug stories is also a powerful influence on community perceptions of drugs and the 'drug problem.' Hidden curricula educate and inform indirectly and through what they don't say and do rather than through what they actually say and do. In focussing on illicit drug use, attention is diverted from the legal drugs which kill approximately 20,000 Australians every year (Commonwealth Department of Health, 1986). In focussing on the pharmacological properties of illicit drugs such as crack, heroin and cocaine, attention is diverted from the other properties of drugs which influence the drug problem. Properties such as legality, heavy promotion through advertising, convenience packaging, social acceptability, and ready availability are alternative criteria for judging a drug as dangerous other than simply rapid addiction and instant death. It is these 'social' properties of drugs as much as their pharmacological properties that can result in a drug problem. This issue is obscured by media awareness programs (or school drug education programs) which focus on illicit drugs and on the biochemical and physiological effects of drug use.

Media and Licit Drugs: A Case in Point

Wine Coolers were introduced with an extensive advertising campaign in February 1985. This study was conducted in November 1986; this preceded the public debate that accompanied the introduction of a 250ml package (January, 1987) and the most recent surveys of drug use among students (e.g., Ministry of Education and Health Commission, Victoria, 1986); this also preceded the inclusion of wine coolers in drug education resources from organisations such as the Alcohol and Drug Foundation, The Road Traffic Authority, and so forth. In general, in November 1986, school health education and drug education programs had not yet caught up with the wine cooler phenomenon.

Student comments about wine coolers displayed considerable misconceptions about composition, alcohol content and the effects of drinking them. Nearly all students believed that wine coolers contained no or very little alcohol and would have very little effect on the drinker. The theme that emerged was that wine coolers are relatively harmless because: (1) they have a low alcohol content; (2) they are diluted with fruit juices (beer is undiluted); (3) they are like soft drinks; and (4) they are natural and good for you (made from 'grapes').

Student attitudes to wine coolers were very positive in terms of taste and packaging.

Students referred to personal vicarious experience and advertisements to illustrate, justify or express their views. Media promotion is particularly important as a source as community knowledge about the 'new drug' was non existent prior to the campaign and the promotion stimulated (created) experience. Misleading advertising and convenience packaging of drugs such as wine coolers are seen by drug educators as among the 'enabling factors' that can lead to increased drug use. On this occasion, the packing and advertising have been subjected to legislative control and the 250ml packages were banned by the Federal and State Governments from July 1st 1987 and the alcoholic content was then set at a maximum of 3.5 percent.

Concern regarding young people and wine coolers arises from two areas of research into drug use: (1) the age at which young people first start using legal drugs, and (2) the concept of 'gateways' in drug use.

Thus, the age of first use of legal drugs such as alcohol and tobacco has been linked to the possibility of misuse of, and/or addiction to, these drugs at a later age. For example, the Royal College of Physicians of London in their report on smoking, stated that 'learning to smoke usually occurs in childhood or in adolescence (Royal College of Physicians of London, 1977). Similarly, in a recent study of alcohol knowledge, attitudes and behavior among year 8 students in Western Australia, Fisher et al. (1987) found that students who were classified as problem drinkers were more likely to have started drinking at an early age. Further, a recent study by Hill et al. (1986) indicated if year 7 students are in some way prevented from using alcohol and tobacco at this early age (approximately 12 years old), they may be more likely to remain non-users throughout their school and perhaps adult life. Thus, one of the aims of the prevention of the misuse of legal drugs has become that of delaying the onset of first use of these drugs among children and adolescents (Fisher et al., 1987; Reid and Massey, 1986).

Wine coolers are more likely to enable early use of alcohol by children because they appeal to the sweeter, less mature taste of children. Children who reject beer, wine or spirits because of their taste are less likely to reject the more appealing tastes of wine coolers. Students made many positive comments about the taste of wine coolers.

Findings from two recent studies of drinking behavior among under-age young people support this assertion. For example, a recent survey by a group of fifth year medical students of drinking patterns among year 10 students in Western Australia found that wine coolers were the most popular drink among female students (Bardsley, Goossens, Hanrahan, & McLellan, 1986).

Similarly, a recent comprehensive survey of alcohol use among young people in South Australia found that: (1) wine coolers were consumed by a significantly higher proportion of under-age drinkers (12 to 17 year olds) than legal-age drinkers (18 to 23 year olds); (2) there was a (non-significant) tendency for the younger under-age drinkers (12 to 14 year olds) to cite wine coolers as their preferred drink in comparison with the older under-age drinkers (15 to 17 year olds); wine coolers were the alcoholic drink most *liked* by under-age drinkers; 'taste' was the most frequently cited reason for liking wine coolers; and 69 percent of under-age drinkers for whom wine coolers were the type of alcohol most drunk stated that soft (non-alcoholic) drinks were the drinks used before they drank wine coolers (the actual question asked was: 'What did you used to drink before you drank wine coolers?').

The authors concluded that:

> Wine coolers have undoubtedly caused a major shift in drinking patterns. Their market share, particularly with the under-age female segment is impressive. There is also evidence of wine coolers being effective in 'recruiting' under-age drinkers (Drug and Alcohol Services Council, 1987).

The concept of 'gateways' or 'routes of entry' in drug use also focuses attention on the early use of legal drugs such as alcohol and tobacco by young people. Several studies have shown that there is a high correlation between licit and illicit drug use and that adolescents who have or will use illicit drugs are those who have already used tobacco and alcohol (McAllister, Makkai, & Jones, 1986; Hamburg, Braemer, & Jahnke, 1975).

Thus, it is believed that delaying the onset of alcohol and tobacco use by young people may help prevent abuse of these drugs in later life and also help prevent the use of illicit drugs (Fisher et al., 1987). This delay in the use of legal drugs is not aided by the promotion and packaging of alcohol and tobacco products which have special appeal to young people.

Students' Predictions of the Causes of Drug Related Deaths in Australia

Students were given a copy of a histogram of the percentage of drug related deaths caused by various drugs, and asked to assign each of the five specific drug groups to the columns of the graph.

Fifty-seven percent of students correctly placed tobacco in column 1 (i.e., causing 81% of drug-related deaths) and 48 percent of students correctly placed alcohol in column 2 (i.e, causing 16.5% of drug-related deaths). Overall, 41 percent of students correctly placed tobacco in column 1 *and* alcohol in column 2.

On the other hand, 32 percent of students assigned alcohol to columns 3, 4 or 5; 19 percent of students placed tobacco in columns 3, 4 or 5; and 29 percent of students placed opiates in columns 1 or 2.

These results are particularly interesting when compared with findings from both Chapman and Homel (1987) and Baker et al. (1987) as the Victorian statistics (57 percent correctly identified tobacco) are notably higher than the New South Wales statistics (35% highest correct).

Differences between the results of the present study and results of the New South Wales study are marked, and several possible explanations for the differences can be proposed. However, once again, it is important to bear in mind that the number of students in the present study was small (63 students completed the graph questions), and that students were not a random sample of all secondary students. Rather, most of the students were from schools which had some form of drug education in the school program. However, a discussion of the proportion of deaths from various drugs was not necessarily included within the school programs, and most students' comments indicated that they had not seen this particular graph (or one like it) before. Thus, they appeared to answer the question on the basis of their general knowledge abut drugs rather than on the basis of a knowledge of the specific statistics.

These findings also raise the possibility that general community awareness of the nature of the drug problem may have changed in recent years, particularly in Victoria where many newspaper articles (and to a lesser extent, television programs) over the past 18 months have stressed that tobacco and alcohol are the major causes of drug-related deaths in Australia.

For whatever reasons, be it individual school drug education programs, or a raised community awareness through more balanced discussions of drug issues (particularly in the print media) it appears that a small non-random sample of Victorian post primary school students in 1986 had a greater awareness of which drugs are responsible for the great majority of drug-related deaths than did a random sample of post primary students in New South Wales in 1987. However, as indicated in Table 1, awareness of tobacco and alcohol as the major causes of drug-related deaths does not necessarily influence students' perceptions of what constitutes a dangerous drug. Thus, speed of addiction and instant death appear to be more important criteria than likelihood of death on a statistical basis, in students' judgements of which drugs are most dangerous; that is, instancy not instances.

Students' Reactions to the Correct Statistics

When students whose estimates were incorrect were given the correct statistics they responded in a range of ways: some related their incorrect estimates to the media; others reflected on the moral values of a society which both permits and promotes the sale of lethal drugs; others dismissed the data and referred to their belief that 'it can't be a drug, it's not illegal'; and others accommodated the new information with no apparent conceptual change (one summed this up as 'it [the knowledge] enlightens you, but it doesn't really change you').

IV. CONCLUSION

It has been argued that meaningful learning can only be achieved through programs that both relate to and build on students' pre-existing understandings, attitudes and experiences. This study exposed a range of student knowledge and some patterns among that knowledge that are of use to drug educators as guides to what students may believe.

The need for any course to begin by eliciting pre-existing beliefs and knowledge is reinforced by findings that the students persisted in perceiving drugs in terms of illicit (hard) drugs. The holding of exemplary or prototypical definitions of drugs makes it harder for students to recognise that substances such as alcohol and tobacco are drugs and can be both addictive and harmful.

Similarly, that students judged relative danger of substances in terms of their pharmacological properties, especially in terms of instancy of addiction and death, makes understanding chronic harm and societal harm difficult. The focus on pharmacology also detracts from explorations of social, political and personal factors in relation to drug use. This was evidenced by the limited criteria the students used to discuss the impact of the substances on the community. The students also saw the issues in reductionist ways—on single dimensions. They did not explore the relationships between factors, or the complexity of drug use and abuse. For example, passive smoking was never discussed nor financial cost to the community of drug induced illness. Rather the emphasis was on the individual and the agent; even then, factors such as drug potency as a function of the amount taken, the individual's weight, tolerance level and health and the manner in which the drug was ingested were not considered. The need for courses to develop the complexity and interaction between factors was clear.

The students in this study did not all see alcohol as a drug and did not seem to understand alcohol and the relationship between potency and quantity, yet they had been learners in courses that 'taught' (96% of them did) about alcohol. Between the 'teaching' and 'learning' lie a whole range of factors, such as pre-existing beliefs, current experiences, cultural pressure and the messages from media sources that lessen and transform the learning.

The fact that in the individual's search to make sense of conflicting cognitions 'school learning' gave way to learning from other sources points to the need for school learning to become more potent. One way to increase potency is to tackle the specific misconceptions held by the group using examples that are plausible in the student's own contexts, another way is to diminish the potency of other sources by analysing their legitimacy. This may involve drug education in a campaign of social action; as the wine cooler legislation and regulations evidences, such action can be effective. There are strong implications that health education must be broadened from the personal decision making model currently used to a model that includes notions of health promotion and advocacy as well as exploration of the ramifications of both the political, ideological, cultural and social factors and the policies of the government that impact on individual health. This is an argument for both a more holistic and a more specific approach and that is not a dissonant argument.

REFERENCES

Ahlgren, A., Norem, A., Hockhauser, M., & Garvin, J. (1982). Antecedents of smoking among pre-adolescents. *Journal of Drug Education*, 12(14): 325-340.

Ausubel, D.P. (1968). *Educational psychology: A cognitive view*. New York: Holt, Rinehart & Winston.

Baker, W., Homel, P., Flaherty, B., & Trebilco, P. (1987). *The 1986 survey of drug use by secondary school students in New South Wales*. Haymarket, NSW: New South Wales Drug and Alcohol Authority.

Bardsley, A., Goossens, C., Hanrahan, J., & McLellan, J.A. (1986). *Drinking patterns in year 10 students*. Department of Medicine, University of Western Australia.

Bell, P. (1985). Drugs and the Media. *Australian Alcohol and Drug Review*, 4(2): 235-242.

Bewley, B.R., Johnson, M.R.D., & Banks, M.H. (1979). Teachers' smoking. *British Journal of Epidemiology and Community Health*, 33, 219-222.

Bjartveit, K., Lochsen, M., & Aaro, L. (1981). Controlling the epidemic: Legislation and restrictive measures. *Canadian Journal of Public Health*, 72, 406-412.

Chapman, S., & Fitzgerald, W. (1982). Brand preference and advertising recall in adolescent smokers: Some implications for health promotion. *American Journal of Public Health*, 72, 491-494.

Chapman, S., & Homel, P. (1987). Smoking prevalence, intentions and knowledge of health risk: Results from a New South Wales school survey. *Supplement to Community Health Studies*, 11(1), 29s-34s.

Commonwealth Department of Health. (1986). *Statistics on drug abuse in Australia*. Government Printing Service, Canberra.

Commonwealth Department of Health. (1987). *Drug Education Programs in Australia*. Government Printing Service, Canberra.

Crow, C.S. (1984). Smoking areas in school grounds. Are we encouraging children to smoke? *Journal of Adolescent Health Care*, 5, 117-119.

Driver, R., Guesne, E., & Tiberghien, A. (1985). *Children's ideas in science*. Milton Keynes, Open University Press.

Drug and Alcohol Services Council. (1987). *S.A. Survey of alcohol use amongst persons aged 12 to 23*. Adelaide, Drug and Alcohol Services Council, Adelaide.

Fisher D.A., Blaze-Temple, D., Cross, D., & Howat, P. (1987). *Alcohol and young people: Australian baseline data for a WHO cross cultural study*. Paper presented at the Second National Drug Educators Workshop, Canberra, 17-21 May.

Garrard, J.E. (1987). *Students' perceptions of health*. Unpublished Ph.D. thesis, Faculty of Education, Monash University.

Garrard, J.E., & Northfield, J. (1987). *Drug education in victorian post-primary schools*. Faculty of Education, Monash University and Victorian Health Department.

Gleitman, L.R., Armstrong, S.L., & Gleitman, H. (1983). On doubting the concept 'concept.' In E.K. Scholnick (Ed.), *New trends in cognitive representation: Challenges to Piaget's theory?* Hillsdale, N.J: Lawrence Erlbaum.

Gunstone, R., & Northfield, J. (1986). *Learner, teacher, researcher: Consistency in implementing conceptual change*. Paper presented at the American Education Research Association, San Francisco.

Hamburg, B.A., Braemer, H.C., & Jahnke, W.A. (1975). Hierarchy of drug use in adolescence. *American Journal of Psychiatry*,1 132, 1155-1167.

Hill, D., Willcox, S., Gardner, G., & Houston, J. (1986). *Cigarette and alcohol consumption among Australian secondary school children in 1984*. Anti-Cancer Council, Carlton.

Jones, K.N. (1981). *Prevention is not easy: Main drugs and society, current perspectives*. Canberra Publishing Company, Canberra.

Long, A. (1975). What does 'hazard' mean? A survey of Sydney school children. *Medical Journal of Australia*, 2 (5): 175-178.

McAllister I., Makkai, T., & Jones, R. (1986). *Attitudes towards drugs and drug use in Australia*. Commonwealth Department of Health, Canberra.

Ministry of Education and Health Commission Victoria. (1986). *Report on the survey of drug use among Victorian post-primary students.* Ministry of Education (Schools Division), Melbourne.

Murray, M., Swan, A.V., & Clarke, G. (1984). Long term effect of a school based antismoking programme. *Journal of Epidemiology and Community Health*, 38, 247-252.

Nolte, A., Smith, B., & O'Rourke, T. (1983). The relative importance of parental attitude and behavior upon youth smoking behavior. *Journal of School Health*, 53 (4): 264-271.

Reid, D., & Massey, D.E. (1986). Can school health education be more effective? *Health Education Journal*, 45 (1): 7-14.

Rowling, L. (1987). Needs based drug education curriculum design. *Drug Education Journal of Australia*, 1 (1): 41-45.

Royal College of Physicians of London. (1977). Smoking for health. Third report from the Royal College of Physicians of London. Pitman Medical, London.

Wallace, S. (1987). *Media as drug peddlers.* Address to the Media Workshop, 5th March. Health Promotion Unit, Health Department Victoria.

Wallack, L., & Corbett, K. (1987). Alcohol, tobacco and marijuana use among youth: An overview of epidemiological, program and policy trends. *Health Education Quarterly*, 14 (2): 223-249.

West, L.H.T., & Pines, A.L. (Eds). (1985). *Cognitive structure and conceptual change.* Academic Press, Sydney.

Wilson, D.H., Wakefield, M.A., Easterman, A., & Baker, C.C. (1987). 15s: They fit in everywhere, especially the school bag, *Supplement to Community Health Studies*, 11 (1): 16s-20s.

A NATIONAL HEALTH STRUCTURE FOR HEALTH EDUCATION AND PROMOTION

Ted T.L. Chen and Alvin E. Winder

Twenty years after the central Chinese government moved to Taiwan from the mainland China, Taiwan began to experience a rapid development. This development took the form of increasing urbanization and industrialization. Public health professionals during these years had also made some remarkable efforts to reduce illness by aggressively carrying out programs in the area of immunization, family planning, and environmental cleanup as well as providing a clean water supply to all families. Additionally, the government established health centers all over the island in order to provide primary health care services to the populace. As a result of these public health practices, Taiwan has achieved some remarkable results in terms of prolonging life expectancy and lowering the infant mortality rate. These changes have led to a change in the major causes of death in Taiwan. Previously deaths were from communicable diseases such as gastro-intestinal diseases, phneumonia, and tuberculosis. Now, however, the major causes of death are attributed to the chronic diseases such as cerebral diseases, cancer and cardiovascular diseases

Research in Human Capital and Development, Volume 7, pages 209-221.

ISBN: 1-55938-132-9

and accidents. In this transition from contagious to chronic causes of death the health status of population in Taiwan is approaching that of the other industrialized nations in the world (Health Statistics, Taiwan, 1987).

In recent years, however, despite a significant increase in medical expenditure, expansion of hospital capacities and an increased supply of physicians and other health professionals, the health status of people in Taiwan has not seen as much improvement as would be expected. Moreover, some of the health insurance programs that the government has developed for the benefit of public employees, laborers and farmers have encountered a number of financial problems. Just like some other industrial nations the health system in Taiwan could benefit from a major overhaul.

As the mortality rate dropped and the life expectancy rate increased, Taiwan is experiencing the average age of its population getting older. It can be expected that this older population will, in the forthcoming years, add more health care demands on the system. As Taiwan has maintained a free-market system for its health care service, it has accumulated some serious problems such as uneven geographical distribution of health manpower, lengthy occupancy of hospital beds, heavy usage of the emergency room for regular visits, lack of a professional drug dispensing system, lack of a referral system, lack of quality control on health care services and lack of a concept and approach to health care cost containment. Moreover, the building of major medical centers and the high-tech research in the area of most advanced medical technology have gradually taking up a larger share of national health budget (Yang et al., 1990). All of these problems have led the health care system in Taiwan to become increasingly disorganized and non-functional. The need to reorganize and reshape the weakened health care system in Taiwan is apparent.

The establishment of a national health insurance plan has thus been proposed as a means to help revitalize the health care system, to redistribute health care resources and to build a forward looking health care system for a population that is becoming older. The national health insurance has also been expected to provide a foundation for establishing a fair and equitable health services opportunity for the population it serves.

However, the national health insurance plan, as it is proposed, has often been looked at as a cure for all health care problems in Taiwan. This is unfortunate because there has been too little discussion that places the national health insurance plan in the context of a national health structure. A structure is necessary that would take cognizance of the changes that have occurred in Taiwan and based on these changes move towards the achievement of national health goals. Moreover, not much discussion is heard about integrating health promotion and disease prevention activities in a national health plan in order to build a healthy foundation for the nation, a foundation from which the national health insurance plan is to operate.

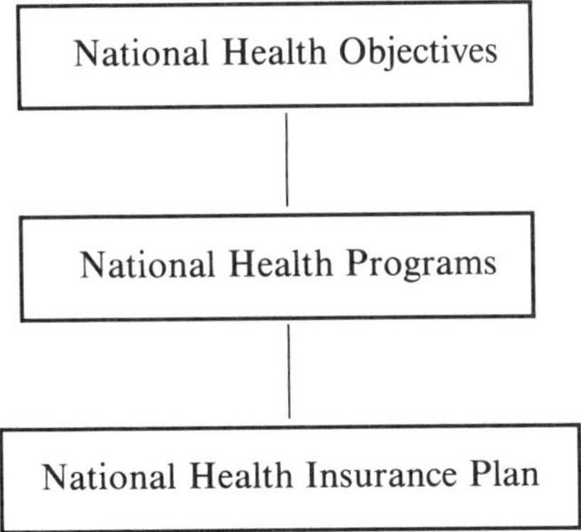

The purpose of this paper is to discuss the role that disease prevention and health promotion should play in a national health insurance program and how health education can be useful to its implementation. This paper will also address the issue of the benefits of prevention and promotion activities in a national health plan. It will also address the role of public health education, prevention and promotion in a structural change in the reimbursement for these activities and the overseeing of both the health plan and health budget allocation.

I. DISEASE PREVENTION AND HEALTH PROMOTION ACTIVITIES

Successful implementation of disease prevention activities is fundamental to the success of any national health program. In the past decades because of the success of disease prevention measures on major diseases such as tuberculosis, typhoid, gastrointestinal diseases, malaria, and measles, the life expectancy in Taiwan was prolonged and the infant mortality rate reduced. Currently, the dominant health problems in Taiwan are chronic diseases such as cancer, heart disease, stroke, and accidents. The health problems of today can no longer be controlled through a single shot of antibiotics or the application of drugs. Most of the current health problems are related to environmental, sociocultural and behavioral origins. These three factors are definitely related to the major health problems experienced by the people of Taiwan today. They express themselves through such behavioral and socioculturally defined acts as cigarette smoking, responses to stress, lack of exercise, obesity and accidents. The prevention and control of these acts, considered risk factors in chronic illness, is a major public health challenge today. Health promotion activities such as smoking cessation, hypertension control and stress management are considered key to the prevention and control of contemporary health problems. Health education methodologies that are effective in bringing about life style or behavior change are the basis for developing relevant health intervention programs.

In the recent years there have been many published reports of effective health promotion and disease prevention programs. There have been some remarkable achievements in this area in the past decades. For example, after many years of antismoking education, the rate of cigarette smoking among Americans has been declining steadily from about 50 percent in 1941 to about 27 percent in 1991 (Center for Disease Control, 1987). Encouraged by this achievement the U.S. National Cancer Institute has recently decided to launch additional community oriented smoking intervention programs throughout the nation in an effort to significantly reduce the cancer mortality rate in the United States. Another example is the U.S. effort in the area of hypertension control and education. Ten years after the national hypertension education project initiated a national survey, the results found that three-fourths of survey respondents indicated that they knew the status of their blood pressure. Of those who were hypertensive, over half were receiving treatment and about one-third of them had their problem of hypertension effectively controlled (Rowland & Roberts, 1982). This result was significantly better than a similar survey conducted before the initiation of the national hypertension education project. Many health professionals attributed the success of the national hypertension education project to the recent significant reduction of cardiovascular diseases and cerebral diseases in the United States.

The promising results of many activities in the area of health promotion and disease prevention, however, have not silenced the critics who challenge the cost-effectiveness of these programs (Cantor, 1985; Russell, 1986). Many critics have argued that these programs are not cost effective in the final analysis because they have failed to contain the rising cost of national health expenditure. They argued that, while these programs prolong life expectancy of the population, they do not necessarily reduce the national health expenditure. Furthermore, extending the life of the population would still require medical expenses to care for them in the later years of their life. On-the-other-hand those who support health promotion and disease prevention programs, argue that the extended healthy life of the population represents people will add to the wealth and productivity of the nation and directly contribute to an increase in the financial base from which the national budget is drawn.

The difference of the two viewpoints, in fact, represent more than a difference in their position on cost containment and expansion of resources. Those who emphasize cost containment put the stress more on calculating all costs related to medical care. These include the cost-benefits of prevention and promotion activities, and the number of additional healthy years due to additional life expectancy. The latter which would lead to additional medical care expenditure needed to support the elderly's additional years of life. For these reasons they argue that cure can often be seen as more cost effective than prevention and promotion.

Those who advocate the benefits of prevention and promotion activities in a national health program often build their argument based on the position that developing a nation with healthy people is primary while concern for expenditure is secondary. They argue that by improving the health status of the nation they will increase the pool of healthy people thereby increasing the national productivity and tax revenues. Eventually the national financial base would be raised and the additional monies would trickle down to benefit the total national health budget.

The position taken in this paper is that a discussion of building a national health program should require an equal emphasis on both cost containment and program effectiveness. There are many prevention and promotion activities that are experimental in nature and remain to be tested. Nevertheless there are many other prevention and promotion activities that have been proved to be effective and cost saving that should be implemented in all communities. Some prevention activities, for example, that have proved to be effective and should be promoted in a national health program include such activities as mandatory immunization programs for the prevention of measles, tetanus and diphtheria. These immunization and vaccination programs have been generally accepted as effective and have been instituted as mandatory practice by law. The ones that generate more debate in terms of their place in a national health program, however, are the health promotion activities such as control and prevention of cigarette smoking, dietary counseling, exercise, accident prevention, and stress management. These activities are promoted because of their identification as the major risk factors to cancer and cardiovascular diseases and are perceived as methodologies developed to reduce these risk factors. The promotion of these activities, however, needs to be reemphasized. The cost effectiveness of these activities have been researched and supported. Smoking control can be seen as an example to illustrate the importance and effectiveness of this kind of activity for the purpose of risk reduction.

The smoking rate among adult males is about 55 percent, among young males about 25 percent, among adult females about 10 percent and young females about 5 percent. In the recent years, because of the importing of foreign cigarettes and increase of family wealth, the rate of cigarette smoking among women and children is on the rise. As a result cigarette smoking is becoming a serious health problem in Taiwan (Chen, 1989).

According to a report released by the former U.S. Surgeon General Koop, cigarette smoking is identified as related to 35 percent of all cancer deaths 40 percent of all deaths from cardiovascular diseases and 82 percent of all lung cancer deaths. There are an estimate of 390,000 deaths per year in the United States that are related to cigarette smoking (U.S. Department of Health and

Human Services, 1989). In Taiwan, it is estimated that 16,000 deaths yearly are related to cigarette smoking (Allukian, 1990). Besides being a major causes of death, cigarette smoking is also related to fire hazard, accidents, indoor air pollution and decreased productivity. The cost of buying cigarettes is an expensive item by itself. All in all the cost of smoking cigarettes to the nation is sizable. According to a report of 1984, there is a loss of 53.7 billion in the United States resulted from smokers medical cost and loss of productivity (Rice, Hodgson, Sinsheimer, Browner, & Kopstein, 1986). In Canada, the loss due to cigarette smoking is 17 times higher than the profit from the sale of cigarettes (Collishaw & Myers, 1984). According to a 1984 study a man in the age range of 35-39 can save $40,829 if he quits smoking for life while a woman can expect to save $404 if she quits smoking for the rest of her life (Schwartz, 1987). The amount saved is higher for males who have potentially higher earning power.

There have been many methods developed to help smokers stop smoking. These include smoking cessation methods, self-help kits, counseling and nicotine gums. The cost of these cessation methods vary, generally in the price range of $20 to several hundred dollars. The effectiveness of these cessation methods also varies, however, they have a 35 percent quit rate one year after quitting (Oster, Golditz, & Kelly, 1984).

In summary, cigarette smoking is a serious health problem, and it can cause a serious financial burden to a nation. Smoking control program can help to reduce the smoking rate of the population. There are many effective smoking cessation methods available for smokers to stop smoking. Implementation of these smoking cessation programs for population in various settings is in the best national interest.

Other health prevention and promotion activities such as the control of hypertension and diabetes are also useful patient education programs that should be promoted. From the point of view of implementing a national health insurance program these health prevention and promotion programs can help to reduce the frequency of clinic visits, increase national productivity and accordingly increase the support base to the national health insurance.

II. PUBLIC EDUCATION

Every system has a function. For a system to work effectively it must be designed to function properly. While necessary, a good design does not ensure adequate functioning. A system must also have the respect of the people and they must know how to use it well.

$$\text{Success} = \frac{\text{Well Designed Plan}}{\text{Well Educated People}}$$

In Taiwan it has taken about three years so far to develop a plan for a national health insurance program. There has not yet, however, been much planning and effort devoted to preparing people to use the system. People in Taiwan have not taken readily to using government health insurance plans such as those developed for public employees, for laborers and for farmers. There have, for example, been a number of abuses. Some of the most notable of these include cheating on insurance claims, and cheating on insurance payments. Additionally, some legislators have used their influence to reduce insurance fee charges, an action that has made it impossible to keep the insurance plan fiscally healthy (Chiang, 1989). These past behaviors, if they are an indication of the future behavior of insurers in Taiwan, suggested that the proposed national health insurance once implemented can be expected to be in real financial trouble. There are two ways to deal with this problem of abuse. One way is to enforce legal acts to prosecute any violations. This approach can be useful only when the violation is incidental and not occurring on a massive scale. Another way is to develop and implement an education process so that the people understand that a national health insurance plan needs the respect and protection of all people. It is analogous to the need for effective protection of environment which to be successful, needs the support of everybody in the nation. The reason that some national health insurance plans work in nations such as Sweden, Germany and Canada is because the people of those countries respect and protect the system. To achieve this respect, it is necessary to develop several fundamental educational measures. These proposed measures should precede the implementation of national health insurance plan in Taiwan.

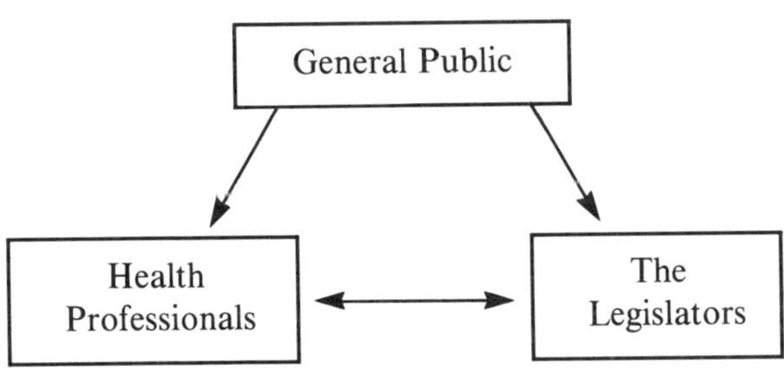

Three categories of people that should be the primary target for education are the general public, health professionals, and the legislators. Legislators who are elected by the general public, make policy decision for health professionals who in turn implement these decisions for the general public. These functions are interrelated. They create a chain of relationship in their operation. They can be positively reinforcing each other's function *or* can create a vicious cycle of operation.

Education of the Legislators

Legislators at all levels should be the first group of people to receive an education in regard to the planning and implementation of a national health insurance plan. They need to be informed and kept up-to-date about the theory and practice of the plan. This can be accomplished through public hearings, seminars and conferences. To achieve this, experts and scholars on the topic should be invited to conduct educational meetings with legislators, at both national and local levels, where they can jointly discuss related issues and problems. Increasing the understanding of the legislators is necessary if they are to both write a workable plan and to allocate budgets to support its implementation.

Education of the General Public

Mass media is the medium through which the public can be educated about the issues and topics of a national health insurance plan. For this purpose both print and electronic media should be designed to educate the public. Moreover, plans should be made to call press conferences, symposia and talk-shows where experts, legislators and scholars would be invited to sit down and discuss issues related to the topic. In this respect the government should take an active role in promoting the plan and not find themselves in a position where they are only willing to respond to criticism.

Education of the Health Professionals

Health professionals are opinion leaders and sometime gate keepers in health practice. Their understanding and support of national health insurance policy and practice will effect how the patients and general public will react to the plan. In this respect schools that train health professionals including those in medicine, dentistry, pharmacy, nursing, and public health should develop plans to have their curricula include both teaching about the health insurance plan and about prevention and promotion concepts. Moreover, in order to earn the respect of the health professionals a high prestige endowment chair should be placed in the school of medicine. Distinguished scholars should be invited to assume the endowed professorship with the understanding that they would lead in teaching and research related to both the national health structure and its relationship to the health insurance plan.

As implementing a national health insurance plan would be a relatively new experience in Taiwan, there would be a need for health professionals of all categories to be prepared and educated. Continuing education programs should be developed at all levels to educate health practitioners including physicians, dentists, public health practitioners, nurses and pharmacists to be familiar with the concept and application of the plan.

Additionally, efforts should be made to work collaborating with an accreditated School of Public Health to design and oversee continuing education programs for current health practitioners in Taiwan. Selected health practitioners in Taiwan should be sent to study oversees on a short-term basis. It would be preferable for foreign study to include a one month intensive workshop followed by two to three months of field training. The UMass program designed for the training of primary health care workers can be used as a model, a model which can be modified for the purpose of developing a manpower training program in the relation to national health insurance plan.

Education of School Children

Students in the schools today are the leaders of the society of tomorrow. Students' knowledge and attitudes in regard to the national health insurance plan and related health prevention and promotion practice should positively effect the implementation of the plan in the years to come. In this respect teaching units should be designed to have the related concepts taught through the school curriculum. Moreover, related courses should be offered to preservice and inservice teacher training programs.

Education of Patients

Patients are the first order beneficiaries of a national health insurance plan. They should be informed thoroughly about their rights and responsibilities in relation to the plan. Moreover, patients should be invited to represent the consumer by serving in an advisory capacity on issues related to the implementation of the insurance plan. Furthermore, patients should be provided with patient education programs in the areas such as smoking cessation, hypertension control and diabetic education to help prevent or reduce the threat to them of related diseases and illness. The success of the patient education program in the reduction of both the incidence and prevalence of chronic illness can further relieve the financial burden of the insurance plan to the state.

Education at Worksites

The worksite is the place where many preventable accidents and injuries occur. Health education activities should be planned at the worksite to help workers learn how to protect their health and how to use health care in case the need arises. Moreover, workers are a captive audience, offering the opportunity for the effective use of education. In addition to traditional health promotion activities such as smoking cessation, alcohol control, stress management, exercise and weight control, other preventive activities such as family planning and injury control programs should be offered. Successful worksite health education programs may be beneficial both in promoting positive health and may also be expected to bring about an increase in workers morale and productivity.

In order to accomplish the educational purposes established for the national health program educational strategies should be carefully designed. The PRECEDE model can be used as a reference for the purpose of planning educational programs. The three major educational activities that should be designed include (1) predisposing activities—activities designed to bring up level of awareness, (2) enabling activities—activities designed to enable positive practice to be performed, and (3) reinforcing activities—activities designed to reinforce positive practice to continue.

For the purpose of this paper practice is defined as to include three kinds of behavior performance. One, practice to use national health insurance properly. Two, practice to do self-help to promote positive health. Three, practice to support national policy on the goal of building a national health program.

Some of the educational activities that should be designed for this purpose include the following.

Awareness Activities

mass media
printed materials
audiovisual materials

Enabling Activities

education of the legislators
education of the health professionals
education of the general public
education of patients
education of workers

Reinforcing Activities

public policy advocacy
incentives for health promotion
enforcing law and regulation
public recognition for positive behavior

III. NATIONAL HEALTH PROGRAM COMMISSION

The national health insurance plan will have great impact on the reorganization of the national health care system. It will also produce significant results leading to the elevation of the health status of the nation. The plan should be carefully designed and proposed. It is critical, however, at the time of planning to also lay out a plan for evaluation. For a plan of this national magnitude, an evaluation plan should collect all kinds of data. These include outcome data, process data, data that are quantitative in nature as well as those that are qualitative in nature. In order to ensure that the planning and implementation of the plan can be done properly, a national commission on the subject matter should be organized in the early stage of the planning. The mission of the commission should be first to develop evaluation steps, and second to analyze and discuss the data collected from such an evaluation plan for improvement purposes. It is proposed to have such a commission composed of 5 to 7 members from both Taiwan and from overseas. The Commission can be organized under the direction of the Director General of the National Department of Health. It should meet twice a year to provide advice to the Director General on the matters regarding the implementation of the plan.

Budget

The proposed activities listed above which include prevention, promotion activities, various educational efforts and the organization of a national commission would require budgetary support to make them work. There are two types of budget that should be considered for the implementation of the listed activities. One type is the insurance reimbursable items and the other type is insurance plan budgeted items.

Budget Plan

Insurance Reimbursable Items
- patient education
- well baby care
- physical check-ups
- immunization and vaccination

Insurance Budgetary Items
- mass media campaign
- school health education
- worksite health promotion

The following is a brief description of these two types of budget.

Insurance Reimbursable Items

Many preventive activities such as immunization and well baby care should be reimbursable by the proposed insurance plan. Moreover, in order to encourage both physicians and patients to carry out preventive health measures such as physical checkups, some kind of incentive system should be considered. An example of this practice is a program in Sweden in which points are given to physicians for conducting physical checkups for their patients and points are given to expectant parents who follow through on prenatal and postal care activities. Such a program should be taken under consideration.

Moreover, selected patient education activities such as smoking cessation, hypertension control, cardiac rehabilitation and diabetic education should be made insurance reimbursable items. Mechanisms should be developed for both physicians and patients to carry through these patient education activities.

Insurance Budgetary Items

Many preventive and promotion activities are not clinic oriented and it would be difficult to arrange payment through health insurance. For example health education for the legislators, for health professionals, at school and at worksite, will not be able to be provided as insurance reimbursable items. Nevertheless, these activities need to be supported financially. A best solution is to allocate a fixed amount of insurance revenue for these activities. A 5 percent fixed income from the national health insurance should be recommended for this purpose.

IV. CONCLUSION

The health care system in Taiwan is outdated. Changes in the past four decades have led to the systems inability to meet the health needs of the population. In order to reorganize the health care system and to revamp the system to make it more responsive to both present pressure and future needs, it is necessary to develop a national health insurance plan in Taiwan that takes into account prevention as well as cure. In order to make the plan work, more attention needs to be paid to prepare and educate both the population and professionals to ensure that the former are healthy and the latter responsive to the system that will be proposed. A structural change to set up a national commission to both evaluate the health insurance plan and to oversee the budget allocations, so that the proposed activities in the area of disease prevention and health promotion can be carried out, is critical. Through careful planning, execution and evaluation, the national health insurance plan in Taiwan can then be expected to carry Taiwan into next stage of becoming a great nation with a modern national health program.

REFERENCES

Allukian, M. (1990). A letter to president Lee Teng Hui.

Cantor, J.C. (1985). Effectiveness of educational interventions to improve patient outcomes in blood pressure control. *Preventive Medicine*, 14 (6): 782-800.

Center for Disease Control. (1987). Public health service. *Morbidity and Morality Weekly Report*, 36(35): 581-000.

Chen, T.L. (1989). *Protecting our children from cigarettes* (pp. 610-627). Hearings before subcommittee on Transportation and Hazardous Materials, U.S. House of Representative.

Chiang, T.L. (1989). *Health Financing Systems in R.O.C.* National Health Insurance Conference, Taipei. December, 18-19, 1989. [in Chinese]

Colligshaw, N.E. & Meyers, G. (1984). Dollar estimates of the consequences of tobacco use in Canada. *Canadian Journal of Public Health*, 75: 192-199.

Health Statistics, Taiwan. (1989). Executive Yuan Publication, R.O.C. [in Chinese]

Oster, G., Golditz, G.A., & Kelly, N.A. (1984). The economic costs of smoking and benefits of quitting for individual smokers. *Preventative Medicine*, 13: 377-389.

Rice, D.P., Hodgson, T.A., Sinsheimer, P., Browner, W., & Kopstein, A.N. (1986). The economic costs of the health effects of smoking. *The Milbank Quarterly*, 64: 489-547.

Rowland, M. & Roberts, J. (1982). Blood pressure levels and hypertension in persons age 6-74 years: United States 1976-80. National Center for Health Statistics Advance Data, No. 84, Table 7.

Russell, L. (1986). *Is prevention better than cure?* Washington, DC: Brookings Institute.

Schwartz, J.L. (1987). *Review and evaluation of smoking cessation methods: The U.S. and Canada, 1978-1985.* NIH Publication NO. 87-2940, Washington, DC.

U.S. Department of Health and Human Services. (1989). *Reducing the Health Consequences of Smoking: 25 Years of Progress.* Report of the Surgeon General. Public Health Service, Centers for Disease Control, Center for Chronic Disease Prevention and Health Promotion, Office on Smoking and Health.

Yang, T.L., T.L. Hsiao & R.F. Lu (1990). National Health Insurance and National Health Care System in Taiwan. *Free China Industry* 73: 581-585. [in Chinese]

PART III

HEALTH AND CHANGING WORK ENVIRONMENT

THE UNITED STATES EXPERIENCE WITH REGULATION OF HEALTH AND SAFETY, 1970-1989

Morton Corn and Jacqueline K. Corn

I. INTRODUCTION

In a real sense, industrialization can be viewed as having completely altered the way in which citizens of the United States live. It has not merely provided the citizenry with goods and services; industrialization has stimulated population migration from rural to urban areas, virtually creating the "American Way of Life." The revolution in mechanized farming now enables 3 percent of the U.S. population to feed the nation and still export food to other nations. The automobile and the airplane, products of mass production techniques, have opened new vistas to the population. If the impact of industrialization on American life has been extensive and pervasive, it follows that its effect on the environment and on the health of the population has also been extensive. However, it is difficult to unravel the threads that tie together health and specific by-products of the industrial revolution. We are, in general, acutely aware of the connections between our environment and our health

Research in Human Capital and Development, Volume 7, pages 225-238.

ISBN: 1-55938-132-9

status, but our efforts to improve this status by altering the environment are often based on imprecise knowledge of the relationships and the complexity of social mechanisms for change.

Public health decisions have two elements—the element of value which determines the degree or extent of health a society wants and is willing to pay for, and a scientific element, which determines how much knowledge a society has upon which to base its health policy. In order for a society to utilize its resources to control disease or ill-health, it must accept disease as undesirable.

Certain facts are clear: life expectancy has increased during the twentieth century, primarily because of the virtual elimination of endemic disease and its toll in infant mortality. With increased longevity, debilitating chronic diseases, such as emphysema and cancer, have increased. The quality of life has improved when judged by the criteria of housing, food, education, and leisure time. In other respects, the quality of life may have deteriorated as a result of industrialization.

This presentation focuses upon one particular aspect of those employed in industry—that is, the areas of concern referred to as occupational safety and health. A unifying theme is the expansion in our utilization of chemicals and chemical by-products. Industry uses enormous quantities of materials, many of which are potentially toxic. Our growing awareness of industrial processes on health, as reflected in occupational safety and health, environmental pollution, and risks to the consumer, is a characteristic of development in occupational safety and health in the United States in the post World War II period.

Background

Broad-based concern for environmental and occupational health coupled with effective action is relatively recent in the United States. Significant political, social, economic and technological changes occurred during the past forty-five years that have affected both the environment and how we respond to the changed environment (Corn, 1978).

After World War II American industry quickly converted to consumer goods. The manufacturer of many of these goods (synthetic fibers, plastics, detergents, and pesticides) created new environmental concerns, contaminated air in factories as well as outside of factories, and polluted both air and water. In general most Americans were either unaware or chose to ignore working conditions and environmental pollution, except in a few instances when addressed by a weak city or county regulation.

Then, in 1948 a temperature inversion that lasted for eight days occurred in the town of Donora, Pennsylvania and caused a severe air pollution episode. Twenty people died and hundreds were hospitalized as a result of that incident. The Donora incident aroused interest in air pollution, alerted the American public and focused attention on the environment. The year 1948 was a turning point. After Donora public concern over the environment continued to increase. By 1955, seven years after Donora, Congress passed a bill authorizing a federal program for air pollution research and training.

By the 1960s Americans were becoming increasingly aware of environmental issues. Federal water pollution and air pollution control programs increased awareness and concern for the environment. At the same time a parallel interest in the work environment slowly developed. Although federal regulation of air and water pollution had begun in the 1960s, it took until 1970 to pass the Occupational Safety and Health Act.

The impact of federal regulation was enormous. It changed the way we view our environment and sensitized the general public and the workforce to occupational and environmental issues. Federal regulation of the workplace and outdoor environment made the American public aware of the relationship between health and environment and made that relationship a public issue.

The chemical industry, because it expanded so rapidly after World War II, is intimately associated with current problems of occupational safety and health and environmental pollution.

The modern American chemical industry covers an enormous span of products and technologies. They include the manufacture of valuable materials used in small quantities for pharmaceuticals and bulk chemicals used in the production of plastics. Chemicals are ubiquitous, providing enormous benefits, but also introducing risks to the health and well-being of workers and the general public. The pervasive nature of the chemical industry causes chemicals to be widespread and often in the wrong place, resulting in illness and pollution. The rapid increase in public awareness of chemicals has made chemical pollution a matter of public policy. The increased pollution of chemicals results in increased exposure of the population to chemical risks, be it in the occupational environment or where effluents to air, water, or solid wastes are encountered by the public; or at the commercial product user stage.

The impact on the population of increased chemical usage is difficult to unravel because there are positive and negative aspects to evaluate. With the exception of the startling revelations of a chemical tragedy such as the industrial misuse of Kepone (Corn & Beck, 1980), a pesticide, in Virginia during 1975-1976 or the exposed population associated with excess cancer from asbestos (Doll & Peto, 1981), there is limited quantitative information on the impact of increased chemical usage in our economy.

Government and private organizations responded slowly to the health problems introduced or aggravated by industry. If statutes and laws are viewed as the instruments of public policy, then broad public policy in these areas crystallized in the 1960-1986 period (Corn & Corn, 1981). The social responses to occupational safety and health and environmental pollution will be traced as illustrative of the societal response to problems of industrialization.

Table 1. Health and Environmental Protection Laws

Law		*Year Enacted*
FDCA	Federal Drug and Cosmetics Act	1938
FIFRA	Federal Insecticide, Fungicide, and Rodenticide Act	1948, 1972, 1975
FHSA	Federal Hazardous Substances Act	1966
NEPA	National Environmental Protection Act	1969
PPPA	Poisonous Packaging Prevention Act	1970
OSHA	Occupational Safety and Health Act	1970
CAA	Clean Air Act	1970, 1977
FWPCA	Federal Water Pollution Control Act (Now Clean Water)	1972, 1977
MPRSA	Marine Protection, Research, and Sanctuaries Act	1972
CPSA	Consumer Product Safety Act	1972
FEPCA	Federal Environmental Pollution Control Act	1972
SDWA	Safe Drinking Water Act	1974, 1977
HMTA	Hazardous Materials Transportation Act	1974
RCRA	Resource Conservation and Recovery Act	1976, 1979
TSCA	Toxic Substance Control Act	1976
SMCRA	Surface Mine Control and Reclamation Act	1977
UMTCA	Uranium Mill Tailings Control Act	1978
CERCLA	Comprehensive Environmental Response, Compensation and Liability Act	1980
SARA	Superfund Amendments and Reauthorization Act	1986
AHERA	Asbestos Hazard Emergency Response Act	1986

In retrospect, the period 1955 through 1986 will be remembered for the large number of federal regulatory standards applicable to our environment, both at work and in the community (Table 1). Some of the U.S. statutes that regulate our chemical environment and that have come into existence since 1959 are The Clean Air Act; The Clean Water Act; The Occupational Safety and Health Act; The Mine Safety and Health Act; The Energy Supply and Environmental Pesticide Control Act; The Federal Insecticide, Fungicide, and Rodenticide Act; The Fish and Wildlife Coordination Act; The Hazardous Materials Transportation Act; The Marine Protection, Research, and Sanctuaries Act; The Resources Conservation Recovery Act; The Solid Waste Disposal Act; The Transportation Safety Act; The Consumer Product Safety Act; The Resources Conservation Recovery Act; The Solid Waste Disposal Act; The Transportation Safety Act; The Consumer Product Safety Act; The Toxic Substances Control Act, and the "Superfund" Act. Each of these statutes legally and ethically obligate professionals to a minimum standard of performance or specifically assign duties to professionals in responsible charge.

In 1970 the Congress enacted sweeping occupational safety and health legislation. The present and future status of occupational health in the United States can only be considered in light of the provisions of the Occupational Safety and Health Act of 1970. In retrospect, the Act, which required twelve years incubation in Congress, was passed because of the increasing trend in the industrial accident rate since approximately 1950 and the threat of health hazards on the job (Corn, 1989). The trend to increased workmen's compensation payments and special government compensation funds (i.e., for Black Lung) were undoubtedly a factor, as was the determined effort of organized labor through its unions. Workers compensation laws covered approximately 37 million workers in 1950 and 67 million in 1975. Total payments increased from $615 million in 1950 to $6.522 billion in 1975. Black Lung benefits to coal miners accounted for over $2 billion in 1989.

The Act is revolutionary because it requires safe and healthful working conditions for approximately 85 million employees in an estimated 5 million establishments affecting interstate commerce. Employers are required to furnish an occupational environment free from recognized hazards and to comply with occupational safety and health standards. The Act represents a legal shift to direct, effective statutory prescriptions and administrative regulations, thus recognizing that the health of the employee is a public rather than a private problem and that the standards to be observed are explicit public policy.

II. SUMMARY OF THE OCCUPATIONAL SAFETY AND HEALTH ACT OF 1970

The Occupational Safety and Health Act of 1970 is an ambitious, even revolutionary regulatory statute (Occupational Safety and Health Act of 1970). The Introduction to the Act states that the "Congress declares it to be its purpose and policy, through the exercise of its power to regulate commerce among several states and with foreign nations and to provide for the general welfare, to assure so far as possible every working man and woman in the Nation safe and healthful working conditions and to preserve our human resources" (Corn, 1989). The Act covers approximately eighty-five million of the one hundred twenty million U.S. workforce. Federal, State and Local government employees and some other smaller categories of the workforce are exempted from provisions of the law.

The Act creates three administrative entities, the Occupational Safety and Health Administration (OSHA), a regulatory agency located in the Department of Labor; The National Institute for Occupational Safety and Health (NIOSH), a research organization in the Department of Health and Human Services; and the Occupational Safety and Health Review Commission (OSHRC), an administrative adjudicative body consisting of three members appointed by and reporting to the President. The role of the Review Commission is to resolve conflicts between regulatees cited for violation and the regulatory agency.

The Act maintains an appeal process for the violator by creating a Review Commission to hear appeals. In addition to the three Commission members, the Review Commission is staffed by administrative law judges distributed throughout the ten Federal regions of the United States. Approximately 5 percent of the 247,000 citations issued last year were contested. About 80 percent of those appealing received relief.

OSHA employs approximately 2,000 persons, and had a $302 million budget in the fiscal year (FY) 1992. The agency employs about 1,200 safety and health compliance officers in approximately 115 regional, area, and field offices. The distribution between headquarters and field staff is approximately 500 in the former and 1,500 in the latter. In addition to private sector compliance activities, OSHA develops safety and health standards and oversees State and Federal programs. OSHA also operates a chemical analytical laboratory and an instrument calibration laboratory. Together they employ about 80 staff.

Occupational Safety and Health Standards

The heart of the Act is the concept of permanent occupational safety and health standards. A health standard in the context of this Act goes far beyond the requirement for a Permissible Exposure Limit (PEL) for the airborne concentration of a toxic chemical for example. Thus, the Act refers to a standard as follows: "any standard promulgated...shall prescribe the use of labels or other appropriate forms of warning as are necessary to ensure that employees are apprised of all hazards to which they are exposed, relevant symptoms and appropriate emergency treatment, and proper conditions and precautions of safe use or exposure. Where appropriate, such standards shall also prescribe suitable protective equipment and control or technological procedures to be used in connection with such hazards and shall provide for monitoring or measuring employee exposure at such locations and intervals, and in such manner as may be necessary for the protection of employees. In addition, where appropriate any such standards shall prescribe the type and frequency of medical examinations or the tests which should be made available by the employer or at his cost, to employees exposed to such hazards in order to most effectively determine whether the health of such employees is adversely affected by such exposure" (Occupational Safety and Health Act of 1970, 1970). Thus, the concept of a standard and its ingredients, as promulgated by the regulatory agency, were prescribed by the Congress. Each of these requirements is very specific and can be the basis for a violation of the standard and an associated citation.

Procedures for adoption of permanent safety and health standards adhere to the Federal Administrative Procedures Act. This Act requires that the agency issue a Notice of Intended Rulemaking and a subsequent Proposal; both must be published in the Federal Register. The Proposal should reflect the agency's

Table 2. Summary of Permanent Health Standards Promulgated Since 1970

Standards Completed	*Standards Proposed, but Not Completed*
Asbestos	Beryllium
Vinyl chloride	Sulfur dioxide
Arsenic	Ketones
Benzene	Toluene
Coke-oven emissions	Ammonia
Fourteen carcinogens	MOCA
Lead	Trichloroethylene
Cotton dust	Generic Monitoring
DBCP	Generic Medical Surveillance
Carcinogen Policy	
Acrylonitrile	
Ethylene oxide	
Asbestos	
Hazard Communication ("Right-to-Know")	
Permissible Exposure Limits (Revised)	
Access to Medical and Exposure Records	
Noise Abatement - Hearing Conservation	
Formaldehyde	
Field Sanitation	

concept of the standard to be promulgated. A Public Hearing and a Public Comment Period follow the publication of the Proposal. All interested parties are permitted an opportunity to comment in writing or orally in public and the agency must consider these comments before promulgating a final standard. Table 2 displays permanent health standards issued by OSHA since its formation. The Toxic Substances Control Act passed in 1977 required registration of chemicals in commercial production. Approximately 65,000 chemicals have been registered. The vast majority of potentially hazardous chemicals in U.S. commerce are still unregulated. OSHA does enforce PELs for approximately 400 additional airborne chemicals, but they do not have the other requirements which are features of a permanent standard.

During the first two years Congress permitted adoption of previously existing Federal Standards and National Consensus Standards. Thus, many federal standards, for example, Walsh-Healey Public Contracts Act, National Construction Act, and many consensus standards, for example, National Fire Protection Association, American National Standards Institute, American Society for Testing Materials, were adopted. These standards caused great difficulties because they were, in effect, guidelines, and not suitable for legal enforcement. Many have been revised in a form appropriate for regulatory effort, for example, safety standards for walking and working surfaces, fire protection, and machine guarding. A significant part of the initial resistance encountered by OSHA and its early, unprofessional reputation were based on the large number of standards adopted during the initial two years of agency effort.

A Supreme Court decision (Donovan *versus* American Society of Textile Manufacturers) (Mintz, 1984) indicated that cost-benefit analysis for standards promulgation is not required of OSHA because the Congress in passing the Act did not have the balancing of benefits to health and costs of control in mind. However, a previous Supreme Court decision (Industrial Union Department *versus* American Petroleum Institute) indicated that the agency must provide substantial evidence that an agent causes a significant risk before a standard is promulgated (Mintz, 1984). The Supreme Court supported the decision of the Fifth Circuit Court to rescind OSHA's lowering of the airborne standard for Benzene from 10 ppm to 1 ppm. These two Supreme Court decisions have established the ground rules for promulgation of OSHA standards; a "significant" risk, defensible by the agency, must be the basis for proposed regulation (National Academy of Sciences, 1983).

Enforcement

The Act establishes a force of health and safety compliance officers (CSHOs), who visit establishments to determine whether they are in compliance with adopted standards. Approximately 60-70,000 workplaces are inspected each year. Inspections can occur because of general scheduling by the agency or as a result of a complaint by an employee. During an inspection the compliance officer walks through the premises and may also obtain samples of the atmosphere (health inspection). Photographs of violations are obtained for documentation and employees are interviewed to determine problem areas. A violation can lead to a civil or criminal penalty; they are classified as "Other Than Serious" or "Serious." A Serious violation is one having a high probability of affecting life or limb. An "Other Than Serious" violation can affect the health of the employee, but not in the manner previously described, Compliance officers are either safety specialists or industrial hygienists. Through cross-over training the agency has given individuals in each of these categories some training and understanding of the discipline of their counterparts. The purpose of this effort was to qualify safety specialists to refer complex situations to hygienists and *vice versa*. Because of the annual inspection numbers and agency jurisdiction for about 5 million establishments, the targeting of compliance inspections has been a controversial aspect of OSHA activities since its formation.

Table 3 summarize OSHA compliance activity for a typical six month period (Occupational Safety and Health Act, 1990).

Table 3. Federal OSHA Compliance Activity From October 1, 1989-September 30, 1990

Total Inspections	45,511
Record Inspections	180
Inspections By Category	36,482
Safety Inspections	9,029
Health Inspections	
Inspections By Type	
Unprogrammed	
Accident	1,358
Complaint	10,833
Referral	4,605
Monitoring	289
Variance	1
Follow-Up	2,559
Unprogrammed Related	7,620
Other	231
Progammed	
Planned	16,542
Programmed Related	1,367
Other	106
Other	
Inspections by Industry	
Construction	24,226
Maritime	567
Manufacturing	12,110
Other	8,608
Inspections by Ownership	
Private Sector	44,350
Public Sector	17
Federal Agency	1,144
Inspection Classification	
Safety Planning Guide	28,918
Health Planning Guide	2,480
Local Emphasis Program	983
National Emphasis Program	2,337
Migrant Farmworker Camp	687
Employee Information	
Employed in Establishment	7,830,129
Covered by Inspection	2,487,166
Average Case Hours Per Inspection	
Safety	15
Health	37

(*continued*)

Table 3. Continued

Violations	
Willful	4,567
Repeat	4,562
Serious	99,929
Other	2,049
F-T-A	2,049
Total	172,663
Penalties	
Willful	31,313,686
Repeat	4,926,879
Serious	27,282,957
Other	264,211
F-T-A	2,789,744
Total	66,577,477
Contested Cases	
Inspections Contested	3,258
Inspections W/Citations Contested (%)	9.4

Role of the States

Section 18 of the Act permits states to assume responsibility for health and safety regulatory programs, consistent with the philosophy in the USA that responsibility should be assigned to the lowest level of government that is capable of discharging the responsibility. The law provides that states "be at least as effective as the Federal program." Federal OSHA is assigned responsibility for monitoring the states. A state desiring to have its own occupational safety and health program must first demonstrate that it has established the structure of a regulatory agency, allocated adequate positions, established standards, appeals mechanism, and so forth. It must then demonstrate success at implementing the program during a minimum period of three years, also with monitoring by Federal OSHA. Finally, the state is given freedom of jurisdiction. The Federal government will pay 50 percent of the cost of such programs during developmental and demonstration periods. Twenty- four states have elected to operate their own programs; several are now operating independent of Federal OSHA. Some of the state programs are more stringent than that of the Federal government for example, California, with respect to both the requirements of standards and the vigor with which standards are enforced. The states perform more inspections, in total, than does Federal OSHA.

Under the Act the Federal government cannot offer consultation. Compliance safety and health officers must cite for violations they see after entering a facility. However, the Federal government has been transferring funds to every state in the Union to permit states to offer consultation services to employers. The Federal government contributes nine dollars to a state for every dollar the state contributes to consultation. The consultation activities of the states are independent of their regulatory activities, unless a serious violation is involved. In that case, the consultant is supposed to inform the regulatory agency in the state of a violation if it is not abated within the time period specified by the consultant. In general, the consultation programs in the United Stares receive high grades from employers; the regulatory programs do not. The number of consultations performed by the states cannot be presented because statistics are not available.

III. NIOSH AND RESEARCH IN OCCUPATIONAL SAFETY AND HEALTH

The Congress conceptualized NIOSH as the research arm of OSHA. During recent years the effective (after accounting for inflation) budget of NIOSH has been drastically cut, from $82 million in 1986 to $84 million in 1990. NIOSH has about 750 employees in offices and laboratories in Atlanta, Georgia, and Cincinnati, Ohio and in ten Regional Offices. NIOSH performs research, administers research grants and contracts, supports professional educational efforts in occupational medicine, safety, nursing, and industrial hygiene primarily through grants to fourteen university-based Educational Resource Centers (ERCs), and performs health hazard evaluations in the field. NIOSH has published the ten leading work-related diseases and injuries in the USA (Table 4). It bases its program priorities and allocates resources on the basis of Table 4 listings.

NIOSH is perhaps best known abroad for the more than three hundred Criteria Documents that is has published. However, its contributions to professional education through the ERCs have been major, adding thousands of qualified practitioners to the field.

Reflections on Future Directions

There is a growing consensus in the United States that the Occupational Safety and Health Act of 1970 should be amended. The following areas of concern have been discussed.

Employee Rights and Responsibilities

Section 5 of the law, the General Duty Clause, assigns full responsibility for the workplace to the employer. The recent trend towards employee right-to-know has led to increased recognition that the employee is key to the

Table 4. The Ten Leading Work-Related Diseased and Injuries—United States 1982-1989*

1. Occupational lung disease: asbestosis, byssinosis, silicosis, coal workers' pneumoconiosis, lung cancer, occupational asthma.
2. Musculoskeletal injuries: disorders of the back, trunk, upper extremity, neck, lower extremity; traumatically induced Raynaud's phenomenon.
3. Occupational cancers (other than lung): leukemia; mesothelioma; cancers of the bladder, nose, and liver.
4. Amputations, fractures, eye loss, lacerations, and traumatic deaths.
5. Cardiovascular diseases: hypertension, coronary artery disease, acute myocardial infarction.
6. Disorders of reproduction: infertility, spontaneous abortion, teratogenesis
7. Neurotoxic disorders: peripheral neuropathy, toxic encephalitis, psychoses, extreme personality changes (exposure-related).
8. Noise-induced loss of hearing.
9. Dermatologic conditions: dermatoses, burns (scaldings), chemical burns, contusions (abrasions).
10. Psychologic disorders: neuroses, personality disorders, alcoholism, drug dependency

Note: * Classification by NIOSH.

achievement of improved safety and health. The employer would like to see more responsibility in the hands of the employee; some sharing of the general duty is the goal of those who wish to change this section of the Act.

Employees, on the other hand, have been discussing the Right-to-Act. The Right-to-Act would give the employee definitive authority to intervene in the production process for safety reasons. This is a very controversial subject.

Enforcement

There has been a tendency in the last 2-3 years to levy egregious fines, some exceeding a million dollars, to drive home the point of OSHA's seriousness. There is also a growing demand for invocation of criminal penalties under the law. The current law requires that the Department of Justice take action to prosecute under the criminal penalties of the Act. There are those who would like to amend the Act to make the criminal prosecution of violators easier. Needless to say, employers are opposed to this amendment.

OSHA and the States

The quality of state programs in the United States is highly varied, with some superb programs and others that are weak. An amendment to strengthen the relationship between state programs and Federal OSHA would result in more effective State programs.

NIOSH

The National Institute of Occupational Safety and Health is not regarded as having been highly effective during the last 20 years. It is difficult to point to major research accomplishments of this agency. There are those who believe that the research agency should be in the Department of Labor under OSHA management. Others believe it should remain in the Department of Health and Human Services, but should be raised to a higher level of visibility and authority in that agency. There is broad dissatisfaction with the funding level for occupational safety and health research in the United States, which in 1990 was about one half of the funding level of 1980.

Standards

The standards promulgation process is thorough but slow. There are demands for speeding up the process and improving its efficiency. The Administrative Procedures Act will most certainly have to be dropped if this goal is to be achieved. The Administrative Procedures Act ensures thorough airing of all proposals; is such a complicated process necessary to promulgate effective, needed standards?

In summary, this has been a period of major change in occupational safety and health in the United States. Since 1970 the nation has brought occupational safety and health to a majority of the workforce, whereas prior to that time the services of professionals in the field reached only a minority. With increased service has come increased demands by the workforce. All of this has been against a backdrop of a complex, evolving social period. It is highly likely that the law governing occupational safety and health in the United States will change in the 1990s to permit further progress. It is predictable that changes in the law will also create greater interactions of OSHA with environmental concerns. In the environmental area recycling and prevention of pollution is now the preferred approach, rather than creating pollution and collecting pollutants prior to environmental discharge. The latter was the approach for several decades. We are now providing incentives for minimization of waste and pollutants. Occupational safety and health concerns will have to be melded with the redesign approaches to waste minimization and recycling.

REFERENCES

Corn, J. (1978). Historical aspects of industrial hygiene 1: Changing altitudes toward occupational health. *American Industrial Hygiene Journal.*

Corn, M. & Beck, P.K. (1980). The Kepone tragedy and its effects. In J. MacLaurey (Ed.), *Protecting people at work.* United States Department of Labor, Government Printing Office, Washington, D.C.

Doll, R. & Peto, R. (1981). The causes of cancer: Quantitative estimates of avoidable risks of cancer in the united states today. *Journal of the National Cancer Institute*, 66:1191-1308.

Corn, M. & Corn, J. (1981). The control of health problems related to industrialization. In Wechler, et al. (Eds.), *The Social Context of Medical Research*. Ballinger Publishing Company.

Corn, M. (1989). The progression of industrial hygiene. *Applied Industrial Hygiene*, 4(6).

Occupational Safety and Health Act of 1970. (1970). Public Law 91-596. 91st Congress. December 29.

Mintz B. (1984). *OSHA: History law and policy* (pp. 269, 313-324). Bureau of National Affairs, Washington, DC.

U.S. National Academy of Sciences Publication. (1983). *Risk assesment in the federal government: Managing the process*. Washington, DC.

CONTRIBUTION OF EPIDEMIOLOGY TO THE UNDERSTANDING OF OCCUPATIONAL HEALTH PROBLEMS

Gilles Theriault

I intend to cover three topics: (1) uses of epidemiology in the study of causal relationship between disease and exposure at work; (2) methodological concerns of special significance for occupational epidemiology; and (3) new trends in occupational epidemiology. In reviewing the several components and principles that would normally fall under those three headings, I quickly realized that this would be too large and too theoretical an enterprise. I therefore decided to be less academic and to share with you some experiences of my own. I do not pretend that my viewpoint is the best nor that other authors have not done better than me, it is simply that I feel so much more comfortable with what I know best and it makes it easier for me to communicate to you my enthusiasm about occupational epidemiology.

Research in Human Capital and Development, Volume 7, pages 239-251.

ISBN: 1-55938-132-9

I. DEFINITION OF OCCUPATIONAL EPIDEMIOLOGY

As it stands, the word epidemiology means the science of epidemics. And this is essentially what it was at its origin, when there existed widespread devastating outbreaks of infectious diseases. Epidemiology was used then to describe the extent of epidemics of infectious diseases and to trace their origin. With the improvement in standards of living, epidemics of infectious diseases have vanished and they have been replaced by chronic diseases such as cancer and heart disease which have reached proportions of 'modern epidemics.' With the wide spread availability of computers and the major development in statistical sciences, epidemiology has progressed significantly. Its object has remained the same, trying to understand the disease by describing its behavior in a population by age, sex, time and space and searching for the agents responsible for it; but its strategies have evolved significantly through designs that are more and more sophisticated. This is why we now adhere to a more refined definition: epidemiology is a science that studies the distribution and the determinants of diseases in a population (MacMahon & Pugh, 1970).

Occupational epidemiology is epidemiology as it applies to the field of occupational health. Workplaces are particularly suitable for epidemiological studies since they regroup cohorts of workers within well delineated limits, keep them together for long periods of time and maintain records of their working activities and health status. Furthermore, very often workers are exposed to discernable and often measurable risks at levels that are sometimes very high. Occupational epidemiology is epidemiology in 'sad to say' laboratory conditions.

II. USES OF EPIDEMIOLOGY IN THE STUDY OF CAUSAL RELATIONSHIP BETWEEN DISEASE AND EXPOSURE AT WORK

One of the most important and most frequent use of occupational epidemiology has been and still is the study of causal relationship between disease and exposure at work. Let me illustrate this to you with an example. In the mid 1970s, occupational health physicians from a large Canadian primary aluminum production company noticed the presence of numerous red spots on the skin of some production workers (Theriault, Cordier, & Harvey, 1980). They were red to red bluish maculae or flat patches (often linear in shape) with a maximum diameter of 3cm. They were painless and non-pruritic, and they disappeared upon finger pressure. These vascular lesions lay within the superficial layers of the dermis and the skin over them had a normal appearance. They were called telangiectasia. These telangiectasia appeared

Table 1. Number of Aluminum Workers with Telangiectasies According to Indices of Exposure

No. Years spent at the plant	*No. workers affected (percent)*	*No. years spent in contact with electrolytic baths*	*No. workers affected (percent)*
3-4	7(16.3)	0	78(32.1)
5-9	34(42.5)	1-4	71(39.0)
10-14	33(37.5)	5-9	36(66.7)
15-19	31(41.9)	10-14	25(86.2)
20-24	27(61.4)	15-19	17(94.4)
25+	153(59.1)	20+	60(96.8)
Total	285(48.5)	total	287(48.8)

mainly on the upper part of the chest, the back and the shoulders. Sometimes, they developed on the face, neck, arms, and backs of the hands. Clothing did not affect their distribution, nor was there an increased concentration of ring pattern found on the neck or wrists. The lesions seem to enlarge with time. We simply looked at the frequency of affected men by time spent in the plant and by time spent in contact with the electrolytic baths (Theriault, Cordier, & Harvey, 1980). The results are illustrated in Table 1. They indicate that working inside the reactor entailed a much higher risk than working elsewhere in the plant and that after some 15 to 20 years of doing so, almost all the workers suffered from this disease. This illustrates, in its most simplistic form, the use of epidemiology in the study of a causal relationship between disease and exposure at work. It is descriptive. By describing the profile of the disease in this working group, we were able to identify the process responsible for its appearance. Things are not always so simple. Identifying a causal relationship between a disease and an exposure is often much more difficult. Health problems such as lung cancer or heart disease which are very prevalent in the general population and for which etiological factors such as cigarette smoking and diet are already known are much more difficult to associate with an exposure at work. It is beyond the scope of this presentation to describe the epidemiological techniques used in such cases, but such techniques exist. They have allowed the discovery of strong associations between exposure to certain chemicals and cancer. Among the most spectacular examples, there are: bladder cancer versus aromatic amines, angiosarcoma of the liver versus vinyl chloridemonomer, mesothelioma versus asbestos exposure, lung cancer versus exposure to polyaromatic hydrocarbons.

III. METHODOLOGICAL CONCERNS OF SPECIAL SIGNIFICANCE FOR OCCUPATIONAL EPIDEMIOLOGY

Like general epidemiology, occupational epidemiology is concerned with case definition, control selection, study design (case-control, cohort, clinical trial), avoidance of biases and confoundants, sample size, power of the study...and so forth, but in addition to these, it is particularly concerned with good estimates of exposure and ways of relating these exposures to the disease. Some of these special concerns can be listed as: (a) job exposure matrices, (b) life time indices of exposure, (c) dose response relationship, (d) interaction, and (e) latency effect. Here is another example to illustrate these methodological issues. One day, we were invited to study the existence of a potential relationship between an excess of bladder cancer and exposure to coal tar pitch volatiles among a cohort of primary aluminum production workers (Theriault, Tremblay, Cordier, & Gringas, 1984). To do so, we computed the risk of bladder cancer according to several indices of exposure. We obtained tables of risk associated with exposure to Benzo-a-Pyrene(BaP) as illustrated in Table 2. It can be observed that the higher the exposure, the higher the risk. This has allowed us to observe that not only was there an association between bladder cancer and working in the primary aluminum production industry but it also showed that the risk was associated to BaP exposure. This is quite a classical example of dose response curves that are sought by occupational epidemiology. They are very instructive and powerful in demonstrating convincingly an association between exposure and disease.These curves may look very simple to the reader, but they hide behind them several methodological techniques. In particular, to construct such curves, one needs not only to measure chemical exposure at each workplace but also to estimate individual cumulative life time exposure to the chemical.

Job Exposure Matrix (JEM)

The first step in constructing a dose response curve is to generate a job exposure matrix. In studying the association between an exposure and a disease, assessment of exposure deserves great care. In the past, many studies have based their results simply on the presence or absence of exposure, comparing globally exposed with non-exposed workers. Although this dicotomization of exposure is sometimes sufficient, most of the time it is too gross and leads to wrong conclusions. Even use of job titles, occupations or tasks may not be sufficient. One needs to quantify each worker's personal estimate. A job exposure matrix is essentially one or several charts whose lines correspond to a job or a task and columns correspond to several periods of time. In a JEM, one wants to estimate with as much accuracy as possible, the level of exposure for each occupation or category of occupations within a work environment. To illustrate the relationship between bladder cancer and exposure to coal tar pitch volatiles, an example of the JEM that we generated (Armstrong, Tremblay, Cyr, & Theriault, 1986) is shown in Table 3. On the left hand column, we listed the several occupations or group of occupations encountered in the aluminum industry. On the X axis, we broke down the entire

Table 2. Risk Associated with Exposure to BaP

Estimated BaPyr	Total			Smokers			Non-smokers		
	Cases	*Controls*	*OR*	*Cases*	*Controls*	*OR*	*Cases*	*Controls*	*OR*
0	6	65	1.00	6	46	1.00	0	19	—
1-9	44	140	3.41	32	406	2.31	2	18	—
10-19	27	43	6.80	22	32	5.27	1	8	—
20+	8	7	12.38	8	5	12.27	0	0	—
Total	85	255		68	189		3	45	

Notes: OR global = 4.50 (CI 1.99-10.19) X_1^2 linear trend = 23.7072 $p = 0.000001$.

period of work into smaller time periods that may have corresponded to technical changes in the industry over time. Each cell indicates the measured or estimated concentrations of BSM for each of the occupation/period cell. To generate such matrices, one needs the help of industrial hygienists and as much historical data as possible. The aim is to obtain with as much precision as it is reasonably achievable the level of contaminant at each workplace and for each period of time. Sometimes, researchers even reopened old sheds and had workers work under past conditions to ascertain that the model for past exposure was reasonably accurate. Obviously, in building up these job exposure matrices, one uses as much actual environmental air measurements of the work place as possible. These matrices are not easy to create and they carry with them a lot of uncertainties and approximations. Depending on the type of data available, the assessment of exposure would range from best to poor. The poor measures of exposure would result in non-differential misclassification and would bias the effect toward the null value (Copeland, Checkoway, McMichael, & Holbrook, 1977). However, they are essential to demonstrate with some degree of credibility an association between an exposure and a disease.

Life Time Indices of Exposure

Once exposure is known for each occupation within a workplace, one needs to estimate for each worker his personal life time exposure taking into consideration the several occupations he has occupied during his working career as well as the several periods during which the exposure took place. Notice that it is not the workplace that will be the object of analysis but the individual. Therefore, one needs to go from workplace estimates to individual estimates of exposure. This is done using the detailed occupational history of each worker in which each occupation performed during his employment is recorded. These work histories are then linked to the previously mentioned job exposure matrix. A life time index of exposure is calculated by summing up the exposure experience in each job taking into account time spent on these

Table 3. Estimated Time-Weighted Average Concentrations of Benzene-Soluble Matter (BSM) and of Benzo-a-Pyrene (BaP): BSM Ratio Determined for Selected Occupations

	BSM Concentration (mg/m3)						*BaP:BSM*
Plant area	*1930-1954*	*1955-1959*	*1960-1964*	*1965-1969*	*1970-1974*	*1975-1979*	*(μg:mg)*
Soderberg							
Potman	1.6	1.0	1.0	0.8	0.8	0.4	8.8
Channel mounter	2.0	2.0	1.8	1.4	1.2	0.54	10.8
Rod raiser	3.5	3.5	2.0	1.4	0.9	0.8	10.1
Stud puller	2.5	2.5	2.1	2.1	0.38	0.38	17.5
Laborer	0.50	0.39	0.39	0.30	0.30	0.15	13.0
Prebake							
Potman	0.10	0.10	0.10	0.10	0.10	0.10	0.0
Alumina unloader	0.05	0.05	0.05	0.05	0.05	0.05	1.2
Laborer	0.10	0.10	0.08	0.08	0.06	0.06	0.4
Potlining area							
Pot replacer	2.5	1.5	0.61	0.47	0.47	0.40	14.1
Pot baker	0.54	0.48	0.48	0.43	0.43	0.43	1.2
Laborer	0.72	0.57	0.57	0.44	0.22	0.17	14.1
Carbon plant							
Conveyer operator	0.71	0.63	0.63	0.56	0.31	0.31	0.3
Crusher operator	1.2	0.1	0.1	0.92	0.46	0.39	1.4
Laborer	0.72	0.57	0.57	0.44	0.22	0.17	1.2
Casting area	0.0	0.0	0.0	0.0	0.0	0.0	0.0
Chemical plant	0.0	0.0	0.0	0.0	0.0	0.0	0.0

Table 4. Calculation of Cumulative Lifetime Exposure to BaP—An Example

Employee no. 1001

Occupation	*Time*	*Duration Years*		*Average Concentration*	*BaP Years*
Potman	1950-1954	4.0	×	1.6	6.4
Rod raiser	1955-1959	4.0	×	3.5	14.0
	1960-1962	2.0	×	2.0	4.0
Casting	1963-1969	6.0	×	0.0	0.0
Total		16.0			24.0

jobs. As an example, look at how we proceeded with bladder cancer cases exposed to Benzo-a-Pyrene in calculating the cumulative life time exposure of a worker (Table 4).

Dose Response Relationship

Once each individual's life time exposure estimate is known, risk according to level of exposure can be computed. It is usually assumed that the higher the exposure the higher the risk. In generating these curves, several models can be tested. In our study of the exposure response regarding bladder cancer in the aluminum industry, we tried several models (Table 5).

Among these we tested time in pot rooms, benzene soluble matters, benzene soluble matters with 10 years latency, benzo-a-pyrene, benzo-a-pyrene with 10 years latency. As can be seen in the table, all those models fit very well but the one that performed best was benzo-a-pyrene with 10 years latency. We therefore recommended that this model be used in further predicting the risk according to exposure.

Interaction

Once an association between an exposure and a disease is found, it is of paramount importance to rule out the possibility that this association is in fact due to a confounder. This is what we call the study of interaction. This is a major concern in occupational epidemiology. The study of bladder cancer associated with coal tar pitch volatiles for example would mean little if we cannot account for cigarette smoking. Everybody knows that smoking in itself causes bladder cancer. In order to state with confidence that CTPV at workplace causes bladder cancer, one has to control for cigarette smoking. There are several ways of doing this. We used a simple 2 × 2 table (Table 6). It showed that the risk for smoking alone was 4.6, the risk for pure exposure to BaP was 2.8, whereas the risk of a combined exposure to BaP and smoking

Table 5. Estimates of the Exposure-Response Models

Exposure index	Relative Risk Slope Parameter		Likelihood ratio chi-squared against $b = 0$(1 df)
	b^a	95% CI	
Time in potroom (years)	0.213	0.08 – 0.47	25.4
Benzene-soluble matter (mg/m^3 · years)	0.131	0.05 – 0.31	22.3
Benzene-soluble matter (mg/m^3 · years) with 10 years' latency	0.177	0.07 – 0.41	25.3
Benzo-a-pyrene (μ g/m^3 · years)	0.0182	0.007 – 0.042	27.4
Benzo-a-pyrene (μ g/m^3 · years) with 10 years' latency	0.023	0.009 – 0.052	29.1

Note: [a] Assuming linear model $R = 1 + bx$; b represents estimated increment in relative risk per unit of exposure.

Table 6. Interaction between Exposure to BaP and Smoking

BaP Exposure	Cigarette Consumption: No	Cigarette Consumption: Yes
No	1.00 (1/21)	4.60 (CI 0.68 – 31.36) (16/73)
Yes	2.80 (CI 0.25 – 32.02) (2/15)	11.26 (CI 2.15 – 58.98) (52/97)

was up to 11.26 indicating a clear interaction between exposure to BaP and smoking in the causation of bladder cancer among aluminum workers. Whatever way is used, the study of interaction between a causal agent and confounders is of paramount importance in occupational epidemiology.

Latency Effect

Finally, a fifth concern of special importance for occupational epidemiology is the latency effect. Environmental carcinogens are usually assumed to require some minimum latency period before producing their effect. How long is this latency period? Is it 5, 10, or 20 years? There is no single response. One can proceed either a priori, deciding on a latency period based on external knowledge to the study and see if, by subtracting this period, the curves fit best. One can also proceed on an a posteriori approach by generating several models and identifying which one fits best. In our study of bladder cancer in aluminum workers (Armstrong, Tremblay, & Theriault, 1988), we have found that the difference between models based on a cumulative exposure and those based on the 10 years prior to diagnosis being ignored was very small, neither suggesting any improvement more than could be accounted for by chance. More formal comparison of different latency models yielded similar inconclusive results. We suggest that the results following from the 10 year minimum latency assumption be preferred on an a priori grounds, because environmental carcinogens generally, and occupational carcinogens more particularly, are usually assumed to require some such minimum latency period.

IV. NEW TRENDS IN OCCUPATIONAL EPIDEMIOLOGY

Here again, let me illustrate some of these new trends using examples.

Risk Assessment

Occupational epidemiology is invited to provide scientific evidence of the risk, scientific evidence upon which standards of exposure can be set. In our example of bladder cancer following exposure to CTPV, we estimated what a safe level of exposure would be. This is risk assessment. By transforming our estimates of life time cumulative indices of exposure into average daily concentrations and by reanalyzing the risk according to these daily concentrations, we calculated the predicted relative risk following an average working life (Table 7).

Notwithstanding all the many uncertainties and limitations inherent to this study and to the model used, we can say that an aluminum smelter worker exposed to coal tar volatiles at the current American Conference of Governmental Industrial Hygienists threshold limit value (TLV) for BSM of 0.2 mg/ m3 for 40 years is predicted from the BSM model to be about 2.5 times as likely to contract bladder cancer as an unexposed person. There is currently no TLV for BaP. In Sweden, an exposure limit of 0.5 mg/ m3 has been recommended for BaP since 1982. Aluminum smelter workers exposed to this concentration for 40 years are predicted to be about five times as likely to contract bladder cancer as an unexposed person. This is an illustration of how occupational epidemiology contributes to establishing risk assessment.

Eligibility for Workmen's Compensation

Another area where occupational epidemiology is called on to make a contribution is deciding which among exposed workers who have developed a disease is entitled to compensation. This question comes down actually to deciding what is the probability that an individual's disease is the result of his exposure at work. This is transforming risk into probability. We did so for bladder cancer in aluminum workers exposed to BaP. The results are shown in Table 8. Essentially, on the basis of the information presented earlier, the Workmen's Compensation Board decided that it would compensate bladder

Table 7. Relative Risks Predicted Following 40 Years of Exposure to Tar Volatiles

BSM			*BaP*		
Concentration (mg/m^3)	*Relative Risk*	*95% CI*	*Concentration* ($\mu g/m^3$)	*Relative Risk*	*95% CI*
1.0	8.1	3.8 − 17.4	10	10.2	4.6 − 21.8
0.5	4.5	2.40 − 9.2	5	5.6	2.8 − 11.4
0.2	2.42	1.56 − 4.3	2	2.84	1.72 − 5.2
0.1	1.71	1.28 − 2.64	1	1.92	1.36 − 2.15
0.05	1.35	1.14 − 1.82	0.5	1.46	1.18 − 2.04
0.02	1.14	1.06 − 1.33	0.2	1.18	1.07 − 1.42
0.01	1.07	1.03 − 1.16	0.1	1.09	1.04 − 1.21

Notes: BSM = benzene-soluble matter, BaP = benzo-a-pyrene.
CI = 95% confidence interval

Table 8. Predicted Relative Risks and Probabilities of Causation* for Bladder Cancer Resulting from Exposure to BaP

Cumulative Exposure in BaP Years	*Relative Risk*	*Probability of Causation*
0	1.00(1.00)	.00(0.00)
5	1.12(1.26)	.10(0.21)
10	1.23(1.52)	.19(0.34)
15	1.35(1.78)	.26(0.44)
20	1.46(2.04)	.32(0.51)
25	1.58(2.30)	.37(0.57)
30	1.69(2.56)	.41(0.61)
35	1.81(2.82)	.45(0.65)
40	1.92(3.08)	.48(0.68)
45	2.04(3.34)	.51(0.70)
50	2.15(3.60)	.53(0.72)
60	2.38(4.12)	.58(0.76)
70	2.61(4.64)	.62(0.78)
80	2.84(5.16)	.65(0.81)
90	3.07(5.68)	.67(0.82)
100	3.30(6.20)	.70(0.84)
110	3.53(6.72)	.72(0.85)
120	3.76(7.24)	.73(0.86)
130	3.99(7.76)	.75(0.87)
140	4.22(8.28)	.76(0.88)
150	4.45(8.80)	.78(0.89)
200	5.60(11.4)	.82(0.91)
250	6.75(14.0)	.85(0.93)
300	7.90(16.6)	.87(0.94)

Note: Numbers in parenthesis indiate upper 95 percent confidence limits.

cancer victims for whom the probability that the cancer was caused by exposure at an aluminum smelter was greater than 50 percent. However, in response to the requirement in the legislation governing workers' compensation in Quebec for the benefit of doubt to be given to the worker in cases of uncertainty, the upper 95 percent confidence limit corresponding to 50 percent risk was used. This criterion resulted in a minimum required exposure to BaP, cumulated until 10 years before diagnosis, of 19 mg/ m3 years to open eligibility to compensation.

Evaluation

Evaluation is another area where occupational epidemiology is in great demand. It is used mainly for two purposes: evaluation of safety intervention (Saari & Nasanen, 1989) and evaluation of health screening programs (Theriault, Tremblay, & Armstrong, 1990). We have recently evaluated the impact of a cytology screening program offered to the aluminum production workers following the discovery of bladder cancer excesses cited previously. We did this evaluation based on information available in the public domain (hospital records, registration at tumor registry, workmen's compensation cases). The outcome we analyzed was the impact of the program on early detection and on survival. The results are shown in Table 9. We concluded that although there was some indication that the cytology screening program allowed some cases to be diagnosed earlier and that survival seemed to improve after the program was instituted, the overall results did not encourage an optimistic view of the effectiveness of the screening in this population.

Biological Monitoring/Molecular Epidemiology

With the development of advanced methods in pharmacology and toxicology, it has been possible to identify and quantify tiny traces of exposure or very early signs of health damage resulting from exposure at work. This has resulted in the development of what is called molecular epidemiology, meaning identifying at the molecular level signs of cellular interaction with the environment. The main use of this new discipline in occupational health has been the rapid spread of biological monitoring. The potential for molecular epidemiology seems very promising. By detecting very early signs of cellular reaction to harmful material and by removing any individual, most particularly sensitive ones from exposure, one hopes to alter any morbid phenomenon in the making and consequently prevent suffering, cancer, and death among exposed people. This discipline (which in fact is not new, occupational health physicians have been measuring lead in blood or cancer cells in urine for many years), has experienced a rebirth with the coming together of biochemists/ toxicologists with occupational health practitioners. The real breakthrough has

Table 9. Bladder Cancer Cases Diagnosed Among Primary Production Aluminum Workers Aged 65 Years or Less, Before and After the Implementation of a Cytology Screening Program

	Time Period			
	1970-1979		*1980-1986*	
Variable	*n*	%	*n*	%
Stage In situ (0)	2	(4.1)	1	(3.3)
A	17	(34.7)	18	(60.0)
B1	4	(8.2)	1	(3.3)
B2	3	(6.1)	2	(6.7)
C	5	(10.2)	3	(10.0)
D1	3	(6.1)		
D2	1	(2.0)	1	(3.3)
Total known	35	(71.4)	26	(86.7)
Unstaged	14	(28.6)	4	(13.3)
Total	49	(100)	30	(100)

come with the development of means to detect markers in biological specimen that reflect either exposure, response or high individual susceptibility. Examples of early markers are proteins and DNA adducts among people exposed to carcinogens such as aromatic amines, PAH, BaP, ethylene oxide and so on. It now appears possible, with valid markers, that it is not necessary to wait for disease before evaluating an association between an exposure and a disease in a group of workers. If, for example, a preclinical change predictive of disease is identified, then the same clinical and epidemiologic method used in traditional epidemiology can be used to determine an association (Schulte, personal cummunication). Molecular epidemiology looks very promising in the fight against health damage and the prevention of it.

V. CONCLUSION

In this paper, I have tried to show how occupational epidemiology has contributed to demonstrate causal relationship between exposure at work and disease. I have indicated some methodological concerns of special significance for occupational epidemiology and I have listed some new trends that are being developed in this discipline. I hope that by so doing, I have been able to illustrate the important contribution that occupational epidemiology has made to the understanding of occupational health problems and to their solution. Although in the context of health, environment and social change, occupational epidemiology may be perceived as a small, and remote discipline, its contribution to the understanding of the interaction between environment and health has been and continues to be of paramount importance.

REFERENCES

Armstrong, B.G., Tremblay, C.G., Cyr, D., & Theriault, G.P. (1986). Estimating the relationship between exposure to tar volatiles and the incidence of bladder cancer in aluminum smelter workers. *Scandanavian Journal of Work, Environment and Health*, 12,486-493.

Armstrong, B.G., Tremblay, C., & Theriault, G. (1988). Compensating bladder cancer victims employed in aluminun reduction plants. *Journal of Occupational Medicine*, 30,771-775.

Copeland, K.T., Checkoway, H., McMichael, A.J., & Holbrook, R.H. (1977). Bias due to misclassification in the estimation of relative risk. *American Journal of Epidemoiology*, 105, 488-495.

MacMahon, B. & Pugh, T.F. (1970). *Epidemiology principles and methods*. Boston: Little, Brown.

Saari, J. & Nasanen, M. (1989) The effect of positive feedback on industrial housekeeping and accidents: A long-term study at a shipyard. *International Journal of Industrial Ergonomics*, 4, 201-211.

Theriault, G., Cordier, S., & Harvey, R. (1980). Skin telangiectases in workers at an aluminum plant. *New England Journal of Medicine*, 303, 1278-1281.

Theriault, G. Tremblay, C.G., & Armstrong, B.G. (1990) Bladder cancer screening among primary aluminum production workers in Quebec. *Journal of Occupational Medicine*, 32, 869-872.

Theriault, G., Tremblay, C.G., Cordier, S., & Gingras, S. (1984). Bladder cancer in the aluminum industry. *Lancet*. 947-950.

LEAD AND CLASSROOM PERFORMANCE AT SEVEN PRIMARY SCHOOLS IN TAIWAN

Michael Rabinowitz, Jung-Der Wang, and Wei-Tsuen Soong

I. INTRODUCTION

Environmental pollution with lead has long been recognized to cause adverse effects on children. Recently, a compilation of many studies on the correlation between child IQ and lead exposure has demonstrated a robust dose-response relationship (Needleman & Gatsonis, 1990). The effect is discernable even at relatively low doses, in many countries, and after considering other confounding risk factors. The pediatric toxicity of lead is not limited to IQ performance, but also other developmental processes (Davis & Svendsgaard, 1987). Recently in Taiwan it has been found that children attending a kindergarten near a lead recycling smelter had elevated blood lead levels and depressed IQ scores, even after considering other risk factors such as parental IQ (Jang, 1989).

Research in Human Capital and Development, Volume 7, pages 253-272.

ISBN: 1-55938-132-9

The present study goes beyond these past efforts in two respects. Children are studied with a wider range of lead exposures, including those near smelters as well as those living in more typical urban and rural conditions, extending downward the range of lead exposures studied. Also, in addition to an IQ test, the present study assesses children with two other instruments in the form of questionnaires which measure the classroom functioning, specific learning handicaps, and behavioral problems.

II. SUBJECTS

Children were recruited into the study by virtue of their attending grades one through three in one of the seven elementary schools, which were chosen because they represented a range of potential lead exposures and served populations with broadly similar ethnic compositions. Some general characteristics of these schools are shown in Tables 1. The age of the first grade children averaged 6.7 years (std dev = 0.4).

In the first week of October 1989 we visited the schools, informing the teachers of the purposes of our study and requesting their help in collecting teeth and completing rating forms for the children. During the next three months the children gave their teachers any teeth that were shed and any earlier teeth which they had saved. The teachers completed a small form to identify the child and location of the tooth. At least one tooth was received from 764 children. A total of 947 teeth were collected, of which 862 (71%) were incisors which were used as measures of lead burden. However, 78 were judged to be too decayed or small to analyze. 122 children submitted more than one tooth; the 862 teeth with lead values represent only 692 children, of whom 518 provided usable incisors. Because of the uncertainty of directly comparing incisors with molar or canine teeth, their having different mean lead levels and periods of growth, only incisors are considered in subsequent analysis. Blood lead measurements were made of sixty children from the two schools near smelters in January 1990. The average blood lead was 13.0 ug/dl (std dev 4.4), the median was 12, and the range was 6 to 24.

Tooth Analysis

Tooth lead levels were determined following earlier methods (Rabinowitz, Bellinger, & Leviton, 1989), in a room with two recirculating HEPA air filters (model 100 Plus, Environmental Air Control, Albuquerque NM). Laboratory air had 1 ng per cubic M of lead. In the sample digestion box, which had an additional HEPA filter, it was 0.03 ng per cu M. The tooth lead was determined in two portions of dentin taken from the zone presumably representative of post-natal deposition. After a cross-sectional sagittal slice, a chisel cut was made

Table 1. Schools Participating in Tooth Collection

School Name	Location	Exposure	Father's Education: Only Primary	Father's Education: Any College	Percent of Teeth with Any Decay
1. Wu Lun	Rural Town Industrial	Lead Smelter 1 km from school	35 %	3 %	46 %
2. Yeh Leo	Coastal Village Fishing, Resort	Control	54	0	41
3. Dong Men	Taipei City Administrative District	City Center	4	42	37
4. Gu Teen	Taipei City Educational District	Urban	9	42	37
5. Hua Jiang	Taipei City Light Industry, Printing	Urban	15	10	39
6. Tzu Ching	Taipei City Jin Mai, Residential	Urban Fringe	13	18	52
7. Chao Leow	Fong Shan, Rural Farming, Industry	Lead Smelter 1.8 km from school	44	3	64

from just below the cementum-enamel junction to midway between the top of the pulp cavity and the crown. For incisors this cut approximates the neonatal line. Any areas which were decayed or within 3 mm of visible decay or which appeared to be reparative dentine was avoided.

Lead was determined in duplicate by anodic stripping voltammetry. These values were averaged if they differed by 2.5 ug/g or less. Otherwise, two more portions of the tooth were prepared, and the three closest values for the tooth averaged, as was necessary for about 15 percent of the teeth. Procedural lead blanks was negligible, averaging 0.1 ng (std dev = 3.4) per sample. The standard deviation, a useful estimate of the uncertainty of the blank, represents about 6 percent of sample lead present. Also, a synthetic standard of lead-enriched calcium chloride was prepared, and its lead concentration was determined by Professor William Manton of the University of Texas using isotope dilution mass spectrometry. The observed mean value of lead in this standard, which accompanied each of the 58 batches of teeth reported here, was 51.8 (std dev = 3.4) ng. The value obtained by isotope dilution, an absolute reference method, was 52.3 (std dev = 0.4). Also, our laboratory participated in the Centers for Disease Control blood lead proficiency testing program. For the 24 samples of blood averaging 30 ug/dl, the mean absolute difference between our value and the target value was 2.5 ug/dl.

Tooth Lead Validity

A further estimate of reliability is to compare several teeth obtained from the same child. For the 68 children who gave two incisors, the Spearman r was 0.77, with a median absolute difference between the incisors of 1.1 ug/g., and for the 22 who gave an incisor and another tooth type, the $r = .68$, not significantly different, but the median difference was larger, 2.4 ug/g. This increased intra-child variability with different tooth types was one of our reasons for using only incisors in our later data analysis (Rabinowitz, Bellinger, Leviton, & Wang, 1991a). There was no difference between maxillary and mandibular incisors (unpaired $p = .89$ for 567 teeth), nor between 123 upper and 161 lower central incisors ($p = .99$). Also, the age of the child when the incisor is shed and its lead content correlate poorly; among the 594 teeth r equals $+.003$, $p = .9$. We surmise that lead values from any incisor are directly comparable without the need for any adjustments for location within the mouth or age when shed.

Questionnaires

The teachers of the 764 children who submitted a tooth were given a one page, 51 item forced choice questionnaire about the child's classroom behavior. These forms includes (1) the 24 yes-no item Boston Teachers Questionnaire (Guild, 1979), (2) a 26 question modified version of the Rutter Child Behavior Check List, and (3) an IQ test score (Raven's Colored Progressive Matrices, CPM), administered near the third month of school during grade 1. Over 97 percent of the teacher forms were completed and returned. Four of the 7 schools achieved response rates of 100 percent. These rates are much greater than the 80 percent rate reported from Dutch teachers or the 93 percent rate from Americans (Achenbach, Verhulst, Baron, & Atlhaus, 1987). For any question, the average number of missing values was 3 out of 726 forms. Also, the parents were given a two page questionnaire about their ages, educations, employment, family composition, moving, language usage, maternal, and child health. Forty potential confounding variables were assessed (Table 2), with a response rate of 90 percent. These high rates suggest a very small bias from selective participation and is indicative of the role of the teacher in a Confucian society such as the Republic of China. After both of the forms were returned to the laboratory, the teachers and students were each given a pair of tooth brushes, with the name of our medical school and department, as a small gift.

Subject Exclusion

With 685 parent and 740 teacher questionnaires were available, only 642 cases had a tooth lead value and both questionnaires. Because of the

Table 2. List of Potential Confounding Factors Assessed with Parental Questionnaire

1. Sex (1 = girl, 2 = boy)	21. Weight of newborn
2. School grade	22. Delivery method
3. Birth order	23. Birth Presentation
4. Total number of siblings	24. Condition of newborn
5. Number of adults at home	25. Incubator usage
6. Father's age now	26. Neonatal Jaundice, severity
7. Father's education	27. Any co-births
8. Father's job classification	28. Any birth defects
9. Mother's age now	29. Encephalitis
10. Mother's education	30. Meningitis
11. Mother's job classification	31. Fever more than 39 C
12. Before birth, mother sick	32. Head injury, not burns
13. When pregnant, any medicine	33. Cerebral palsy
14. When pregnant, any bleeding	34. Seizures
15. Hormone to halt miscarriage	35. Child's longest hospital stay
16. When pregnant, any drinking	36. Child ever seriously ill
17. When pregnant, ever drunk	37. Handedness of child
18. When pregnant, any tobacco	38. In past year, moved home
19. Any pregnancy complication	39. Languages used by family
20. Length of gestation	40. Age when tooth shed

uncertainty of directly comparing incisors with molar or canine teeth, their having different mean lead levels (see Results) and periods of growth, a further restriction was that only children who gave incisors be considered, yielding 515 children. Also, a few cases were excluded from further analysis because the child had a risk factor which would place the child at extremely high risk of a learning disorder. These included having cerebral palsy (3 cases), meningitis (2 cases), birth weight less than 2000 grams (5 cases) or having ever been hospitalized for more than 10 nights on one occasion not including child birth (16 cases). Taken together these criteria reduce the number of subjects by 22 (11 of each gender) yielding 493 cases with complete data sets. There was no tendency for the excluded cases to be over-representative of higher or lower incisor lead levels.

Data Reduction Strategy

Confounders, other factors besides lead that can affect IQ, must be considered. Data was collected for 40 separate variables to help describe each case (Table 2). Depending on the nature of the variable (bivariate, continuous, or categorical), different statistical tests of its association with lead and the outcomes were performed. A potential confounder was retained for further consideration if the two-tailed p values between it and lead and also between it and the outcome of interest was less than 0.25. These retained confounders form a shorter list.

Modeling of the outcome was done by multiple regression for continuous outcomes such as IQ and logistic regression for discrete outcomes such as the handicap clusters. All potential confounders and lead were used in the initial model, and then individual variables with the highest p value were deleted. This deletion was continued until all remaining variables had significance levels less than 0.20. Then the lead term was deleted and the models with and without lead were compared for goodness of fit and any changes in each variable's parameter estimate, indicative of interactions. Also, step-up modeling was used to examine the stability of the lead parameter estimate as each confounder is introduced.

Because parental education and tooth lead were inversely correlated, using the education term simultaneously with the lead term in models of child IQ, produced considerable shared variance and the risk of over-controlling for the exposure variable. To minimize this problem, the sample was stratified into three groups according to parental education. The association between lead and IQ was then explored in each strata of parental education taking into account other risk factors such as sex, current grade, being ambidextrous, and the number of siblings.

III. RESULTS

Tooth Lead Values

Incisors had more lead than canines or molars: N, mean (SD) respectively are: 642, 4.5 (3.3) ug/g; 129, 4.1 ug/g (3.9) ug/g; and 94, 3.0 (2.5) ug/g. Only incisors are used in the further analyses, as previously explained. Lead levels were significantly different among the seven schools, as were some social factors (Table 1). Schools 1 and 7 were near smelters. Number 2 is a rural, coastal school, about 8 km from number 1, with lower lead exposure. Numbers 3, 4, 5 and 6 are urban schools, exposed to various sources of ambient lead, including considerable automobile traffic. Schools 1 and 7 have significantly more lead, and number 3 less lead than the overall mean. Compared to incisors from Boston and analyzed following exactly the same procedure, the children in Taiwan have a higher lead level (Lewandowski et al., 1987): Taipei City mean (SD) 4.4 (3.5) vs Boston 3.3 (2.5) ug/g, $p < .001$. Children from near the smelters had even higher lead levels, 6.3 (3.2), $p < .0001$.

Behavioral Handicap Clusters

The teachers' response regarding classroom behavior were grouped into seven clusters of dysfunction following exactly the advice of Guild (1979): reading, behavior (easily frustrated and peer problems), tasks (not persistent, independent, or flexible in work), directions (difficulty following simple or sequential instructions), mathematics, daydreaming, and hyperactivity. To be classified as positive for a cluster, the child must have been considered positive for all the question items in the cluster. This might avoid misclassification into the dysfunctional group. The additional reference category "none" is composed of children with no individual questions rated as problems. Cases were arranged in terms of the prevalence of each poor teacher's rating cluster in each quartile category of tooth. The total numbers of children of each gender in each lead quartile with and without each handicap cluster is shown in Table 3. Hyperactivity among boys shows a trend of increasing frequency with increasing lead. The chi-square for trend is 6.9, $p = .009$. The relative risk in the highest quartile is 4.2 (1.2-19.1, 95% confidence interval) relative to the rate in the lowest quartile. Similarly the task handicap among boys is lead related: chi-square for trend 8.4 , $p = .004$, relative risk is 14.9 (1.9-318, 95% confidence interval). Reading difficulties among girls shows a modest increase with increasing lead levels; the chi-square for trend is 2.8, $p = .09$, but the relative risk for the highest exposure quartile compared to the lowest quartile is 2.8 with a confidence interval including 1. The prevalence of each handicap cluster is not different among the sub-group whose teeth were too decayed to measure, compared to children who yielded a measurable tooth.

The two behavioral handicap clusters which appear to be somewhat related to lead, at least in a bivariate fashion are task among boys and hyperactivity among both genders, but particularly among boys. A search for covariates of these two clusters among the available parental, pregnancy and childhood factors revealed only a few factors which were associated with poor outcomes. Among the 32 boys with the task handicap, 15 percent of all of the boys, being ambidextrous, but not left handed, was associated with an increased risk. Among the 8 percent of the boys who were ambidextrous, 6 or 43 percent had the task syndrome, yielding a p-value of 0.01 from a chi-squared test. The risk ratio of having task difficulties is 3.3 for ambidextrous boys compared to the right handed. Also, task difficulties were related to the father's education, job, and the mother's education. Hyperactivity was associated with the number of adults in the home, but neither handedness nor head injury were related to hyperactivity or to reading difficulties. Reading difficulties were related to the number of adults and siblings in the home and the parents' education and employment. In logistic modelling of the several syndromes (Table 4), these risk factors need to be considered along with lead. Lead appears to have a

Table 3. Number of Cases of Various Learning Handicaps Among Four Quartile of Incisor Lead Levels

	Incisor Lead Level (ug/g)						
Cluster	<2.9	*3.0-3.9*	*4.0-5.5*	>5.6	*Total*	*Chi-Sqrd*	*p*
			Girls				
Behavior	3	3	0	5	11	4.7	.2
Hyperactive	3	6	4	7	20	2.8	.4
Reading	5	7	6	10	28	2.8	.1
Math	10	8	10	14	42	1.8	.6
Directions	2	2	2	1	7	.5	.9
Daydreaming	6	4	5	7	22	.6	.9
Tasks	8	5	6	4	23	1.1	.8
None	23	22	14	14	73	5.4	.1
Total	73	59	62	66	260		
			Boys				
Behavior	1	7	4	7	19	5.2	.16
Hyperactive	4	11	13	14	42	6.2	.10*
Reading	4	12	13	6	35	5.7	.13
Math	5	12	8	7	32	2.4	.5
Directions	4	1	4	4	13	2.7	.4
Daydreaming	5	7	9	7	28	0.8	.9
Tasks	1	9	16	12	38	13.5	.004**
None	11	17	10	11	49	2.3	.5
Total	53	63	62	56	234		

Notes: To be classified as positive for a handicap, all questions related to a syndrome must be positive. "None" refers to having no questions positive of any cluster. P value refers to chi-squared test, with 3 degrees of freedom. Chi-square for trend is also shown.

* chi squared for trend < .01

** chi squared for trend < .005.

role in the task behavior, even after controlling for other risk factors. The lead term is significantly non-zero, and adding the lead term improves the model.

There was an association between gender and handedness. Boys are more likely to be left-handed than girls, chi-squared 8.3, $p = 0.015$. Only 3.4 percent of girls are left-handed, compared to 10 percent of the boys, a risk ratio of 2.9. Being ambidextrous was not associated with gender.

A comparison of the handicap cluster in Taiwan with the finding from the same questionnaire in a cohort of normal Boston children is shown in Table 5. In general the results are similar regarding gender trends and frequencies, except for hyperactivity and tasks.

Some children show multiple handicaps clusters. Although 338 children (68% of the cases) were in no handicap cluster, 85 cases (17%) had one handicap, 42 cases (9%) had two, 21 cases (4%) had three handicaps, and 9 children (2%) had four of the seven handicaps. Compared to no handicaps, having only one

Table 4. Logistic Models of Two Handicaps With and Without a Lead Term

Model Term	*Without Lead Term*			*With Lead Term*		
	Beta Estimate	*Standard Error*	*p Value*	*Beta Estimate*	*Standard Error*	*p Value*
1. Task Syndrome (lack of persistence, independence, and flexibility): 31 with handicap out of 206 boys						
Intercept	−.33	.59	.58	−1.85	1.04	.08
Ambidextrous	1.71	.61	.005	1.66	.60	.006
Fathers' Education	−.37	.14	.008	−.28	.15	.05
Log Incisor Lead				.78	.43	.07
Model Chi-Square	14.3 $p = .0008$			17.8 $p = .0005$		
Change in Model Chi-Square 3.5, $p = .06$						
Model r-square	6.6%			8.1%		
2. Hyperactivity Syndrome: 47 with syndrome out of 399 children						
Intercept	−4.9	.71	.0000	−5.5	.85	.0000
Sex	1.2	.35	.0005	1.2	.35	.0005
Number of Adults	.35	.12	.004	.34	.12	.006
Log Incisor Lead				.45	.30	.13
Model Chi-Square	21.3 $p = .0000$			23.6 $p = .0000$		
Change in Model Chi-Square 2.3, $p = .13$						
Model r-square	5.1%			5.6%		

Note: After adjusting for other risk factors, the association between lead and task difficulties among boys persists. The lead term is significant, and adding the lead term improves the model. That is not the case for hyperactivity.

Table 5. The Prevalence of Learning Handicaps from Teachers' Questionnaires in Boston and Taiwan, number of cases and percentages

Cluster	*Boston*				*Taiwan*			
	Girls		*Boys*		*Girls*		*Boys*	
Behavior	38	4.0%	92	9.5%	21	5.4%	23	7.1%
Hyperactive	14	1.5	59	6.1	31	7.9	64	19.5
Reading	73	7.7	113	11.6	39	10.0	44	13.6
Math	98	10.3	110	11.3	60	15.3	44	13.6
Directions	45	4.7	50	5.1	13	3.4	18	5.5
Daydreaming	109	11.5	180	18.5	36	9.4	43	13.5
Tasks	51	5.4	53	5.4	33	8.5	52	16.1
Total Children	948		973		387		322	

Note: To be considered as a case, all component questions of a cluster must be positive.

handicap is associated with a significantly higher lead level. Lead levels are significantly elevated among the 85 children who have any one learning handicap compared to the 337 with no handicaps (5.5 std err 0.5 vs 4.4 std err .2, $p = .004$). However, having multiple handicaps is not related to having more lead, implying a rather specific nature to the lead associated difficulties.

Behavioral Problems

More severe behavior problems were examined with a 26 item section of the teachers' questionnaire which closely follows the work of Rutter (1967). However, in the Chinese version, instead of offering the teacher three choices for each item (doesn't apply, applies somewhat, and certainly applies), four choices are offered (never, seldom, often, and always). This was found to be more appropriate in a Chinese setting to overcome the strong tendency for Chinese to respond with a middle choice. The collected data is then collapsed into three categories by combining never and seldom. Following Rutter's recommendations, this data was considered in three ways: a total sum score with double weighing for responses in the most severe category and two subscales, neurotic and antisocial.

Rutter proposed cut-off for these three measures for screening and diagnostic purposes, but no children exceeded the cut-off value for neurosis, and only 2 cases were in the anti-social category. For exploratory purposes we created a moderate cut-off also, forming three categories, but still there were no associations between lead and neurotic or anti-social behavior in this population. Regarding the total behavioral problem score, only 11 children, 8 boys, had total scores exceeding the cut-off value, and there was no association between their occurrence and their incisor lead expressed as quartile categories (chi-squared 2.6, $p = .5$). Considering the full scale behavior scores, the Pearson correlation coefficient between the total behavior score and incisor lead, each expressed as the logarithm, was only 0.061, p value 0.18, for 477 pairs. For 249 girls the coefficient was 0.039, p is 0.54; for 228 boys the coefficient was 0.07, p equals 0.27. Apparently there is no bivariate association between lead and behavior scores. To verify this, multiple regression models of the total score with and without lead terms showed that lead plays no appreciable role in severe behavioral disorders.

Intelligence Scores

Intelligence was measured with the Raven's Colored Progressive Matrices test, CPM, during first grade, as part of their normal school activity. The scores for this test, the number of correct answers out of 36, correlate well with the lead content of their incisors, as shown in Table 6 which is grouped by gender, school grade, and parental education. The relationship was stronger among

Table 6. Correlation Coefficients Between Incisor Lead Levels (log transformed) and the Performance of the Raven's Progressive Matrices Test

Sub-group of Children	*Pearson r*	*Number*	*p-value*
All	−.193	443	.0001
Girls	−.255	232	.0001
Boys	−.118	221	.087
Grade 1	−.274	252	.0001
Grade 2	−.161	136	.06
Grade 3	+.054	55	.7
Fathers' Education:			
Less than High School	−.146	107	.13
High or Vocational	−.123	197	.09
Any College	+.004	127	.9

girls than boys, and it is weaker when second and third graders were considered. Also, it varies considerably according to parental education.

The CPM Test is particularly useful because it measures "fluid intelligence and cognitive ability," correlates well with WISC (median correlation 0.51), its utility is unaffected by hearing difficulties, and it is free of obvious cultural content (Sattler, 1974). A test score of 32 corresponds to the top 5 percent of the overall Taipei school population, which is approximately equivalent to a Stanford-Binet IQ of 127, 25 is the median IQ of 100, and 16 for boys and 14 for girls is the lowest decile, approximating an IQ of 80. The quartile categories of CPM test scores by incisor lead categories is shown in Table 7, chi-square test showing a highly significant trend. With increasing lead levels, there is a marked decrease in the proportion of children scoring well and an increase in low scoring children.

Multivariate Analysis of Intelligence

It is necessary to examine the intelligence-lead relationship in light of other factors which are related to both intelligence and lead exposure (Rabinowitz, Wang, & Soong, 1991). Each of the variables shown in Table 2 was considered a potential confounder. The factors which are related to both tooth lead and IQ, using a p value of 0.15 as the criteria, form a short list of only ten variables, which include the number of siblings, birth order, paternal and maternal education and employment, having had a vaginal or Cesarean delivery, and being ambidextrous. Most of these parental factors are strongly inter-correlated. For example, the correlation of maternal and paternal education is 0.81 for 471 pairs, and between paternal education and paternal job classification is 0.67 for 439 pairs. Also, birth order and family size are

Table 7. Prevalence of Intelligence Scores Among Children in Different Quartiles of Incisor Lead

	Incisor Lead Levels (ppm)									
CPM Test Score	*<3.0*		*3.0-3.9*		*4.0-5.5*		*>5.5*		*Total*	
All Children										
> 29	38	35%	26	23%	22	20%	19	18%	105	24%
26-29	29	26	29	25	30	27	26	24	114	26%
22-25	20	18	30	26	33	30	19	18	102	23%
< 22	23	21	29	25	26	23	44	41	122	28%
Total	110		114		111		108		443	
Chi-Square = 22.77 p =.0067										
	Incisor Lead Levels (ppm)									
CPM Test Score	*<2.8*		*2.8-3.7*		*3.8-5.4*		*>5.4*		*Total*	
Girls										
> 29	21	38%	16	28%	12	21%	11	18%	60	26%
25-28	18	32	21	36	11	19	13	22	63	27%
21-24	7	13	8	14	20	35	13	22	48	21%
< 21	10	18	13	22	15	26	23	38	61	26%
Total	56		58		58		58		232	
Chi-Square = 22.95 p =.0063.										

Note: Categories of IQ and lead were constructed to form nearly equal quartiles for each variable. Number of cases and column percentages are shown.

interrelated ($r = 0.60, p = .0001$, 459 pairs). Therefore, considerable care needs to be exercised when these variables are considered in a multivariate analysis of IQ.

Rather than using fathers' and mothers' education and employment as four independent variables, it was decided to use only the education variables, because in Taiwan it has been shown that the response to questions about employment categories are highly dependent on the size of the company and on the perceived purpose of the questioning (Chang & Wang, 1988). Also, the mode of delivery was eliminated because of the high number of missing cases and the small r-square (0.6%). This resulted in a shorter list, which is also shown in Table 8: sex, grade, birth order, number of siblings, fathers and mother's education, and being ambidextrous. Also, the separate fathers' and mothers' education variables were combined by averaging to form "parental education" because they are strongly collinear and averaging available data reduces by nine the number of cases with missing data. The parental education variable was then reduced into three nearly equal size categories: any middle school attendance or less, high school or vocational schooling, or any college. Furthermore, we feel that in a Confucian society, where a high premium is

Table 8. Short List of Significant Confounders: each relates to both IQ and Lead with $p < 0.15$.

Confounder Variable	** missing Values*	*simple r-squared from Simultaneous Regression*
Sex (1 = girl, 2 = boy)	0	.9 %
Grade (1,2, or 3)	0	3
Birth order	8	3
Total number of siblings	21	5
Parental education	0	15
Ambidextrous child (yes or no)	35	1

Notes: * cases with missing values is out of 431 cases with incisor lead, IQ and parent's education. R-squared is from a simultaneous regression model with 393 cases with complete data for all 8 variables.

placed on scholarship and examinations are the historically accepted determinants of advancement, the parental education variable is an especially strong marker for broader family social status and child-rearing practices.

Parental education and tooth lead are inversely correlated in the entire study population ($r = -.315$, $N = 435$, $p = .0001$) and even in only the four lower lead, Taipei City schools ($r = -.231$, $N = 315$, $p = .0001$). Putting this education variable in a model along with lead would over-control for any influence of lead. So, further multivariate analysis was done in three separate populations, stratifying for parental education (Table 9). A general model is shown for each group as well as models with reduced numbers of variables. Only in the lowest parental education category and among girls does lead achieve nominal statistical significance, after adjusting for other risk factors. The magnitude of the lead effect is about as large as the effect associated with being ambidextrous.

Another strategy is to start with the lead term and add potential confounders one by one, as shown in Table 10, separately for all children and for only girls. As confounding terms are added, the parameter estimate for lead decreases somewhat from its initial value, although it does not change significantly. However, the standard error does not decrease, so the p value for the lead term becomes larger and no longer statistically significant. The pattern seen for girls is similar, except the parameter estimate starts larger, and falls less as new terms are added.

IV. DISCUSSION

One of the limitations of this study was that we relied on the students to donate their teeth and assist in obtaining parental information. Children who were very disorganized or troublesome may not have given us their teeth. Thus our sample may systematically be excluding children with behavioral problems.

Table 9. Multiple Regression Models of IQ in Each Category of Parental Education

Variable	*Parameter Estimate*	*Standard Error*	*Value*	*R-Sqr Term*	*Model F Ratio*	*R-Sqr*
PARENTAL EDUCATION: Some Middle School or Less, N=135						
1. Sex	−.19	1.07	.87	.0002		
Grade	−.51	.71	.48	.006		
Siblings	−.19	.53	.71	.002		
Ambidextrous	−4.2	1.7	.01	.05		
Tooth Lead	−1.88	.92	.042	.038	2.37	8.9 %
2. Ambidextrous	−4.19	1.61	.010	.048		
Tooth Lead	−2.07	.88	.021	.039	6.23	8.6 %
PARENTAL EDUCATION: Some High School or Vocational						
1. Sex	1.43	.80	.077	.018		
Grade	−1.47	.57	.01	.041		
Siblings	−.80	.61	.19	.013		
Ambidextrous	−.73	1.74	.67	.0002		
Tooth Lead	−.36	.77	.65	.004	2.42	7.6 %
2. Sex	1.68	.76	.029	.025		
Grade	−1.41	.54	.01	.037		
Siblings	−.91	.56	.10	.016		
Tooth Lead	−.51	.73	.48	.006	3.71	8.4 %
PARENTAL EDUCATION: Some College or More, N = 113						
1. Sex	.98	.95	.30	.012		
Grade	−1.94	.72	.008	.070		
Siblings	−.34	.77	.65	.0002		
Ambidextrous	.21	1.9	.91	.0008		
Tooth Lead	.149	1.12	.89	.0000	1.72	8.5 %
2. Sex	1.01	1.81	.23	.014		
Grade	−2.05	.64	.002	.085		
Tooth Lead	.147	1.01	.89	.0000	3.98	9.9 %

Note: For each category several models are shown: a general model with many terms and a simplified model which retains only significant terms. The model F ratio, r-square, and number of cases is shown for each model. The logarithm of incisor lead is used.

Also, since our population was selected from public primary school children, we necessarily did not include severely handicapped or retarded children.

Lead levels showed a marked difference between ambient urban levels and the children near the smelters. Although the ranges of lead at all schools overlapped, children who lived near the smelters had median incisor lead levels 61 percent higher than the urban children. It is likely that the smelters raise the children's lead level by more than 60 percent above what they would be if there were no smelter at these rural, otherwise less contaminated locations.

Table 10. Stability of Parameter Estimate of Lead in Multiple Regression Models of IQ Scale for All Children and for Only Girls

	Lead Term				*Model*	
Terms in Model	*Parameter Estimate*	*Standard Error*	*p-value*	*R-Square Lead Term*	*R-Square*	*N*
		All Children				
Tooth Lead Term Only	−2.04	.50	.0000	3.7%	3.7%	443
above + Parents Educat	−0.94	.49	.056	4.3	16.2	435
above + Grade	−0.79	.49	.11	4.3	18.6	435
above + Ambidextrous	−0.77	.51	.13	4.6	19.6	399
above + Sex	−0.83	.51	.10	4.6	20.2	399
above + Birth Order	−0.85	.51	.10	4.4	19.5	393
above + Cesarean Deliv	−0.68	.53	.20	3.8	19.4	372
above + Head Injury	−0.86	.57	.13	4.1	20.0	344
		Girls Only				
Lead Only	−2.59	.65	.0001	6.5 %	6.5%	232
above + Parents Educat	−1.73	.68	.011	7.1	13.7	228
above + Grade	−1.58	.67	.018	7.1	16.3	228
above + Ambidextrous	−1.68	.69	.015	7.9	17.7	210
above + Birth Order	−1.74	.70	.013	7.6	16.3	205
above + Cesarean Deliv	−1.52	.74	.041	6.2	15.0	194
above + Head Injury	−1.80	.78	.022	7.0	15.5	80

Note: In this step-up procedure, one additional new term is added on each line. After the addition of the parental education term, the parameter estimate for lead is relatively stable.

The blood lead levels of the 60 children near the smelters, averaging 13 ug/dl, support this.

We chose to use only the incisors as markers of body burden, disregarding any molar or canine teeth (Rabinowitz et al., 1991a). Other surveys (Patterson et al., 1988; Fergusson, Fergusson, Horwood, & Kinzett, 1988) have reported systematic differences according to tooth type, some with molars having higher lead levels. We did not feel confident with any scheme of adjusting the lead values of different teeth, which calcify at different times. So, we elected to limit our analyses to only incisors, which resulted in a smaller, but more orderly, cohort.

The demographic factors associated with a higher tooth lead level included more siblings, not being the oldest sibling, less parental education, having a younger mother, and having been delivered by Cesarean section. Similar patterns were seen in Boston, where higher cord blood lead levels were also associated with less educated and younger mothers. However, in Boston higher parity was associated with lower lead levels (Rabinowitz & Needleman, 1984).

The prevalence of learning problems as reported by Taiwanese teachers was generally very similar to the rates reported in Boston using the same form.

Taiwanese teachers were more likely to report problems with hyperactivity, mathematics, and tasks than their Boston counterparts. These small differences may be as much caused by different levels of sensitivities of the teachers as by real behavioral differences in the two cohorts. Boston teachers are loath to report hyperactivity because that triggers administrative action. However, in Taiwan with no such mechanism in place, teachers are less hesitant to report perceived hyperactivity, and they report it more than three times as often.

Logistic models of hyperactivity and task problems were constructed to see if lead is a significant predictor after taking other risk factors into account, such as family size, parental education, gender, and being ambidextrous. There is ample evidence from the published literature that excessive lead exposure is related to both hyperactivity (David, Hoffman, Clark, & Sverd, 1983) and school difficulties (Needleman, Schell, Bellinger, Leviton, & Allred, 1990). However, here the coefficient of the covariate adjusted lead terms are not significantly different from zero, except for task difficulties. Also, there was no association between lead and the scores from Rutter's child behavior problems checklist expressed as the neurotic, anti-social or total problem scores, either in bivariate of multivariate analysis (Rabinowitz, Wang, & Soong, 1992a) .

The very strong association of child intelligence with parental eduction is a common finding (Yeates, MacPhee, Campbell, & Karney, 1983). Parental education may have a direct or genetic effect as well as being a marker for other factors for development such as the stimulating quality of the home environment. Indeed, in Taiwan the influence of parental education on a child's reading skills is even stronger than comparable children in Japan or the United States (Stevenson, Lucker, Lee, Stigler, Kitamura, & Hsu, 1987). We suspect that in a Confucian society such as China, where education is highly valued and access to higher education is limited by success in examinations, parental education variables are stronger correlates of family status and child rearing behavior than in a more socially mobile and egalitarian society such as America.

The bivariate association between lead and IQ score from the Raven's Colored Progressive Matrices Test is strong. For 443 children with incisor lead and IQ test results the correlation is $-.193$, $p = .0001$. Among the 232 girls the coefficient is higher, $-.255$. Also, the strength of the association is stronger among children whose parents had the least education. This tendency of lower social class children to be more susceptible to lead has been noted by others (Hawk, Schroeder, Robinson, & Otto, 1986 and Bellinger, Leviton, Waternaux, Needleman, & Rabinowitz , 1989). Even after adjustments for other risk factors, the lead term remains significantly different from zero, especially among girls.

An apparent threshold for lead's effect on intelligence can be deduced from this study (Rabinowitz, Wang, & Soong, 1992b). For each child a predicted

CPM test score may be calculated from the best parsimonious multiple regression model of IQ (CPM Score), without a lead term (r-squared 21%, $F = 25.5$, $p < .0001$). The parental education variable was the most potent predictor of the child's test score and alone accounted for 17 percent of the variance in the child's IQ. Our model was: The Predicted Score = 18.6 + 0.84*Gender (1 or 2) + 1.7*Parental Education (1 to 7) − 1.7*Ambidextrous (0 or 1) −1.2*Grade (1 to 3). This provided a predicted score for each child which was subtracted from their actual test results to obtain an intelligence deficit, which might be attributable to lead (Bellinger & Needleman 1983). This deficit averaged zero (std dev 5.1, normality 0.98, skewness 0.25) and ranged from −13.3 to 15.5. The correlation between lead and this deficit is weak (Pearson $r = 0.094$, $n = 380$, $p = .06$).

Because we were interested in detecting any threshold of lead's effect, we tried various limits and compared the mean deficits above and below each trial limit using the non-parametric Mann-Whitney test. Thc lowest lead level across which there is a difference would be the threshold of lead's effect. There was no difference in mean dcficits for children below or above the lower trial limits, such as 2 or 3 ug/g. Any threshold must be at higher lead levels. However, the mean deficit of children above 3.5 ug/g was statistically greater than those below 3.5 ug/g. Similarly when even higher lead levels are chosen as test thresholds, 4 or 6 ug/g, for example, the difference in IQ deficits is still significant. This sets an upper bound on the threshold near or below 3.5 ug/g. The siginificance of this threshold may be judged by noting that, althought there is considerable overlap, children above and below 3.5 ug/g display different degrees of IQ deficits. The higher lead children are 1.3 times more likely to have a deficit of more than 2 CPM units, 38 versus 29 percent, for example.

The usual measure of lead exposure is blood lead concentration. Tooth lead levels of shed incisors from Boston correlate well with blood lead at 57 months of age, r − .56 among 88 children (Rabinowitz, Bellinger, & Leviton, 1989). Using that calibration line, a tooth lead of 3.25 ug/g corresponds to a blood lead of approximately 8 (q 2) ug/dl, below the currently accepted safe level of blood lead. (Centers for Disease Control, 1985).

The association between lead and intelligence seen in this study is consistent with trends observed in other studies. Table 11 shows a compilation of studies from five other countries which have used teeth to assess lead burden. This study has the lowest mean lead level, 4.6, versus an average of 7.3 for the others which range from 5.1 to 12.7 ppm. Also, this study uses the Raven Progressive Matrices Test rather than the Wechsler Scale. Despite these differences, all of these studies show that lead is correlated significantly with intelligence even at these lower levels, both in bivariate analysis and after adjusting for covariates. The effect size for lead on IQ scores is about twice as strong among girls as boys. Based on their standardized estimates, the lead effect is about

Table 11. Compilation of Studies of Tooth Lead and Intelligence of Children

Study Author	*Population*	*Number*	*Lead Level Mean (SD)*	*Intelligence Outcome Measure*
1. Needleman 1985	Boston, USA: urban	218	12.7	WISC-R:V,F
2. Hansen 1989	Aarhus, Denmark: urban	156	10.7	WISC-R:V,F
3. Winneke 1983	Stolberg, Germany: smelter	115	6.2	WISC-R:V,F
4. Pocock 1987	London, England: urban	317	5.1 (2.8)	WISC-R:F
5. Fergusson 1988	Christchurch, NZ: urban	724	6.2 (3.8)	WISC-R:V,F
6. This Study 1990	Taipei, WuLun, and FongShan: smelter and urban	399	4.6 (3.3)	CPM

Study	*Multiple Regression Lead Coefficient (Std Err)* *Unadjusted*	*Adjusted*	*p*	*Partial r*	*Number of Covariates*	*Total Model r-squared*
1.	NA	−0.21 (.07)	.001	−.20	5	.35
2.	NA	−4.27(1.21)	.01	−.18	7	.20
3.	NA	−0.13 (.47)	.49	−.003	4	.13
4.	* −2.66 (.86)	−0.77 (.63)	.11	−.06	6	NA
5.	* NA	−1.46(1.25)	.12	−.04	8	NA
6.	* −2.04 (.50)	−0.83 (.51)	.05	−.19	4	.20 all =399
6.	* −2.59 (.65)	−1.68 (.69)	.007	−.26	3	.18 only girls n=210

Note: Full scale IQ test results are displayed. Note here 1 tailed p values are used.
p is one tailed in this table only.
* log transformed lead value.
NA not available from published data.

as strong as being ambidextrous or the child's gender, but much smaller than influence of parental education (.081 vs .080,.082, and .33 respectively). Using all of the measured variables in a model, we were able to account for only about 20 percent of the variance in IQ scores, about 15 percent among girls. The lead factor alone accounts for only about 4 percent of the variance, 7 percent among girls. Although the influence of lead represents a small part of the populations variation in IQ scores, it should be remembered that of all of the variables measured, only lead represents a factor that can be changed by stricter pollution laws.

ACKNOWLEDGMENTS

This research was funded by a grant from the National Science Council of the Republic of China (NSC 79-0421-B002-1Z). Excellent technical support was provided by Chao

Wen-ying, Lu Chin-siung, and Chao Kun-yu. Statistical advice was kindly provided by Chen Chen-hsin. We are very thankful to the school principles and classroom teachers who fully supported this research effort.

REFERENCES

Achenbach T., Verhulst, F., Baron, G., & Althaus, M. (1987). Epidemiological comparisons of American and Dutch children. *Journal of American Academy Child Adolescent Psychiatry* 26, 326-332.

Bellinger, D., Leviton, A., Waternaux, C., Needleman, H., & Rabinowitz, M. (1989). Low-level lead exposure, social class and development. *Neurotoxicology and Teratology*. 10, 497-503.

Centers for Disease Control. (1985). *Preventing Lead Poisoning in Young Children*. Atlanta, Georgia. United States Department of Health and Human Services. No. 992230.

Chang P., & Wang J. (1988). The accuracy of occupational histories obtained from spouse. *Prog. Occupat. Epidem.*, 53-62.

David, O., Hoffman, S., Clark, G., & Sverd, J. (1983). The relationship of hyper-activity to moderately elevated lead levels. Arch. *Environmental Health* 38, 341-346. Davis, J. and Svendsgaard, D.(1987). Lead and child development. *Nature 329*, 297-298.

Fergusson, D., Fergusson, J., Horwood, L., & Kinzett, N. (1988). A longitudinal study of dentine lead levels, intelligence school performance, and behavior. *Journal of Child Psychology and Psychiatry? 29*, 793-809.

Guild, M. (1979). A case study of questionnaire reliability and validity. Thesis: Graduate School of Education, Harvard University, Cambridge.

Hansen, O., Trillingsgaard, A., Beese, I., Lyngbye, T., & Grandjean, P. (1989). A neuropsychological study of children with elevated dentine lead level. *Neurotoxicolgy and Teratology. 11*, 205-213.

Hawk, B., Schroeder, S., Robinson, G., & Otto, D. (1986). Relation of lead and social factors to IQ of Low-SES children. *American Journal of Mental Defiency 91*, 178-83.

Jang C.S. (1989). Study of a lead recycling factory's occupational and environmental disease (in Chinese). Masters Thesis, National Taiwan University, Department of Public Health, Taipei, Taiwan.

Landsdown, R., Yule, W., Urbanowicz, M., & Hunter, J. (1986). The relationship between blood lead concentrations, intelligence, attainment and behavior. *International Archives Occupational Enviromental Health 57*, 225-35.

Lewandowski, A., Rabinowitz, M., Leviton, A., Iverson, K., & Rose, S. (1987). Initial results of lead measurements of deciduous teeth. *Biological Bulletin 173*, 442.

Needleman, H. & Gatsonis, C. (1990). Low-level lead exposure and the IQ of children. *Journal of American Medical Association 263*, 673-678.

Needleman, H., Greiger, S., & Frank, R. (1985). Lead and IQ scores. *Science 227*, 701-704.

Needleman, H., Schell, A., Bellinger, D., Leviton, A., & Allred, E.(1990). The long-term effects of exposure to low doses of lead in childhood. *New England Journal of Medicine 322*, 83-88.

Patterson, L., Raab, G., Hunter, R., Laxen, D., Fulton, M., Fell, G., Halls, D., & Sutcliffe, P. (1988). Factors influencing lead concentrations in shed deciduous teeth. *Science of the Total Environment. 74*, 219-233.

Pocock, S., Ashby, D., & Smith, V. (1987). Lead exposure and children's intelligence. *International Journal of Epidemiology 16*, 57-67.

Rabinowitz, M., & Needleman, H. (1984). Demographic, medical, and environmental factors related to cord blood lead. *Biological Trace Element Research.* 6, 57-67.

Rabinowitz, M., Bellinger, D., & Leviton, A. (1989). The blood lead—tooth lead relationship among Boston children. *Bulletin of Environmental Contamination Toxicology.* 43, 485-492.

Rabinowitz, M., Wang, J.D., & Soong, W.T. (1991). Dentine lead and child intelligence in Taiwan. *Archives of Environmental Health.* 46: 351-360.

Rabinowitz, M., Bellinger, D., Leviton, A., & Wang, J. (1991a). Lead levels among various deciduous tooth types. *Bulletin of Environmental Contamination and Toxicology.* 47: 602-608.

Rabinowitz, M., Wang, J.D., & Soong, W.T. (1991b). Children's classroom performance and lead in Taiwan. *Bulletin of Environmental Contamination and Toxicology.* 48: 282-288.

Rabinowitz, M., Wang, J.D., & Soong, W.T. (1991c). Apparent threshold of lead's effect on intelligence in Taiwan. *Bulletin of Environmental Contamination and Toxicology.* 48: 688-695.

Rutter, M. (1967). A children's behavior questionnaire for completion by teachers. *Journal of Child Psychology, Psychiatry and Applied Disciplines.* 8, 1-11.

Sattler, J. (1974). *Assessment of children's intelligence* (pp. 44, 82, 155). Saunders, Philadelphia.

Stevenson, H., Lucker, G., Lee, S., Stigler, J., Kitamura, S., & Hsu, C. (1987). Poor readers in three cultures (pp. 157-177). In *The role of culture in developmental disorders*, edited by C. Super. San Diego: Academic Press.

Winneke, G., Kraemer, U., Brockhaus, A, Ewers, U., Kujanek, G., Lechner, H., & Janke, W. (1983). Neuropsychological studies in children with elevated tooth-lead concentrations. *International Archives of Occupational and Environmental Health.* *51*: 231-252.

Yeates, K., MacPhee, D., Campbell, F., & Ramey, C. (1983). Maternal IQ and home environment as determinants of early childhood intellectual Ccmpetence. *Developmental Psychology.* *19*: 731-739.

ENVIRONMENTAL BIOTECHNOLOGY:
BIOTECHNOLOGY SOLUTIONS FOR A GLOBAL ENVIRONMENTAL HEALTH PROBLEM, HAZARDOUS CHEMICAL WASTES

Gilbert S. Omenn

Our Planet Earth appears to be a marvelously resilient natural system. It has survived numerous Natural upheavals, including earthquakes, tsunamis, and violent storms, as well as huge temperature shifts over geologic time. On the other hand, our generation is the first to have seen its own planet from a distance, photographed most memorably as the "Earthshot" by Apollo 8 astronaut William Anders. In this photograph, we see a tiny fragile globe floating in the vastness of space—a closed, vulnerable system upon which all our lives depend. The impact on human thinking, as noted by The World Commission on Environment and Development, The Brundtland Commission (1987), may surpass even the sixteenth-century discovery that the Earth is not the center of the Universe.

Research in Human Capital and Development, Volume 7, pages 273-283.

ISBN: 1-55938-132-9

The intrusion of human civilizations has presented increasing challenges to Planet Earth. These challenges include retention of infrared radiation or global warming due to greenhouse gases, depletion of stratospheric ozone, loss of biological diversity, deforestation, desertification, acid precipitation, threat of major epidemics among humans (AIDS) or crops, and threat of nuclear war. Among the risks to life on this Planet, the chemical contamination of soils and water systems deserves our attention, since water is the most distinctive and enabling feature for life on Earth. In the densely populated countries of Asia, land and water are especially precious resources.

Since the 1940s, rapid growth of the chemical industry has fueled economic growth and improvements in standards of living and has produced millions of tons of hazardous and toxic wastes—petroleum products, lubricants, protective coatings, pesticides, dielectric fluids, flame retardants, refrigerants, and heat transfer fluids. Natural resources, once abundant and forgiving, have become threatened by "out of sight, out of mind" attitudes toward disposal of these chemicals, their residues, and off-grade mixtures. These chemical wastes accumulate in landfills, holding ponds, lakes, rivers, groundwater and soil environments, and the atmosphere. The generation of chemical wastes is highly correlated with population and with standard of living, as we heard from Dr. Chien of the Environmental Protection Administration. We have some similar problems in the United States, of course.

Industrialization in Third World countries has brought hazardous chemical problems to often-unprepared societies (Castleman & Navarro, 1987). As the Bhopal accident demonstrated, hazardous chemical processes are more likely to be managed inadequately. Prevention of worker exposures and prevention of emissions to air and water are considered luxuries, or not considered at all. Furthermore, many chemicals, especially pesticides, that have been banned or restricted in industrialized countries are being exported to Third World countries. Ill-advised subsidies for purchase of pesticides stimulate gross overuse, with a worldwide epidemic of acute poisonings and with adverse agricultural effects (Repetto, 1985).

In 1982, the United Nations General Assembly approved a resolution (with one dissent) that "Products which have been banned for domestic consumption and/or sale because they have been judged to endanger health and environment should be sold abroad by companies, corporations, or individuals only when a request for such products is received from an importing country or when the consumption of such products is officially permitted in the importing country." In theory, these nations may wish to accept certain (low-level) risks, which other countries choose to avoid, but they seldom make such explicit decisions and they lack the expertise to make detailed risk assessments. Less developed countries may also be recipients of wastes from more developed countries needing disposal sites. The Eastern European countries have abused their land and water resources in this way.

The ever-growing human population forces us to ask "How can we help Nature's cycles keep up with the waste streams we introduce on Planet Earth?" Throughout the world efforts are increasing to recycle wastes and reduce the amounts of municipal and industrial wastes produced (World Resources Institute, 1989).

The guiding principle in managing accumulated hazardous wastes must be to detoxify them, preferably at the sites where they exist. We cannot continue to rely on removal of wastes to disposal sites, usually landfills, at those places we collectively call "Elsewhere."

I. ON-SITE REMEDIATION

On-site remediation requires extensive knowledge of the hydrogeology of the site, the ecology of the soil and water compartments, and the effectiveness of various alternative and complementary technologies. Technologies for clean-up of soils and groundwater contaminated with hazardous chemicals include several types of incineration, chemical and physical treatment to solidify or vitrify and thereby immobilize the chemicals, vapor extraction and air stripping with absorption, and a variety of bioremediation approaches.

Biotechnology has a growing place in the remediation of hazardous waste sites in the United States and, surely, in Taiwan and other countries throughout the Asia-Pacific region. The main bioremediation technologies in the field today involve engineering applications of basic principles of aerobic metabolism: optimizing the concentrations of oxygen and nutrients and assuring adequate moisture within a given environment to enhance the indigenous microbial population. Generally, there is little or no knowledge of the organisms present at the site. Better understanding of microbial ecology and genetic enhancement of biodegradation should accelerate progress in this field.

Brief Principles of Bioremediation: Environmental Biotechnology

Microorganisms can use many chemicals as food and energy sources. With full aerobic metabolism, using oxygen as final electron acceptor, the end products are carbon dioxide and water. With some chemicals, especially man-made chemicals, oxidation may be incomplete or may be better carried out by anaerobic organisms, which use nitrate or sulfate as final electron acceptor. Some organisms can biotransform chemicals but obtain no energy yield; these organisms need additional substrate to grow, a co-metabolic scheme.

To assess the feasibility of biotreatment, three aspects must be combined (see Gibson, 1984; Omenn & Hollaender, 1984; Omenn, 1988; Bourquin, 1989):

- Microbial physiology, biochemistry, and genetics, to understand the metabolic processes leading to detoxification and the genetics controlling the enzymc functions involved;
- microbial ecology, to appreciate the microenvironments in which the treatment may be performed and the structure and function of indigenous or inoculated microbial communities; and
- field site engineering, to implement the desired biodegradation scheme, maintaining optimal growth conditions and combining with physical or chemical methods, as necessary.

Table 1 outlines some of the most prevalent and important chemicals contaminating soils or groundwater and the present capability of biotechnology to detoxify these chemicals *in situ*.

In general, aerobic biodegradation is best suited for remediation of sites contaminated with petroleum hydrocarbons and polar solvents, such as alcohols and ketones. Anaerobic biodegradation is best applied to reductive dechlorination of chlorinated aliphatic and aromatic hydrocarbons, such as tetrachloroethane. Because anaerobic degradation may result in the accumulation of partially oxidized organic compounds, this treatment technique is often coupled with aerobic biological treatment. Metals are not usually good targets for bioremediation—or for physical methods, either; however, the redox state of certain metals, including cadmium, chromium, arsenic, and mercury, can be transformed by microorganisms to a state better suited to separation or isolation, or less toxic.

II. SOLID-PHASE BIOREMEDIATION FOR CONTAMINATED SOIL

The traditional form of bioremediation of contaminated soil has been known for years as "land farming", often little more than dumping contaminated waste onto land and letting Nature work its way, as in the biocycling of natural compounds. The main advances in modern "solid-phase bioremediation" come from optimization of conditions, by addition of nutrients, active aeration, and enhanced release of chemicals adsorbed to soil particles. This technique has been used to clean up fuel oils, diesel fuels, pesticides, and other types of easily degraded substrates. Solid-phase biotreatment of petroleum-contaminated and creosote-contaminated soils is the most widely used and most cost effective biotreatment technology at the present time.

For example, at a site with extensive hydrocarbon contamination of soil (up to 16,000 ppm), indigenous organisms were activated by spraying with nitrogen and phosphate, and oxygenating, reducing all components below the target of 100 ppm total concentration. This action was sufficient to permit disposal

Table 1. High-Priority Chemicals by Type of Contamination

Soils	*Groundwater*	*Biotechnology*
Petroleum hydrocarbons		++++
aliphatic (alkanes)		
aromatic (benzene, etc)		
chloro-aromatics (PCP)		
Polychlorobiphenyls (PCBs)		+/−
	Chlorinated Solvents (TCE)	+++
Chlorinated Pesticides		−
Organophosphate pesticides		++
	Gasoline (BTX)	++++
	Triazine herbicides	+
Heavy Metals	Heavy Metals	−/?+

Notes: Rating of Biotechnology Effectiveness: −, ineffective; +, limited effectiveness, to ++++, demonstrated highly effective. Sentinel compounds indicated: PCP, polychlorophenols; TCE, trichloroethylene, BTX, benzene/toluene/xylene.

at a Class III landfill, rather than Class I (most hazardous) landfill, as previously scheduled to be done. Complete biodegradation was demonstrated in the laboratory to be feasible, but was not called for in this case.

A more complicated case was a site with substantial amounts of 4-6 ring polycyclic aromatic hydrocarbons (PAHs). It was necessary to add an organism capable of biodegrading these more recalcitrant, higher molecular weight PAH compounds. Constitutive strain B600 of Beijerinckia B1, isolated by Gibson and Mahaffey, was useful in degrading phenanthrene and other high MW ring compounds, especially since it did not require induction of activity by low MW PAH substrates (Bourquin, 1989). Similarly, Pseudomonas strain DBM101 with constitutive biodegradative activity against polycyclic aromatic hydrocarbons, including dibenzofuran and benzo(a)pyrene, was isolated from a creosote-contaminated site, evaluated in the laboratory, and inoculated in the field at a test site in California.

The solid phase system can be modified to control volatiles and leachate. For example, a treatment bed has been lined with an 80 mm high-density liner having heat-welded seams (Bourquin, 1989) (Figure 1).

The liner is covered with sand, which protects it and provides proper drainage for contaminated water leaching from soils placed on the treatment bed. Lateral perforated drainage pipes on top of the synthetic liner in the sand bed collect the soil leachate. The whole treatment bed is covered by a modified plastic film greenhouse. An overhead spray irrigation system within the greenhouse provides moisture and distributes nutrients and microbial inocula, as needed, as large batches of soil are brought into the treatment bed for detoxification. The soil treatment facility is attached to an air management system for the volatiles, with a vapor-phase bioreactor and then activated carbon, in series.

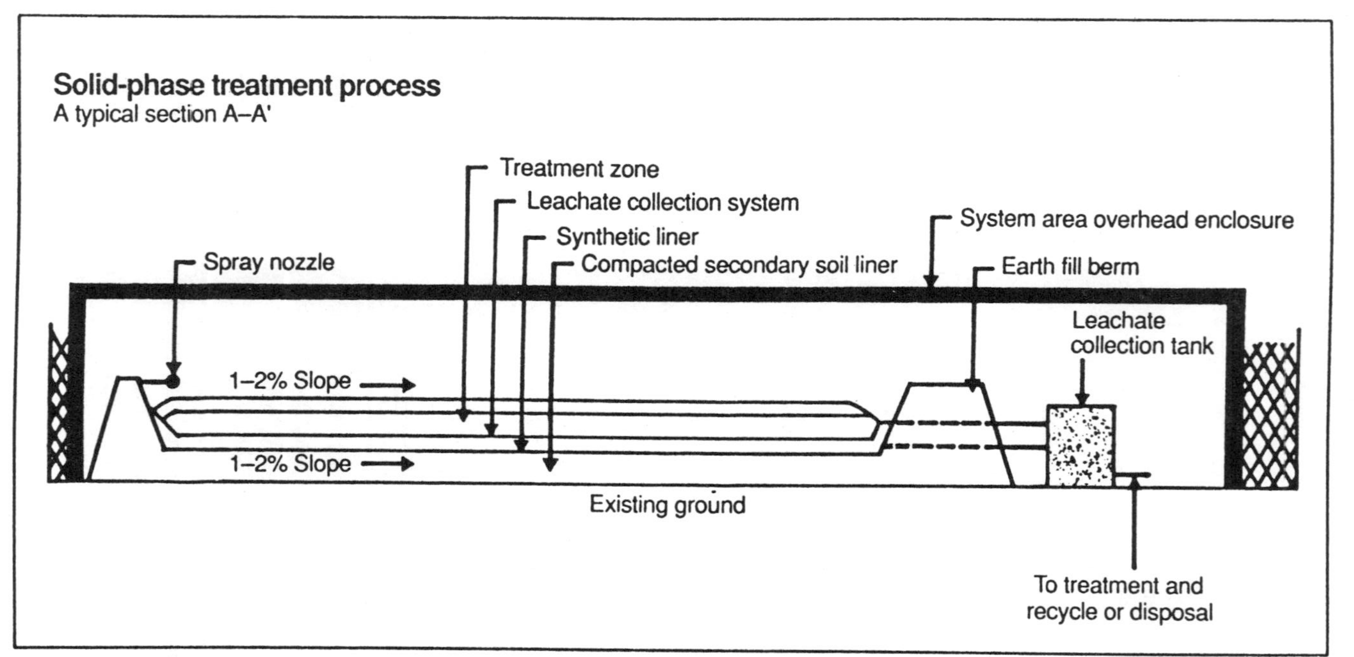

Figure 1. Scheme for Solid-phase Bioremediating of Contaminated Soils Brought into a Controlled Environment On-site. From Bourquin (1989).

Contaminated leachate is collected in a sump, then pumped to an on-site bioreactor.

The nature and concentration of the contaminants and the regulatory requirements in a given country or state will determine whether elaborate closed systems are required, or some emissions of volatiles into the air would be permissible.

III. SLURRY-PHASE BIOREMEDIATION OF CONTAMINATED SOIL

Another approach with soils is solid-phase treatment in an aqueous slurry, essentially a large bioreactor. This approach is especially appropriate for control of manufacturing effluents and for groundwater clean-up. An example is treatment of a field contaminated with polychlorophenols up to 8000 ppm. In this case aeration and nutrients had little effect over 13 days, but inoculation of the soil slurries with a consortium of five organisms selected by chemostat yielded prompt reduction of PCP levels. There was stoichiometric release of chloride, demonstrating full detoxification. Addition of organisms was essential and was effective in reducing levels to below 0.5 ppb. Similar good results were obtained in a soil-slurry biotreatment for trichloroethylene (TCE).

The bioreactor scheme decreases acclimation time, increases biodegradation rates, allows greater process control, increases contact between microorganisms and contaminants, and facilitates inoculation with specific cultures. The percent solids in the aqueous slurry can be adjusted based on the concentration of contaminants, the rate of biodegradation in feasibility studies, and the physical nature of the soils. The per-unit cost of treatment using slurry-phase bioremediation is higher than that of other biotreatments, but much less expensive than incineration.

It is important to monitor the biodegradation process to prove that detoxification has actually been accomplished. Also it is necessary to assess adsorption of compounds, such as benzo(a)pyrene, in high-clay soils, since microorganisms may be unable to attack compounds unless desorption is facilitated.

IV. BIOTREATMENT OF CONTAMINATED GROUNDWATER

Natural microorganisms may be employed either by direct injection or incorporated into bioreactors. Bioreactors provide a practical means of assuring a controlled environment for biodegradation, thereby avoiding questions about release of organisms into the general environment. Such questions are still an obstacle for use of genetically-engineered organisms in the United States (Tiedje et al., 1989; National Academy of Sciences Council, 1987).

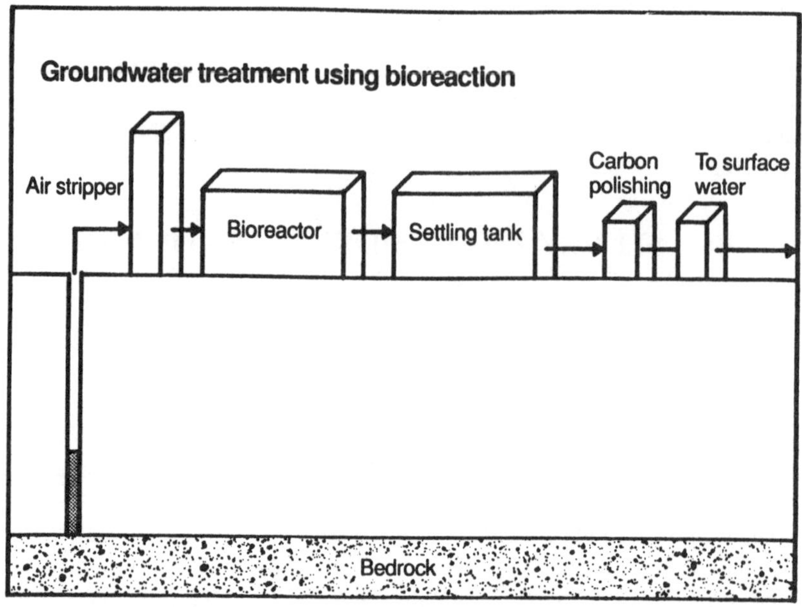

Figure 2. Scheme for Biotreatment of Contaminated Groundwater from Bourquin (1989).

For groundwater sites contaminated with chlorinated or mixed solvents, a typical approach involves empirical development in the laboratory of a site-specific bioreactor with a consortium of indigenous organisms plus laboratory stock cultures. Then the bioreactor can be taken into the field in combination with an air stripper, so that non-biodegradable solvents are air-stripped while the biodegradable solvents are treated in a continuous stir bioreactor (Figure 2).

For example, a Superfund site in California was contaminated with short-chain chlorinated hydrocarbons and soluble organic compounds such as acetone, 2-butanone, alcohols, and glycols. The contaminated groundwater was pumped into first an air stripper at 50 gallons/minute and then into a 10,000 gallon bioreactor, with a site-specific microbial consortium. The effluent from the bioreactor is directly discharged under national permits. Discharge levels less than 5 ppb for chlorinated hydrocarbons, 500 ppb for acetone and ketones, and 1 ppm for alcohols and glycols have been achieved continuously during more than three years of operation of the system.

This case illustrates the use of combined technologies. Neither air stripping nor biotreatment alone was effective in reducing the contaminants to acceptable levels. The combination was cost-effective and prevented any movement of the groundwater plume.

A particularly common groundwater contaminant is trichloroethylene (TCE). Nelson, Pritchard, & Bourquin (1988), while at the U.S. Environmental Protection Agency, isolated a Pseudomonas strain G4 which grows on phenol and in which phenol induces a monooxygenase which biodegrades TCE, as well as phenol. This organism has been employed in a bioreactor through which TCE-contaminated groundwater is pumped. It would not be permissible to add phenol, a toxic compound, as a "nutrient" for this strain in the environmental compartment. However, Nelson and Bourquin, now at Ecova Corporation, a leading environmental biotechnology company, have discovered a non-toxic, fully metabolized substitute substrate/inducer to replace phenol. With this proprietary system, they have been able to utilize the G4 strain by direct injection in a suitable well-demarcated groundwater site (Bourquin, personal communication).

These kinds of metabolic manipulations presage genetic manipulations. An alternative genetically-engineered solution, which eliminates the need for phenol or another inducer altogether, is the construction of a constitutive toluene monooxygenase producing *E. coli* strain; Winter, Yen, & Ensley (1989) at Amgen, Inc, used recombinant DNA techniques to introduce the toluene-oxidizing pathway genes from *Pseudomonas mendocina* KR-1 into the *E. coli* host. This organism has not yet been utilized in field trials.

V. PROSPECTS FOR GENETICALLY-ENGINEERED ORGANISMS

The modern manipulations feasible with recombinant DNA biotechnology permit modifications of existing strains of bacteria to assure higher biodegradative activity of key enzyme steps, to overcome substrate inhibition, to combine enzymes from unrelated metabolic pathways, to broaden substrate specificity, and to ensure complete mineralization of toxic intermediates. [See Timmis and others discussed in Omenn, 1988, and Chakrabarty, Kamely, & Omenn, 1990.] Recombinant environmental biotechnology is an exciting area for basic and applied research. Molecular, microbiological, and ecological tools are available for empirical studies that should steadily advance our knowledge and narrow our uncertainties about the behavior and effects of both genetically engineered and indigenous organisms. Systematic risk assessment can be carried out (Omenn & Borquin, 1990).

I confidently predict major advances in biotechnological solutions to these many kinds of hazardous waste clean-up challenges. And I urge that here in Taiwan, in the United States and Europe, and in Third World Countries we stimulate the use of biological systems in cleaning up polluted soil and water before these accumulations in the aggregate poison life on our Planet.

International Cooperation

As Rene Dubos stated, "Trend is not destiny." Those of us with capabilities of biotechnology and engineering have the opportunity to modify severely negative trends in environmental contamination. Dubos also stated, "Think globally; act locally." We must not be deterred by the huge scale of some of the environmental challenges; every desirable local act is a step in the right direction.

This Symposium and many analogous international conferences have recognized that multinational actions are required to address global environmental risks. Significant cooperative efforts can be cited (Matthews, 1987). Nine countries cooperate in the Nile River Basin; 18 in the Mediterranean Regional Sea Agreement, the model for what are now 11 regional sea agreements with 120 participating countries; 34 in the Long-Range Transboundary Air Pollution Agreement; 61 nations in the London Dumping Convention; and hopefully all countries in the Montreal Accord on restriction of chlorofluorocarbons. The Law of the Sea, Outer Space, and Antarctica Treaties are other major cooperative efforts.

The World Health Organization has established in this Western Pacific Region a Centre for Promotion of Environmental Planning and Applied Studies (PEPAS), now 14 years old, located in Kuala Lumpur. Finally, there is an ongoing struggle to make environmental assessments a routine and effective part of World Bank and other economic development efforts under the important theme of "sustainable development" (Clark & Munn, 1986; World Commission, 1987; World Resources Institute, 1989).

Albert Schweitzer, in his introduction to Rachel Carson's famous book *Silent Spring*, wrote in 1962 that "Man has lost the capacity to foresee and forestall." His gloomy conclusion was that "Man will end by destroying the Earth." We have the mission to respond to Schweitzer's challenge: to show that we can at least try to foresee and forestall adverse consequences, while gaining benefits for the people, the economies, and the eco-systems of Planet Earth through Environmental Biotechnology.

ADDENDUM

An up-to-date listing of field applications of bioremediation in the United States was published by the EPA Office of Solid Waste and Emergency Response and Office of Research and Development in August, 1991 (EPA/540/2-91//018): "Bioremediation in the Field."

ACKNOWLEDGMENTS

I am grateful to Dr. Al W. Bourquin, Vice President and Chief Scientist, Ecova Corporation, Redmond, Washington, and affiliate professor, Dept of Environmental Health, School of Public Health, University of Washington, for the two figures and field studies demonstrating applications of environmental biotechnology.

REFERENCES

Bourquin A.W. (1989). Bioremediation of hazardous waste. *Hazardous Materials*, 16-23, 48-59.

Castleman B.I. & Navarro, V. (1987). International mobility of hazardous products, industries, and wastes. *Annual Review Public Health* 7, 1-19.

Chakrabarty, A.M., Kamely D., & Omenn G.S. (eds). (1990). Biotechnology and Biodegradation. Woodlands, TX: Portfolio Publishing.

Clark, W.C. & Munn R.E. (1986). Sustainable Development of the Biosphere. Cambridge Univeristy Press, Cambridge.

Gibson, D.T. (1984). *Microbial Degradation of Organic Compounds*. Microbiology Series, 13. New York: Marcel Dekker, Inc.

Guo, P.H. (1989). Promoting a health environment, the Centre for Promotion of Environmental Planning and Applied Research. *World Health*, 10-11.

Mathews, J.T. (1987). International cooperation in environmentally sound economic development. In Report of Salzburg Seminar No. 259, Managing Global Environmental Risks, Salzburg, Austria.

Nelson, M.J.K., Pritchard, P.H., & Bourquin A.W. (1988). Preliminary development of a bench-scale treatment system for aerobic degradation of trichloroethylene. In G.S. Omenn (ed), *Environmental Biotechnology: Reducing Risks of Environmental Chemicals through Biotechnology* (pp. 203-209). Plenum Press, New York.

National Academy of Sciences Council. (1987). Introduction of Recombinant DNA-Engineered Organisms into the Environment: Key Issues. National Academy Press, Washington DC.

Omenn, G.S. (ed). (1988). Environmental Biotechnology, Reducing Risks from Environmental Chemicals through Biotechnology. New York: Plenum Press.

Omenn, G.S. & Bourquin, A.W. (1990). Risk assessment for biodegradation in pollution control and pollution clean-up. In A.M. Chakrabarty, D. Kamely, & G.S. Omenn (eds), *Biotechnology and Biodegradation*. Portfolio Publishing Co., Woodlands, TX.

Omenn, G.S. & Hollaender, A. (eds). (1984). Genetic control of environmental pollutants. New York: Plenum Press.

Repetto R. (1985). Paying the price: Pesticide subsidies in developing countries. Washington DC: World Resources Institute.

Tiedje, J.M., Colwell, R.R., Grossman, Y.L., Hodson, R.E., Lenski, R.E., Mack, R.N., & Regal, P.J. (1989). The planned introduction of genetically engineered organisms: Ecological considerations and recommendations. A report of the Ecological Society of America. *Ecology* 70, 298-315.

Winter, R.B., Yen, K.M., & Ensley, B.D. (1989). Efficient degradation of trichloroethylene by a recombinant. *Escherichia coli. Biotech* 7, 282-285.

World Commission on Environment and Development (Brundtland Commission). (1987). Final Report, Our Common Future. Geneva, Switzerland.

World Resources Institute, International Institute for Environment and Development, and United Nations Environment Programme. (1989). World Resources 1988-89, An Assessment of the Resource Base that Supports the Global Economy. New York: Basic Books.

PART IV

THE ECONOMICS OF HEALTH CARE

HEALTH INSURANCE AND ACCESS TO HEALTH CARE

Karen Davis

The U.S. health system is increasingly the subject of critical reexamination and calls for major reform. After pursuing a policy of promoting access to health care services in the 1960s and 1970s, the emphasis shifted to curbing rising health care costs in the 1980s. Many have come to feel that the United States fails to achieve either objective—leaving millions of Americans without health insurance coverage yet spending far more than any other industrialized nation on health care.

As the nation enters a new decade and nears the beginning of a new century, it is an important time of reassessment for national health policy. Several efforts are currently underway in the United States to develop major health care reform proposals. This paper summarizes the experience to date with assuring access to health care in the United States and describes the Pepper Commission comprehensive health financing reform proposal currently under consideration. It concludes with an analysis of this proposal and its merits for shaping the future of U.S. health financing policy.

Research in Human Capital and Development, Volume 7, pages 287-306.

ISBN: 1-55938-132-9

I. THE GREAT SOCIETY AND EXPANDED HEALTH INSURANCE COVERAGE

Commitment to ensuring access to health care has never been complete in the United States. Beginning in the early 1950s, employers have voluntarily provided private health insurance to workers and their dependents. Today, most of those who work receive some private health insurance coverage through their employment (CBO, 1979; Congressional Research Service, 1988; Davis, 1975). However, not all firms provide such coverage. Many small businesses, and businesses in the agriculture, construction, retail trade, and service sectors of the economy do not cover their workers.

In 1965 the federal government enacted Medicare and Medicaid to provide coverage under public programs for many of those without access to employer health benefits—the aged and certain groups of poor (Davis & Schoen, 1978). Medicare is a federal health financing program that covers those who are permanently and totally disabled as well as nearly all individuals age 65 and above. Medicaid is a federal-state government program that covers low-income women, children, elderly, and disabled individuals. Many poor people are excluded, however, because of strict limits on income and assets to qualify for eligibility and because of exclusion of most working age men and adults without children.

Other federal programs enacted in the mid-1960s and early 1970s expanded the availability of health resources in rural and high poverty inner city areas. State and local governments have traditionally sponsored public community hospitals and clinics to provide services as a last resort to those unable to pay. Some private, voluntary hospitals and most teaching hospitals have been a major source of charity care (Feder, Hadley, & Mullner, 1984).

The accumulated evidence suggests that these governmental health programs have been an important contributing factor to major gains in health in the last 25 years (Davis, 1973, 1976; Davis & Schoen, 1978; Rogers & Blendon, 1977; Rogers, Blendon, & Moloney, 1982). These gains have been especially noteworthy for the aged and for minorities. As shown in Table 1, life expectancy at birth in the United States has jumped a total of 5 years from 1960 to 1987—from 69.7 years to 74.9 years. Blacks experienced greater gains in life expectancy at birth than whites, with especially marked improvements for black women (an increase of 8 years in life expectancy at birth).

Longer life expectancy at birth reflects lower infant mortality and lower death rates in middle age. However, a substantial portion of the improvement in life expectancy is accounted for by improvements in health of the aged. As shown in Table 1, life expectancy at age 65 increased 2.6 years between 1960 and 1987. Leading the gains in improved life expectancy among the aged were white women, who upon reaching the age of 65 in 1987 live an average of 18.7

Table 1. Life expectancy, by race and sex, 1960-1987, selected years (in years)

	1960	*1970*	*1975*	*1980*	*1987*	*% Change 1960-1987*
Life expectancy at birth						
Total	69.7	70.9	72.6	73.7	74.9	7.5%
White men	67.4	68.0	69.5	70.7	72.1	7.0
White women	74.1	75.6	77.3	78.1	78.8	6.3
Black men	60.7	60.0	62.4	63.7	65.4	7.7
Black women	65.9	68.3	71.3	72.3	73.8	12.0
Life expectancy at age 65						
Total	14.3	15.2	16.1	16.4	16.9	18.9%
White men	12.9	13.1	13.8	14.2	14.9	15.5
White women	15.9	17.1	18.2	18.5	18.7	17.6
Black men	12.7	12.5	13.1	12.9	13.6	7.1
Black women	15.1	15.7	16.7	16.5	17.2	13.9

Source: U.S. Department of Health and Human Services, National Center for Health Statistics, *Health, United States, 1988*, p. 53.

more years, three years longer than in 1960. Medicare deserves at least a portion of the credit for the increased life expectancy experienced by those 65 and above.

Gains in health status have been especially rapid for those causes of death amenable to medical care intervention and which historically have been higher among the poor. As shown in Table 2, age-adjusted death rates for the entire population declined 29 percent from 1960 to 1986. Deaths from strokes dropped by 61 percent over this period—reflecting both the lower rate of uncontrolled hypertension in the population and improved health services. Deaths from pneumonia and influenza were cut in half between 1960 and 1986; historically the poor have died from these causes at a greater rate than higher income individuals. Heart disease death rates fell by 39 percent; while the exact reasons for this decline are uncertain better availability of sophisticated health services and emergency medical care may be an important factor. Death from diabetes declined moderately over the period, as did accidental deaths. Upward trends were evident in deaths from cancer, especially respiratory cancer, suicide, and homicide. These increases are more related to smoking, stress, and crime levels and could not be expected to be especially sensitive to the availability of improved health services.

Infant health has also improved over the last 25 years. Infant mortality, as shown in Table 3, has dropped by 62 percent between 1960 and 1987, dropping from 26 deaths per 1000 live births in 1960 to 10.0 deaths per 1000 live births in 1987. This is especially significant in light of the fact that infant mortality rates were virtually unchanged in the ten years preceding passage of Medicaid

Table 2. Age-adjusted death rates, by cause, 1960-1986, selected years (Deaths per 100,000 population)

	1960	*1970*	*1980*	*1986*	*Percent Change 1960-1987*
All causes	760.9	714.3	585.8	541.7	−28.8%
Diseases of the heart	286.2	253.6	202.0	175.0	−38.9
Cerebrovascular disease	79.7	66.3	40.8	31.0	−61.1
Cancer	125.8	129.9	132.8	133.2	5.9
Respiratory	19.2	28.4	36.4	39.0	103.1
Colorectal	17.7	16.8	15.5	14.4	−18.6
Breast	22.3	23.1	22.7	23.1	3.6
Pneumonia and influenza	28.0	22.1	12.9	13.5	−51.8
Cirrhosis and liver disease	10.5	14.7	12.2	9.2	−12.4
Diabetes mellitus	13.6	14.1	10.1	9.6	−29.4
Accidents	49.9	53.7	42.3	35.2	−29.5
Suicide	10.6	11.8	11.4	11.9	12.3
Homicide	5.2	9.1	10.8	9.0	73.1

Source: U.S. Department of Health and Human Services, National Center for Health Statistics, Health, United States, 1988, p. 62.

and other Great Society health programs for the poor. Rates for both whites and blacks have declined at similar rates—with black infant mortality rates continuing to be about twice as high as those of whites throughout the period. Some progress has also been made in reducing the proportion of low birth weight infants. The percent of infants weighing less than 2,500 grams has declined from 7.9 percent in 1970 to 6.8 percent in 1986 (see Table 3).

More women are getting care early in pregnancy. Studies have shown that receiving prenatal care in the first trimester is important in reducing infant mortality and low birth weight infants—by identifying high risk mothers and getting chronic health problems that can have an adverse effect on birth outcomes under control (e.g., diabetes, anemia) (Institute of Medicine, 1985). The proportion of white women receiving prenatal care in the first trimester increased from 72.4 percent in 1970 to 79.2 percent in 1986. For black women the gains were even more striking. The proportion of black women receiving prenatal care in the first trimester increased from 44.4 percent in 1970 to 61.6 percent in 1986.

Perhaps the most compelling evidence on the success of the Great Society programs for the poor has been the improved access to physician services. The poor, now as in the past, are much more likely than high income persons to have fair or poor health and to suffer from chronic health conditions (Davis & Schoen, 1978). Despite their poorer health status, low-income persons in 1964 were twice as likely not to have seen a physician in the previous two years as high income persons (Table 4). By 1987 the proportion of the low-income population not seeing a physician in the last two years was only 20 percent greater than that of the high income population.

Table 3. Infant health, 1960-1981, Selected Years

	1960	*1970*	*1975*	*1980*	*1986*	*Percent Change 1960-1986*
Infant deaths per 1000 live births						
Total	26.0	20.0	16.1	12.6	10.1[1]	−61.5%[2]
White	22.9	17.8	14.2	11.0	8.9	−61.1
Black	44.3	32.6	26.2	21.4	18.0	−59.4
Percent of live births with birth weight of 2,500 grams or less						
Total	n.a.	7.94%	7.39%	6.84%	6.81%	−14.2%[3]
White	n.a.	6.84	6.26	5.70	5.64	−17.5[3]
Black	n.a.	13.86	13.09	12.49	12.53	−9.6[3]
Percent of live births with prenatal care beginning in first trimester						
Total	n.a.	68.0%	72.4%	76.3%	75.9%	11.6%[3]
White	n.a.	72.4	75.9	79.3	79.2	9.4[3]
Black	n.a.	44.4	55.8	62.7	61.6	38.7[3]

Notes: [1] 1987
[2] Percent change, 1960-1987
[3] Percent Change 1970-1986.

Source: U.S. Department of Health and Human Services, National Center for Health Statistics, *Health, United States, 1988*, p. 47, 54.

Table 4. Percent with Interval of Two Years or More Since Last Physician Contact, by Family Income, 1964, 1982, and 1987

	1964	*1982*	*1987*	*Percent change 1964-1987*
Percent not seeing a physician in previous two years				
All family income[1]	19.1	13.2	12.8	−33.0%
Under $10,000	28.2	12.5	12.8	−54.6
$10,000-14,999	23.3	13.9	14.9	−36.0
$15,000-19,999	18.7	14.9	14.9	−20.3
$20,000-34,999	15.7	13.7	12.9	−17.8
$35,000 and over	13.5	11.8	10.8	−20.0

Note: [1] Family income categories for 1987. Income categories in 1964 are: less than $2,000-$3,999; $4,000-$6,999; $7,000-$9,999; and $10,000 or more; and, in 1982 are: less than $7,000; $7,000-$9,999; $10,000-$14,999; $15,000-$24,999 and $25,000 or more.

Source: U.S. Department of Health and Human Services, National Center for Health Statistics, *Health, United States*, 1988, p. 107.

The introduction of Medicaid and other Great Society health programs had a major impact in assisting those covered with gaining access to physician services at levels comparable to those of higher income persons with similar health problems. This is particularly evident when the rate of physician visits of poor people with and without Medicaid are compared. As shown in Table 5, in

Table 5. Adjusted Mean Annual Physician Contacts According to Poverty and Medicaid Status, United States, 1982

		Below Poverty	
	Above Poverty	*With Medicaid*	*Without Medicaid*
All Ages	5.3	5.7[1]	3.9[3]
Under 17 Years	4.4	4.2[1]	3.3[3]
17-44 Years	4.8	6.3[2]	3.9[3]
45-64 Years	6.5	4.0[1]	1.6[3]
65+ Years	7.9	9.2[1]	7.1[1]

Notes: [1] Not Significant ($p \geq 0.05$)
[2] $< .05$
[3] $< .01$

Source: Newacheck, P.W. 1988. "Access to Ambulatory Care for Poor Persons." *HSR: Health Services Research*, 23:3. August. p. 411.

Table 6. Hospital discharges per 1000 population, by age and family income, 1964, 1981, and 1987

	1964	*1982*	*1987*	*Percent change 1964-1987*
Total	109.1	121.7	96.5	−9.6%
By age				
< 15 yrs	67.6	64.3	48.6	−28.1
15-44	100.6	97.0	69.2	−31.2
45-64	146.2	175.1	143.3	−2.1
65 yrs and over	190.0	283.6	255.6	34.5
By family income[1,2]				
Under $10,000	102.4	165.1	143.7	40.3
$10,000-14,999	116.4	137.5	132.6	13.9
$15,000-19,999	110.7	124.5	102.4	−7.5
$20,000-34,999	109.2	119.8	87.9	−19.5
$35,000 or more	110.7	104.6	77.1	−30.4

Notes: [1] Age Adjusted.
[2] Family income categories for 1987. Income categories in 1964 are: less than $2,000; $2,000-$3,999; $4,000-$6,999; $7,000-$9,999, and $10,000 or more; and, in 1981 are: less than $7,000; $7,000-$9,999; $10,000-$14,999; $15,000-$24,999; and $25,000 or more.

Source: U.S. Department of Health and Human Services, National Center for Health Statistics, *Health, United States, 1988*, p. 111.

1982 poor people on Medicaid saw physicians an average of 5.7 times per year, compared to 5.3 times for nonpoor persons—adjusting for differences in health status. Poor people not covered by Medicaid, however, lagged well behind in use of physician services—averaging 3.9 physician visits per person annually.

Hospital utilization among the general population has declined over the period since the introduction of the Great Society. In 1964 hospital discharges per 1000 population averaged 109.1; by 1987 this had dropped to 96.5 (see Table 6). With shortening hospital stays over this period, days of hospital care dropped even more rapidly. Important increases in hospital utilization did occur, however, for the poor and for the aged. As shown in Table 6, hospital discharges for the aged increased from 190 per 1000 in 1964 to 256 per 1000 in 1987. Studies have demonstrated that much of this gain in hospital use reflects an improved quality of life for the elderly—with major increases in cataract surgery and hip replacements (Davis & Schoen, 1978). Medicare has made this use of modern medical technology affordable for the old and their families.

II. RETRENCHMENT IN THE REAGAN ERA

The U.S. health financing system came under considerable strain in the 1980s. Federal and state government budgetary restraint has curbed the growth in outlays under Medicaid (Rowland, Lyons, & Edwards, 1988). The changing nature of employment and pressure from international competition have contributed to cutbacks in employee health benefits (Davis, et al., 1990). Competition among health care providers has reduced the availability of charity care (Rowland, 1987).

These changes began in 1981 as the Reagan Administration ushered in a major shift in health policy. Unlike previous administrations, it did not propose expanded coverage through a national health insurance plan. Rather, it called for major cutbacks in Medicare and Medicaid, and governmental funding for direct primary care delivery programs (Davis, 1981).

The U.S. Congress responded by attempting to protect the poor and elderly from harmful cuts in health programs. Medicare deductibles for hospital and physician services were increased, but Reagan budget proposals to institute a 10 percent hospital copayment and to increase the Medicare premium paid by beneficiaries to cover a greater share of outlays for physician services were not enacted. Similarly, coverage of the working poor under Medicaid was restricted in 1981, but the Congress subsequently expanded coverage for poor pregnant women, children, elderly, and disabled. Reagan Administration proposals for New Federalism to set a cap on federal payments for Medicaid or to turn the program over to state governments were defeated. Reagan Administration proposals to reduce funding for primary care delivery programs by 25 percent and fold into state block grants were similarly rejected. Instead Congress increased funding for primary care centers moderately and explicitly exempted them from Gramm-Rudman automatic budget cuts. However, the need to find budgetary savings to counter Reagan administration proposals led to a number of legislative changes to tighten hospital and physician payment rates under Medicare and to give states greater flexibility to set payment limits under Medicaid.

Table 7. Percent of Persons under 65 Years of Age without Health Insurance Coverage, by Family Income, 1980 and 1986

	1980	*1986*	*Percent Change 1980-1986*
Total, all family incomes[1]	12.5%	15.3%	22.4%
Less than $10,000	31.0	37.0	19.4
$10,000-$14,999	25.9	31.3	20.8
$15,000-$19,999	15.0	21.2	41.3
$20,000-$34,999	6.2	8.4	35.5
$35,000 or more	3.9	3.9	0.0

Note: [1] Family income categories for 1980 are: less than $7,000; $7,000-$9,999, $10,000-$14,999; $15,000-$24,999; $25,000 or more.

Source: U.S. Department of Health and Human Services, National Center for Health Statistics, *Health, United States, 1987*, p. 171.

The preoccupation with cutting Medicare, Medicaid, and primary care budgetary outlays and the absence of any Presidential leadership in support of national health insurance, however, have stymied serious efforts to make further progress in improving access to health care. The result has been a marked slowdown in further improvements in improving health of the poor, and mounting evidence of a deterioration in access to health care services.

The number of uninsured has increased steadily throughout the 1980s. As shown in Table 7, the proportion of the population under age 65 without health insurance coverage from either a private plan or a public program increased from 12.5 percent in 1980 to 15.3 percent in 1986—or from about 29 million people in 1980 to 37 million people in 1986.

The majority of nonelderly Americans receive health insurance coverage through their employers. Consequently, the common impression is that the uninsured are outside the work force—mostly young adults who have not yet found jobs. This is not the case. Surprisingly, over half of the uninsured, 19.6 million people, are in families where at least one member has a full-time job working 35 or more hours per week. Two-thirds of the uninsured are in families where at least one member works at least 17 1/2 or more hours per week (Congressional Research Service, 1988).

Gaps in employer-provided health insurance coverage occur because such coverage is optional for employers. About half of all employed uninsured persons work in firms with fewer than 25 employees. Employer-provided health insurance coverage is particularly low in certain industries—including agriculture, construction, retail trade, and services. Coverage of workers is lower in the South and West than in the North and Central regions of the country.

About one-third of the uninsured are children under age 18. Half of the uninsured are parents or other adults between the ages of 17 and 45. The remaining sixteen percent of the uninsured are split equally between older adults between the ages of 45 and 54 and between the ages of 55 and 64. Many of these older adults are widows or spouses of retired persons who do not yet qualify for Medicare.

Nearly all of the uninsured have modest incomes. About one-third have incomes below the poverty level. Only 20 percent have incomes greater than three times the poverty level. Individual purchase of private health insurance is not economically feasible for most of the uninsured. Individual plans typically have inadequate benefits and charge premiums well in excess of actual benefit outlays (Congressional Research Service, 1988).

Although Medicaid provides a safety net for many low-income families, it fails to cover the majority of the poor. Absence of Medicaid coverage among the poor occurs because states set income eligibility levels well below the federal poverty level and because categorical restrictions limit coverage largely to one-parent families—excluding two parent poor families, childless couples, and single individuals (Congressional Research Service, 1988; Schoen, 1984).

To a considerable extent health insurance coverage in the United States is a matter of luck. Those fortunate enough to be employed by large, unionized, manufacturing firms are also likely to be fortunate enough to have good health insurance coverage. Those who have modest incomes, live in the South and West or in rural areas, and those who are black or minority group members are more likely to bear the personal and economic effects of lack of insurance and the consequent financial barriers to health care.

Several factors account for deterioration in health insurance coverage in the 1980s:

- The growth of jobs in the service sector which tend not to have health insurance coverage.
- The growth of jobs in smaller firms.
- The increasing tendency for employers to require employee contributions to health insurance premiums, including paying the full cost of dependent coverage.
- The growth in one-parent families, who are less likely to have health insurance coverage than two-worker families.
- The growth in the number of adults between the ages of 17 and 45 who are less likely to have health insurance coverage.
- Financial pressures on government and employers that have led to a reduction in coverage.

While considerable further analysis and research will be required to sort out the independent contribution of these and other factors, it is clear that gaps in employer-provided health insurance are responsible for a large portion of the uninsured population.

The reversal of trends in health insurance coverage have important implications for trends in improving health of the disadvantaged and in access to health care services. A close examination of the trends in health status shown in Tables 1-3 reveals that most of the gains in improved health occurred in the period from 1960 to 1980, with relatively little further progress during the 1980s. Life expectancy at birth and at age 65 have increased only moderately since 1980. Age adjusted deaths from pneumonia and influenza are up slightly in the 1980s, although further improvements have occurred in death rates from diseases of the heart and cerebrovascular diseases. Infant mortality rates have declined slowly in the 1980s (Griffith & Cislowski, 1986). However, the percent of black babies weighing less than 2500 grams is up slightly, and the percent of black women receiving care in the first trimester of pregnancy is down somewhat. These data suggest that progress in improving health of poor and minority population groups has certainly slowed or halted, if not actually reversed.

A 1986 report supported by the Robert Wood Johnson Foundation contained evidence on the deterioration in access to health care in the 1980s (Freeman, et al., 1988). According to the survey, the years 1982 through 1986 witnessed a reversal in the trends over several prior decades of improving access to health services for low-income groups. For example, the rate of physician visits by low-income and black individuals in fair or poor health decreased between 1982 and 1986 (Table 8). On the other hand, physician visits by nonpoor and white individuals with similar health status increased over the same period, widening a gap that had virtually disappeared prior to the last decade.

The uninsured are one-third more likely to be in fair or poor health than the nonelderly insured. Yet despite their poorer health status, in 1986 the uninsured received 27 percent fewer physician services (Table 8) and were hospitalized 19 percent less frequently than the insured. Further, one-fifth of the uninsured with chronic illnesses did not see a physician during the year. Fully two-thirds of the uninsured with serious symptoms (e.g., bleeding, loss of consciousness, chest pain, shortness of breath, weight loss unrelated to diet) did not see or contact a physician. One-fifth of uninsured pregnant women did not receive care in the first trimester of pregnancy. Twenty-two percent of the uninsured with hypertension did not receive a blood pressure check in the year (Freeman, et al., 1987).

Clearly, lack of health insurance coverage presents a significant threat to maintaining health and economic security. In all, 13.5 million people reported not receiving medical care for financial reasons in 1986. An estimated one million individuals actually tried to obtain needed care but were turned away. Millions of Americans are at risk of death and disability because of an inability to pay for needed health care (Freeman, et al., 1987).

Table 8. Mean Number of Physician Visits by Insurance Coverage, Race, and Income, 1982 and 1986

	1982	*1986*	*Percent Change*
Uninsured	3.8	3.2	−16.8%
Insured	4.7	4.4	−6.4
% Difference	−19.0	−27.0	
Black[1]	7.6	6.8	−10.5
White[1]	8.6	10.1	17.4
% Difference	−12.0	−33.0	
Poor and near poor[1]	9.1	8.4	−7.7
Nonpoor[1]	8.1	11.5	42.0
% Difference	+12.0	−27.0	

Note: [1] Includes only individuals reporting their health as fair or poor.
Source: Freeman, et al. (1987. pp. 10-13).

III. LOOKING FORWARD TO THE TWENTY-FIRST CENTURY

The United States moves toward the twenty-first century with several major problems in its system of financing health care for its citizens. Over 35 million Americans have no health insurance coverage—and evidence of the failure to get needed medical care as a result is a national embarrassment. The private health insurance market is becoming increasingly selective—with insurers declining to cover or restricting benefits for individuals viewed to be poor health risks. AIDS and biomedical advances in genetic screening that make it possible to identify individuals at risk for a wide range of health conditions will exacerbate this trend.

In addition, as the U.S. population ages markedly in the next several decades the inadequacy of financing long-term care will become more serious. Over 30 percent of the nation's elderly live alone—many without a child nearby to provide assistance when their ability to care for themselves becomes impaired (Commonwealth Commission, 1987). Substitutes for family care in the form of formal personal care are not widely available, not covered by Medicare or private health insurance, and of very uneven reliability and quality where they exist.

At the same time the United States spends 11 percent of its GNP on health care—40 percent more than the next closest country (Schieber & Poullier, 1989). Further, health as a percent of GNP has been increasing steadily throughout the 1980s—while it has stabilized at about 7 to 8 percent of GNP in most other industrialized nations. Medicare and Medicaid represent the most rapidly increasing segments of federal and state government budgets.

To further complicate matters, Medicare will enter the next century on the brink of insolvency. The hospital portion of Medicare is financed by a payroll tax set at 2.9 percent of earnings (including both the employer and employee share). By 1995 outlays under the hospital portion of Medicare will exceed payroll tax revenues flowing into the Hospital Insurance Trust Fund—beginning the depletion of accumulated reserves (Ways and Means, 1989). By the year 2006 under the most realistic economic assumptions, the Trust Fund will be bankrupt. This is just before the impact of the post World War II baby boom bulge begins to affect retirement and growth in Medicare enrollment.

The magnitude of the problem the United States faces is beginning to be reflected in calls for a fundamental reform of our health care financing system. In March of this year, a Bipartisan Commission on Health Care Reform—called the Pepper Commission in honor of the late Senator Claude Pepper who proposed legislation establishing the Commission—issued a report calling for universal health insurance coverage and long-term care financing for all Americans (Pepper, 1990). While the recommendations of this Commission are controversial and by no means certain of adoption, it seems likely that they will have an important influence on the shape of future health financing legislation.

Universal Health Insurance

The Pepper Commission proposal for assuring universal health insurance coverage has the following elements:

- All businesses with more than 100 employees would be required to provide all employees and nonworking dependents with private health insurance with specified minimum benefits or make a payroll tax contribution to a public plan. Employers would have to pay at least 80 percent of the private insurance premium. The minimum benefit plan includes hospital and physician services subject to a $500 family deductible and a 20 percent coinsurance with a maximum $3,000 annual ceiling on out-of-pocket spending. Preventive services such as prenatal care, well-child care, mammograms, and Pap smears are covered with no cost-sharing.
- Businesses with less than 100 employees would receive incentives to provide coverage voluntarily to employees and dependents. This includes a tax credit/subsidy of 40 percent of private health insurance premiums, reforms to make such insurance more affordable, and the option of purchasing coverage for employees under a public plan by making a payroll tax contribution. If, after five years, at least 80 percent of small businesses did not provide coverage to workers voluntarily, such coverage would be mandatory.

- The Pepper plan calls for replacing Medicaid with a new public plan with provider payment rates set at Medicare levels. It would eliminate all premiums and coinsurance for persons with incomes below the poverty level and provide subsidies for those with incomes between 100 percent and 200 percent of the federal poverty income level.
- Finally, the Pepper plan would permit any individual not covered by an employer plan to purchase such coverage from a public plan. Premiums would be eliminated for those with incomes below the poverty level, and subsidized for those with incomes between 100 and 200 percent of the poverty income level.
- The plan is phased in gradually over seven years, beginning with coverage of larger firms and public plan coverage for poor pregnant women and children.

Long-Term Care Financing

The Pepper Commission also contains major recommendations to improve financing for long term care services for disabled individuals of all ages. These recommendations include:

- Providing up to 400 hours of home care for disabled individuals annually. Adult day care services may be substituted on a two-for-one basis with hours of home care coverage.
- Coverage of the first three months of nursing home care.
- Coverage of nursing home expenses after an individual has contributed all except $30,000 of assets excluding the home and 30 percent of income.

Health System Reform

The Pepper Commission also set forth recommendations for major reforms in the health system:

- Private health insurance sold to small businesses would be regulated to guarantee community rating, prohibit refusing coverage to high-risk groups or individuals, or excluding coverage for pre-existing health conditions.
- Managed care options such as health maintenance organizations and preferred provider organizations would be made available to all persons covered by private or public plans.
- Private plans would be encouraged to pay physicians and hospitals according to Medicare payment rules which provide for compensation to physicians on the basis of a resource-based relative value fee schedule tied to a target on total outlays and to hospitals on the basis of Diagnosis-Related Group prospective per patient payment rates. The new public

plan for employment groups and individuals would also follow Medicare provider payment rules.

- The two Congressional Commissions charged with developing recommendations for the Congress on payment of hospitals (Prospective Payment Assessment Commission) and physicians (Physician Payment Review Commission) under Medicare would be asked to develop recommendations with regard to provider payment under private health insurance plans.
- Primary care services in underserved rural and inner-city poverty communities would be expanded.
- Funding for health promotion, disease prevention, risk reduction, and health education programs would be expanded by $1 billion.
- Development of national practice guidelines and standards of care, expanded funding of effectiveness and health outcomes research, development of more effective methods of quality assessment and assurance, and a uniform health care data system would be facilitated.

Cost

The Pepper Commission estimated that the total cost of the plan when fully implemented would be $66.2 billion in net new annual federal expenditures. This includes $23.4 billion for universal health insurance coverage and $42.8 billion for long-term care financing. Some of these costs represent the replacement of federal government expenditures for services that are now financed privately—typically directly by patients who would be subsidized under the plan. The net new spending in the health system for acute health care services is estimated at $15 billion.

These costs—while modest compared to the $600 billion the United States spends on health care—have proved to be the most controversial feature of the plan. The plan did not make recommendations about specific new taxes to finance the public cost of the plan, but rather stipulated that any financing source should be progressive, adequate to cover expenditures both initially and over time, and applied to persons of all ages—rather than financed by only the working population or the elderly population, for example.

Evaluation

The Pepper plan has several key characteristics that are particularly designed for the U.S. economic and political system. It builds on the American tradition of employer-provided health insurance coverage for workers and their families and public plan coverage for those falling outside the workplace. Building on this structure, it proposes a fundamental strengthening and integration of our mixed private-public system of health insurance coverage to guarantee coverage to all Americans. There are many innovative features of this plan which deserve special attention.

Insurance Market Reform

The private health insurance market is becoming increasingly selective—with insurers declining to cover individuals viewed to be poor health risks or instituting restrictions or waiting periods for pre-existing conditions. Small businesses, in particular, risk having their coverage dropped if a worker or family member gets ill, or have certain individuals excluded from coverage, or find premiums raised to exorbitant levels.

One of the most important features of the Pepper plan is the reform of the insurance market. It would prohibit excluding individuals or pre-existing conditions in small group plans. It would require that the same coverage be offered to all firms on the same terms. A voluntary reinsurance mechanism for high-risk individuals would be established. These changes would go far to curb the worst abuses in the small employer insurance market, and forestall even greater trends toward denying coverage to high risk individuals.

Option of Purchasing Medicare-Type Public Coverage

Another extremely innovative feature of the Pepper plan is the option it gives all employers and all non-working individuals to purchase coverage from a Medicare-type public plan. Employers could make a payroll tax contribution to cover all workers, or part-time workers only. This would eliminate the necessity for small businesses to provide and administer an adequate private insurance plan. It would provide subsidies for low-wage firms who found the private health insurance premium excessive. It would provide a stable source of insurance coverage for part-time, temporary, and seasonal workers who are in and out of the workplace. Unemployed workers could continue their coverage by picking up the premiums based on their ability to pay.

Most importantly, retired individuals or other non-working adults under age 65 would have the opportunity of buying-in to a Medicare type plan before age 65. Employers would have the option of purchasing this coverage for retirees rather than attempting to purchase such coverage from very expensive private plans. In other cases retirees do not receive any employer-provided health insurance. For these older adults the option of purchasing Medicare-type coverage would be particularly attractive. Even disabled individuals must wait at least two years for Medicare coverage. Spouses or widows of Medicare beneficiaries who are under 65 do not quality for Medicare. Such individuals could purchase coverage with subsidies for those with incomes below 200 percent of poverty.

Medicaid Reform

The Pepper plan would replace the current Medicaid program with a universal low-income entitlement program that is not tied to the welfare system—either in terms of eligibility or in terms of administration. All poor persons would receive coverage without charge under this new federal public plan. Near-poor persons would contribute up to 3 percent of income.

This new low-income plan would reverse some of the deterioration in the Medicaid program that has occurred as the result of budgetary cutbacks in the 1980s. Physicians and hospitals would be paid at Medicare payment rates—replacing the substandard Medicaid payment rates but incorporating the cost containment and efficiency incentives of Medicare. This should encourage greater provider participation and reverse the trend toward refusing care to Medicaid beneficiaries.

Cost Containment and Health System Reform

The Pepper plan also contains a number of innovative features to encourage efficiency in the health care system. The most important in my view is extending Medicare's provider payment principles to a broader beneficiary base. The recently enacted Medicare physician payment reform represents a fundamental reform of physician payment in this country. It would reverse the bias toward high-cost specialty care and provide greater rewards for primary care. It would limit the financial burden to beneficiaries through limits on balance billing. It would establish targets on total Medicare physician outlays known as Volume Performance Standards to curb rising expenditures.

The Pepper plan would extend this system of payment as well as the Medicare hospital prospective payment system to all beneficiaries covered under the public plan including employment groups and nonworking individuals electing to purchase such public plan coverage. This would greatly expand the scope and effectiveness of Medicare's cost containment measures. It would also strongly encourage private plans to adopt similar provider payment methods.

The one lesson from the experience of other industrialized nations that is most compelling is the effectiveness of cost containment in those systems with a strong government role in setting or negotiating provider payment rates. The Pepper plan is a significant step toward such an approach. Expanding the mandate of the Prospective Payment Assessment Commission and the Physician Payment Review Commission to develop recommendations on effective cost containment measures for both the public and private sectors is especially laudable.

Other recommendations that include support for effectiveness research, data systems including physician profiling and practice patterns for care of all patients not just Medicare beneficiaries, choices of managed care systems, funding of prevention, health education, outreach, and primary care, and quality assurance mechanisms are also extremely important.

Phasing

The Pepper plan would begin by insuring all our nation's children followed by phased implementation of insurance coverage for adults. This phasing places top priority on investing in the health of future generations by immediately assuring universal coverage of pregnant women and young children, with complete coverage of pre-natal, well-baby care, and other preventive services such as Pap smears and mammography. All uninsured pregnant women and children under age 6 would be eligible for public plan coverage, with full subsidies for those in families with incomes below 185 percent of the federal poverty level.

Coverage of working families and adults outside the workforce would be phased in beginning with incentives for smaller firms to offer coverage voluntarily, and following with mandatory coverage for larger firms and then smaller firms if coverage targets are not met voluntarily. In the final phases non-working adults would be permitted to purchase public plan coverage, with subsidies for poor and near poor adults.

This phasing enhances both the economic and administrative feasibility of the plan. It gives employers opportunities to plan for coverage of workers, and subsidizes the start-up of coverage by firms. It would give employers time to make adjustments in total compensation packages to minimize unemployment and economic disruption effects.

Another advantage of the phasing approach is that it permits mid-course corrections to be made if economic conditions change or if the demands on the federal budget or health system should prove different than anticipated. Subsequent phases can be delayed or accelerated, for example, if initial cost estimates prove high or low. Experience with the cost-containment provisions can indicate whether more stringent measures are required, or whether private and public plans are building on the best elements of managed care and provider payment currently incorporated in Medicare and employer plans. Coverage of an initial set of preventive services will provide evidence of the desirability of a broader preventive care benefit package.

Summary

In summary the Pepper plan both as a comprehensive package and as innovative improvements in existing programs has much to commend it. It represents an equitable sharing of the burden of the cost of financing health care among large and small employers, among workers, those able to afford to contribute individually to their own coverage, and federal and state governments. It builds on the administrative expertise in the private health insurance industry, while eliminating practices that have made health insurance unaffordable for many businesses. It institutes many much needed health system reform measures to curtail rising health care costs, and shifts the emphasis in our health system toward prevention and primary care. It moves immediately to address our underinvestment in the health of our children.

The Pepper Commission estimates that expanded health services for the uninsured would lead to a total increase in health spending of $15 billion annually—about 2.5 percent of current national health expenditures. With the expanding supply of physicians and hospital occupancy rates at record low levels, this new demand for health services should be easily accommodated without inflationary pressures.

While the cost and economic impact would be small relative to our nation's economic resources, the improved access to health care services would have a major impact on solving one of our nation's most pressing social problems. It would contribute to improved health of the population by removing financial barriers to medical care and increasing funding for prevention and primary care. Maternity and infant care services would be covered without cost-sharing for those covered by both employer plans and the new public plan that replaces Medicaid. Improved access to acute care for the uninsured will improve health and give children a better chance at productive lives.

The proposal would lead to a more equitable distribution of the financial burden of health care expenses. Maximum out-of-pocket ceilings on health care expenses would be instituted in all plans. Incentives to control costs and improve efficiency would be provided through numerous provider payment and system reform provisions. Quality standards would be developed and monitored through the public plan, private health insurance plans, and health maintenance organizations. Provider payment rates would be set to ensure continued room for technological progress and development.

While the fate of the Pepper Commission recommendations remains in doubt, it has stimulated serious debate in the United States about alternative directions for the health system. It is becomingly increasingly clear that the United States can not afford to continue on its present course—with a costly health system that lets many of its most vulnerable citizens fall through the safety net. Our problems will only be compounded as we experience an aging population—with growing needs for both acute and long-term care. We clearly have the economic and intellectual resources to meet this challenge. What we need is a national commitment to do so.

REFERENCES

Commonwealth Fund Commission on Elderly People Living Alone. (1987). M*edicare's Poor: Filling the Gaps in Medical Coverage for Low-Income Elderly Americans*, prepared by Diane Rowland & Barbara Lyons. Baltimore, MD: The Commonwealth Fund Commission on Elderly People Living Alone.

Commonwealth Fund Commission on Elderly People Living Alone. (1989). *Help at Home: Long-Term Care Assistance for Impaired Elderly People*, prepared by Diane Rowland. Baltimore, MD: The Commonwealth Fund Commission on Elderly People Living Alone.

Congressional Budget Office. (1979). *A Profile of the Uninsured: The Haves and Have Nots.* Washington, D.C.

Congressional Research Service. (1988). *Health Insurance and the Uninsured: Background Data and Analysis.* A Report prepared for the U.S. House of Representatives, Energy and Commerce Committee, Subcommittee on Health and the Environment, Committee Print Serial 100 X. Washington, DC: U. S. Government Printing Office.

Davis, K. (1973). Lessons of medicare and medicaid for national health insurance. Hearings on National Health Insurance, Subcommittee on Public Health and Environment, Committee on Interstate and Foreign Commerce, U.S. Congress, Washington, D.C.

Davis, K. (1975). *National health insurance: Benefits, costs, and consequences.* Washington, DC: The Brookings Institution.

Davis, K. (1976). "Achievements and Problems of Medicaid." *Public Health Reports*, 912(4): 309-316.

Davis, K. 1981. "Reagan Administration Health Policy." *Journal of Public Health Policy*, 2(4): 312-322.

Davis, K. 1983. "The Cost of Health Care for Families." Testimony before the Select Committee on Children, Youth, and Families, House of Representatives, U.S. Congress, Washington, D.C.

Davis, K., G. Anderson, D. Rowland, & E. Steinberg. (1990). *Health care cost containment.* Baltimore, MD: The Johns Hopkins Press.

Davis, K., & D. Rowland. (1983). "Uninsured and underserved: Inequities in health care in the United States." *Milbank Memorial Fund Quarterly/Health and Society*, 61(2).

Davis, K., & D. Rowland. (1986). *Medicare Policy: New Directions for Health and Long-Term Care.* Baltimore, MD: The Johns Hopkins Press.

Davis, K., & C. Schoen. (1978). *Health and the War on Poverty: A Ten Year Appraisal.* Washington, DC: The Brookings Institution.

Feder, J., Hadley J., & Mullner, R. (1984). "Falling Through the Cracks: Poverty, Insurance Coverage, and Hospital Care for the Poor, 1980 and 1982." *Milbank Memorial Fund Quarterly.*

Freeman, H.E., R. Blendon, L. Aiken, S. Sudman, C. Mullinix, & C. Corey. (1987). "Americans Report on Their Access to Health Care." *Health Affairs* 6(1): 6-18.

Griffith, J.E., & J.A. Cislowski. (1986). Infant mortality: Are We making progress? *Congressional Research Service Review*, January.

Iglehart, J.K. (1985). "Medical care of the poor: A growing problem." *New England Journal of Medicine*, 313(1): 59-63.

Institute of Medicine, Committee to Study the Prevention of Low Birthweight. (1985). *Preventing low birthweight.* Washington, DC: National Academy Press.

Lurie, N., Ward, N.B., Shapiro, M.F., & R.H. Brook. (1984). "Termination from medical: Does it affect health?" *New England Journal of Medicine*, 311(7): 480-484.

Newacheck, P.W. (1988). "Access to Ambulatory Care for Poor Persons." *Health Services Research*, 12(3): 401-419.

Pepper Commission. (1990). *Report of the bipartisan commission on comprehensive health care*. Washington, DC: U.S. Government Printing Office.

Rogers, D.E., & Blendon, R.J. (1977). "The Changing American Health Scene: Sometimes Things Get Better." *Journal of the American Medical Association*, 237: 1710-1714.

Rogers, D.E., Blendon, R.J., & Moloney, T.W. (1982). "Who Needs Medicaid?" *New England Journal of Medicine,* 307: 13-18.

Rowland, D. (1987). *Hospital care for the poor.* Doctoral dissertation, Johns Hopkins School of Hygiene and Public Health, Baltimore, MD.

Rowland, D., Lyons, B., & Edwards, J. (1988). "Medicaid: Health Care for the Poor in the Reagan Era." *Annual Review of Public Health*, 9: 427-50.

Schieber, G., & Poullier, J.P. (1989). "International Health Care Spending." *Health Affairs*, 8.

Schoen, C. (1984). "Medicaid and the Poor: Medicaid Myths and Reality and the Impact of Recent Legislative Changes." *Bulletin of the New York Academy of Medicine*, 60(1).

Woolhandler, S., & Himmelstein, D.U. (1988). "Reverse targeting of preventive care due to lack of health insurance." *Journal of the American Medical Association*, 256: 2872-2874.

FINANCING THE MEDICARE AND MEDICAID PROGRAMS IN THE UNITED STATES

Alan L. Sorkin

The Medicare Program of the United States, enacted in 1965, was designed to finance acute medical care primarily for elderly Americans. It also covers some categories of the disabled and those with end-stage renal disease. The program is divided into two parts: Part A, which provides hospital insurance (HI), and Part B, which covers supplementary medical insurance (SMI). The HI component includes short term hospitalization, skilled nursing care, and home health services, while the SMI portion covers physician's services, outpatient hospital care, and laboratory fees, as well as home health care. The program does not cover long-term nursing home care, dental care, or outpatient drugs.

Cost sharing is imposed on Medicare beneficiaries who use medical services. Under HI, a deductible amount approximately equal to the cost of one day in a hospital ($560 in 1989) must be paid by beneficiaries who are hospitalized. Aside from this deductible, the HI program pays in full the cost of the first sixty days of hospitalization for an episode of illness. From the sixty-first day through the ninetieth day, a 25 percent coinsurance payment of $140 per day

Research in Human Capital and Development, Volume 7, pages 307-327.

ISBN: 1-55938-132-9

was required as of 1989. For stays of more than 90 days, each beneficiary has a life time reserve of 60 additional days, but must pay $270 for each day that is used (Hsiao & Kelly, 1984).

HI also covers up to 100 posthospital days in a skilled nursing facility (SNF). After 20 days, the beneficiary is required to pay an amount per day that is equal to 20 percent of the average charge in a skilled nursing facility.

Under SMI, as of 1989, beneficiaries paid $27.90 per month plus an annual deducible of $75, beyond which Medicare would pay 80 percent of the "reasonable charges" for covered services. If the provider's charges were reasonable according to Medicare standards, then the patient's share was the remaining 20 percent of the total. If the charges exceeded such standards, the beneficiary was liable for the excess amount in addition to his 20 percent share (except when the physician accepted assignment).

State Medicaid programs frequently serve to complement Medicare for low-income elderly persons (Burwell, Clauser, Hall, & Simon, 1987). Medicaid may finance cost sharing amounts as well as other noncovered services for eligible Medicare beneficiaries who are too poor to pay these bills.

A major weakness of Medicare's benefit structure is that it violates the primary purpose of insurance, which is to protect the beneficiary from destitution. The cost-sharing provisions of the HI and SMI mean that elderly people face unlimited liabilities if a catastrophic illness occurs. Under HI, patients are required to pay the entire hospital cost after 150 days of hospitalization. Moreover, they have already paid relatively high coinsurance rates beginning on the ninety-first day. Furthermore, SMI requires patients to pay 20 percent of reasonable charges for physician visits as well as other outpatient services. For expensive surgery, the 20 percent coinsurance rate would be a costly financial burden on an elderly patient. Consequently, even though the probability of a large financial outlay is low, there is an incentive for beneficiaries to buy supplementary insurance coverage. This weakness in Medicare's benefit structure helped to create the demand for what is presently called Medigap insurance.

Medigap insurance pays a substantial portion of the health care costs that are not covered by Medicare. It permits those elderly persons who can afford this insurance roughly the same degree of insurance protection as that obtained by employed nonaged persons.

The Medicare Catastrophic Coverage Act of 1988 protected older and disabled Americans from a wide range of high health care costs. Medicare beneficiaries were protected against multiple costly hospitalizations, frequent doctor visits, or high annual prescription expenses.

The costs for the catastrophic benefits were borne by all Medicare beneficiaries. However, higher income individuals (annual taxable income greater than $10,000) paid proportionately more than lower income individuals. Because of the extreme unpopularity of the latter provision with nonpoor elderly persons, Congress repealed the Act in 1989.

I. MEDICARE COST CONTROLS

Both overall national health expenditures and Medicare expenditures have been rising since enactment of the latter in 1965 (see Table 1). In 1989, Medicare's HI expenditures were almost 12 times the 1970 level, and SMI expenses were more than 13 times the 1970 level. Over the same period, non-Medicare hospital expenditures (total expenses less expenditures under Medicare's HI) rose slightly more than 7 times, and expenses for non-Medicare physician's services increased more than 9 times. Part of the reason why Medicare expenditures have risen more rapidly than non-Medicare expenditures is the growth and aging of the elderly population. Another reason for the differential expenditure growth results from covering the disabled and persons with end-stage renal disease under Medicare after 1972. Finally, increases in Medicare utilization rates and prices explain a small portion of the differential growth between Medicare and non-Medicare expenditures.

Medicare Cost Containment

The Tax Equity and Financial Responsibility Act (TEFRA) was the first federal legislation explicitly designed to reduce Medicare costs. The law, passed in 1982, profoundly changed Medicare's hospital reimbursement method (Lave, 1984). First, the basis of reimbursement was shifted from an implicit per diem system to an explicit case system; second, case mix was incorporated into the payment system; and third, a limit was placed on the rate of allowable increase in costs per case (Dobson, Langenbrunner, Pelovitz, & Willis, 1986). While reimbursement continued to be based on reasonable costs, the application of this concept was radically altered. Costs per case, which were higher than 120 percent of the average (adjusted for wages and case mix for comparable hospitals), or which rose by more than the target rate over the past year, were no longer considered reasonable. TEFRA also required that a prospective payment system be developed by the Secretary of the Department of Health and Human Services (HHS).

The 1983 Social Security legislation included the substitution of a hospital prospective payment system for the former reasonable cost basis of reimbursement. This action represents the largest change in reimbursement policy since the establishment of Medicare. Significantly, the cost-control aspect of this policy focuses on hospitals, not beneficiaries.

The prospective payment system only applies to the Medicare program. Thus, despite limits on Medicare payments, hospitals have the opportunity to earn additional revenue from non-Medicare patients. This opportunity for cost shifting enables the hospitals to offset losses in revenue resulting from treating Medicare patients.

Table 1. National Health Expenditures, Hospital and Physician Insurance Expenditures, and Medicare Expenditures, 1960-1989*
(Billions of Dollars)

Year	*Total Health Expenditures*	*Percentage of GNP*	*Hospital Insurance*	*Insurance for Physicians Services*	*Total Medicare*	*Medicare Hospital Insurance*	*Supplementary Medical Insurance*
1960	$ 26.9	5.3	7.3	2.0	—	—	—
1965	41.7	6.1	11.6	3.3	—	—	—
1970	74.7	7.6	24.8	7.8	7.4	5.3	2.1
1975	132.7	8.6	48.3	18.5	16.0	11.6	4.4
1980	249.0	9.4	93.7	32.6	36.8	25.6	10.7
1981	286.6	9.8	108.7	38.5	43.6	30.7	12.9
1982	322.3	10.5	124.6	44.0	51.1	36.7	11.4
1983	355.4	10.7	133.6	49.1	57.8	40.4	13.4
1984	387.4	10.6	142.0	54.5	64.6	44.4	14.6
1985	419.0	10.4	151.4	59.7	69.3	48.2	16.7
1986	455.7	10.7	161.7	67.9	74.6	50.4	19.3
1987	500.3	11.1	176.2	76.4	81.2	53.3	22.3
1988	544.0	11.2	190.1	85.0	88.5	57.5	24.2
1989	604.1	11.6	208.7	95.3	99.8	62.1	27.5

Note: * For periods ending June 30.

Sources: Katherine Levit, Helen Lazenby, Daniel Waldo and Lawrence Davidoff, "National Health Expenditures, 1985," *Health Care Financing Review*, 7, No. 1 (1985): 3, 17, 18, 20; Suzanne Letsch, Katherine Levit and Daniel Waldo, "National Health Expenditures, 1987," *Health Care Financing Review*, 10, No. 2 (1988): 112, 113, 116, and 117; Helen Lazenby and Suzanne Letsch, "National Health Expenditures, 1989," *Health Care Financing Review*, Vol. 12, no. 2, Winter, 1990, pp. 1, 17, 19 and 20.

Because the new system applies on a per case basis, it generally results in the same payment regardless of the length of stay or the volume of services provided. This provides an incentive for hospitals to discharge patients as quickly as medically possible.

II. THE DRG PROSPECTIVE PAYMENT SYSTEM

The basic features of the Medicare prospective payment system are: (1) all patients are classified into one of 468 diagnosis-related groups (DRGs); (2) with few exceptions, the hospital receives a fixed payment per DRG to cover operating costs; (3) the payment per DRG received by a hospital is a function of regional wages, whether the facility is located in a rural or urban area, and the number of full-time interns and residents on its staff; and (4) capital costs and direct education are excluded, but the Secretary of HHS is to report to Congress on methods of including these costs in the prospective rates. There was a three year phase-in period during which the payment rates shifted from being essentially based on retrospective reimbursement to being set prospectively on a national basis with adjustments based on region, staff size, and local wage rates. Thus, by 1987, reimbursement to an individual hospital to pay for the operating costs of producing services to Medicare beneficiaries became fully based on a national prospective payment system.

The current law explicitly determines how payment rates should be increased. Basically, payment rates on the average are to increase by the "market basket plus one." The market basket is a measure of the rate of increase in the prices that hospitals have to pay for their inputs, and the additional one percentage point (the intensity factor) is to provide some room for "technological change." Because the market basket price index has consistently increased more than the overall consumer price index, the new law insures that the payment rate for a Medicare illness episode will continue to increase at a faster rate than that of goods and services in general.

Although one might have expected an increase in Medicare hospital admissions after the implementation of the DRG system (Russell, 1989), (as hospitals attempted to offset expected declines in per patient revenues) this in fact was not the case. Hospital admissions per Medicare enrollee fell 15.9 percent between 1983 and 1987; admissions fell 11.3 percent for the population as a whole (Feinglass & Holloway, 1991).

Much of the decline can be traced to the shift to outpatient surgery encouraged by the Peer Review Organizations, and especially to a massive shift in the location of cataract surgery. A study of 646 hospitals over the period from 1980-1985 found that admissions for lens procedures fell from 15,000 in 1983 to 2,000 in 1985; (Harnais, Chesney, & Fleming, 1987) this category alone accounted for 54 percent of the decline in admissions for these hospitals between 1984 and 1985.

Similar trends occurred for procedures like carpal tunnel release and dilation and curettage. Much of the increase in outpatient surgery was related to intensive marketing and advertising by new, for profit, ambulatory surgery centers, which increased fourfold between 1983 and 1988. Outpatient surgery on the oldest, old—patients over age 80—increased 21 percent in the first two years of PPS (Guterman, Eggers, Riley, Greene, & Terrell, 1988).

United States hospitals reacted swiftly to the 1982 TEFRA limits and PPS incentives. Average hospital length of stay for Medicare patients behaved exactly as predicted, dropping a total of 14.6 percent between 1982 and 1985, before leveling off over the next three years. Medicare patients average length of stay was 25 percent lower in 1985 than in 1980. A more modest length of stay decrease of about 5 percent occurred for non-Medicare patients under age 65 (Feinglass & Holloway, 1991).

From 1984-1988 the average length of stay was unchanged. The occupancy rate—the average percentage of beds filled with patients during the year—fell from 74 percent in 1983 to 65 percent in 1987. The number of hospital employees dropped slightly in 1983 and more sharply in 1984 and 1985.

In response to the demand for alternatives to inpatient care, hospitals have rapidly added new outpatient facilities and expanded existing ones (Cromwell & Pope, 1988). In 1986, 63 percent had organized outpatient departments, up from 38 percent in 1982 and the percentage with home health programs had tripled to 35 percent in 1986, compared with only 12 percent in 1982. Some of the unused beds were converted for use by long term, rehabilitation, and other patients not covered under prospective payment.

Quality of Care

To date, there is little generalizable evidence that PPS has reduced the quality of care for Medicare patients. Hospital use and mortality rates for potentially unprofitable patients such as the oldest old, minorities, self-paying, uninsured, or nursing home patients covered by both Medicare and Medicaid has decreased at the same rate as the rest of the population (Schramm & Gabel, 1988, 1989). A three hospital study of Medicare patient users of intensive care before and after PPS found no differences in discharge illness severity despite declines in intensive care beds and occupancy rates (Mayer-Oakes, Oye, Leake, & Brook, 1988). Hospital readmissions within 7, 30 and 60 days of initial discharge are monitored by the PRO's and the federal Prospective Payment Assessment Commission. These rates have grown at a lower annual rate since 1983, despite some contrary reports from individual states (Gay, Kronfeld, Baker, & Amidon, 1989). There is little consistent evidence to confirm fears that hospitals have increased "dumping"—that is inappropriately transferring severely ill, unprofitable Medicare patients.

However, a study of Medicare PPS on hip fracture care provides disquieting results (Fitzgerald, Fagan, Tiemey, & Dittus, 1987). Although mean length of hospitalization fell (from 16.6 to 10.3 days) post-PPS, the number of physical therapy sessions received also decreased (from 9.7 to 4.9) and the proportion of patients discharged to nursing home care increased (from 21% to 48%). More revealing about effects on patient well-being is that, after six months, 39 percent of patients remained in nursing homes post PPS as opposed to 13 percent pre-PPS. According to the authors, these results suggest worsening care and an overall cost increase.

Weinberger et. al. showed DRGs for non-insulin dependent diabetics hospitalized for glycemic control resulted in shorter hospital stays and fewer tests but led to adverse long-term effects in terms of care and in terms of medical outcomes (Weinberger, Ault, & Vinicor, 1988).

The slower growth of *total* hospital expenditures in the 1983-1987 period is one indicator that reductions in Medicare hospital spending were not associated with large-scale cost-shifting to other, non-Medicare hospital patients. A Blue Cross study carefully investigated the issue of cost-shifting in the 1983-1986 period (Sheffler, Gibbs, & Gurnick, 1988). It reported over $1.3 billion in savings directly related to PPS, above and beyond savings related to Blue Cross's own utilization management. Financial incentives to shift care to nonhospital settings have permanently changed physician patterns of hospital use for all patients, irrespective of patient age or payer per se.

The Current Method of Paying Physicians

With few exceptions, Medicare uses the customary-prevailing reasonable (CPR) charge method to determine how much it will pay for each service provided by a physician (Bovbjerg, Held, & Pauly, 1982). About 6,000 different services are identified, and payment for each is determined by comparing the amount of physician charges with both physician and area-specific ceilings for that service.

On each claim, physicians have the option of accepting or rejecting assignment of the benefit due. Accepting Medicare assignment limits the amount the physician can charge the beneficiary in exchange for a federal guarantee to pay part of the bill (usually 80%). Rejecting assignment allows the physician to charge the beneficiary as much as he wants, but Medicare does not guarantee collection of the billed amount.

The 1972 Social Security amendments included a provision to limit the growth in community-wide prevailing charges to a rate determined by an economic index that reflects national increases in incomes and physician

Table 2. Medicare's Spending for Hospital Care and Physician Services: Amounts and Rates of Growth, 1975-89

	Hospital Care		Physicians Services	
Year	*Dollars (billions)*	*Percent of Total Medicare Spending*	*Dollars (billions)*	*Percent of Total Medicare Spending*
1975	11.6	74.4	3.3	21.4
1979	21.7	73.8	6.4	21.8
1980	26.0	72.8	7.8	21.8
1981	31.0	72.0	9.7	22.3
1982	36.8	72.0	11.4	23.1
1983	40.5	70.6	13.4	23.3
1984	44.4	70.4	14.6	23.1
1985	44.7	63.4	17.3	24.5
1986	45.8	61.9	18.8	25.4
1987	53.7	62.5	21.6	26.5
1988	57.5	63.8	24.2	27.0
1989	62.1	62.1	27.5	7.5

Percentage Growth

Years	*Hospital Care*	*Physician Services*
1981-89	100.3	183.5
1975-89	435.3	733.3

Sources: Robert Gibson "National Health Expenditures, 1979," *Health Care Financing Review*, 2, No. 1 (Summer, 1980): 29-32; Robert Gibson, Daniel Waldo and Katherine Levit, "National Health Expenditures, 1982," *Health Care Financing Review*, 5, No. 1 (Fall, 1983): 13-15; Katherine Levit, Helen Lazenby, Daniel Waldo and Lawrence Davidoff, "National Health Expenditures, 1984," *Health Care Financing Review*, 7, No. 1 (Fall, 1985): 28-29; *Medicare and Medicaid Data Book*, 1988 (U.S. Department of Health and Human Services, Washington, D.C., 1988): 8. Helen Lazenby and Suzanne Letsch, "National Health Expenditures, 1989," *Health Care Financing Review*, Vol. 12, no. 2, p. 12.

practice costs. In spite of this index, Medicare's payments for physician services have grown faster than its payments for hospital services (See Table 2). The share of Medicare's total spending for personal health care allocated to physicians services increased from 21.4 percent in 1975 to 27.5 percent in 1989. Although much smaller than hospital care's 1989 share of 62.1 percent, payments for physician services are substantial.

A major criticism of physician payment under Medicare is that it provides little incentive for physicians to utilize cost- effective treatment methods. First, as a fee-for-service system it provides an incentive to provide more rather than fewer services. Second, CPR-determined fees for procedures do not decline as the cost of providing those services fall over time due to technological change. Third, the CPR system provides more favorable reimbursement for complex procedures performed by specialists as opposed to less costly primary care services.

Medicare Financing

Revenues for the funding of HI come primarily from a portion of the Social Security payroll tax. Employers and employees covered by the program each contribute 1.45 percent of earnings (1989). Under current law, general revenues cannot be used to make up any shortfall between outlays required to pay benefits and the balance in the trust fund (Ginsburg & Moon, 1984).

In the early 1980s, the HI trust fund seemed headed for total depletion in 1989 or 1990. When the prospective payment system (DRG) was first introduced in 1983, it was expected that the expected savings in Medicare cost would delay depletion of the HI trust fund until 1992 or 1993. However, actual expenditures from 1984-1988 and the most recent projections show a saving in 1990 dollars of $18 billion per year due primarily to the prospective payment system. The trust fund is expected to be able to cover its costs until the years 2002-2005 (Russell, 1989).

SMI Financing

Between 1975 and 1987, Medicare spending for *physician services per beneficiary* increased at a compound rate of 15 percent per year. About half of this increase was due to increases in physicians' fees while the other half was due to increases in the volume and intensity of their services.

In 1983, Congress took two important steps to limit the growth in physician payments. These included imposition of a freeze on Medicare payment rates from July 1, 1984 to January 1, 1987. Moreover, the freeze was followed by imposition of limits—called "maximum allowable actual charges" on fee increases.

However, total SMI expenditures have continued to increase rapidly. While the annual growth rate was 9.4 percent from 1979-1982, it rose to 10.3 percent from 1984-1987 (Russell, 1989) perhaps reflecting some shift in expenditures from hospitals to physicians services after the imposition of the DRGs.

The proportion of general revenues required to finance the SMI trust fund rose from 3.7 percent to 5.7 percent from 1982 to 1988. If both revenues and SMI outlays were to continue growing at present rates from 1988-1995, then SMI would require a transfer of more than 11 percent of general revenues now allocated to other purposes in 1995.

III. THE MEDICARE COMPETITION DEMONSTRATIONS

A total of 26 HMOs and competitive medical plans (CMP's) participated in the Medicare competition study. These organizations entered the Medicare market from 1982 through 1984 and were studied through 1986.

The analysis of the impact of the Medicare competition demonstrations indicates that HMOs and CMPs had little or no effect on hospital use in the first year that they served the Medicare population but, by the second year, there was a measurable and significant reduction in the use of hospital services. Higher skilled nursing facility use patterns observed for the post-enrollment period enrollees suggest that HMOs are, to some extent, successful in substituting skilled nursing facility services for a more costly hospital day (Langwell & Hadley, 1989).

There is strong evidence that the demonstration HMOs experienced favorable selection in enrollment. The extent of favorable selection appears to have been greater for group and staff model HMOs than for IPAs but evidence of favorable selection is present even in the latter case.

The results of the evaluation of the impact of the Medicare Competition Demonstrations on costs to the Medicare program indicate that risk contracting may have actually increased Medicare program costs. It appears that the Medicare program has paid more to HMOs on behalf of enrollees than the costs that would have been incurred had the beneficiary chosen to remain in the fee-for-service sector (Longwell & Hadley, 1989).

The Resource Based Relative Value Scale

In 1987, Congress responded to rising costs for physicians under SMI by asking the Health Care Financing Administration (HCFA) to develop a resource-based relative value scale (RBRVS) as an alternative to the present Medicare physician reimbursement system.

A relative value scale is a method of standardizing fees among providers in a community. Such scales assign specified weights to certain physician services.

HCFA contracted with Dr. William Hsiao and his colleagues at Harvard University to develop a relative value scale. The study was completed in late 1988.

In the Hsiao model, a resource based relative value for a particular medical service comprises three factors: the total work of the service (both the time involved and the intensity with which it is spent); practice costs; and the opportunity cost of physician training (Hsiao, Yntema, Braum, Dunn, & Christine, 1988).

A resource-based relative value scale (RBRVS) attempts to reflect the average resource inputs, measured primarily in terms of physician work effort, used to produce services. Because it focuses on resource inputs, the RBRVS does not incorporate all the factors relevant to pricing a product or service. For example, the RBRVS approach ignores the role of demand in determining price. It does not reflect the benefits of, or the value patients attach to, particular services or classes of service (Roper, 1988). Moreover, the RBRVS does not take into account physician willingness to supply services. For example, physicians may have preferences to supply a service that requires three times the work effort of another for something less than three times the payment amount.

Finally, using the average work for a procedure as the basis of its relative value does not take into account any systematic differences among physicians in the severity of the cases they treat. Thus, the effort of physicians who typically treat patients who are sicker and presumably require more work will be understated and those physicians will be underpaid.

An RBRVS-based fee schedule, implemented in a budget neutral manner will redistribute Medicare payments among physicians by service, specialty, and geographic area. Hsiao, Braun, and Kelly (1988), provide some preliminary analyses of the redistributive impacts of their RBRVS for selected procedures and for the major types of service, assuming budget neutrality and no behavioral responses. They show that, on average, payments for invasive procedures would be reduced by 42 percent and that payments for evaluation and management procedures would be increased by 56 percent (Hsiao, Braun, & Kelly, 1988).

An RBRVS would result in significant redistributions of Medicare revenues across specialties, and it is unlikely that the "losers" would not respond. For example, physicians who would be adversely affected, could increase the volume and intensity of their services, increasing Medicare outlays. Moreover, physicians whose fees are reduced may simply treat fewer Medicare patients or provide more services to non-Medicare patients, thus reducing access for Medicare beneficiaries.

The resource-based relative value scale was implemented in January, 1992.

III. MEDICAID

Medicaid is a combined federal and state program that provides medical assistance to certain categories of low-income persons, including those on welfare and some of the medically indigent (persons whose incomes are too low to pay for medical care). The program is administered and roughly half the costs are absorbed by the state and local governments.

Medicaid, like Medicare, has traditionally based reimbursement of providers on market prices or costs, paying hospitals according to the Medicare cost-based standard. However, they were permitted to pay physicians at rates below Medicare reimbursement levels. Mandatory covered services (which could not be subject to patient copayment or deductible) included hospital care, physician's services, diagnostic services, family planning advice, and nursing home care in skilled nursing facilities. Screening and treatment of children were subsequently added to the mandatory coverage category. Optional coverage items included services in intermediate care facilities, dental care, drugs, eyeglasses, and some other medical services. Cost sharing was eventually permitted for some of these optional services and for hospital and physicians services provided to the medically indigent (Stevens & Stevens, 1974).

Mandatory eligibility is now required for persons receiving cash assistance under federally funded income transfer programs. Therefore, persons eligible for income transfers under Aid to Families with Dependent Children (AFDC) are automatically eligible for Medicaid. States have considerable flexibility in establishing income levels or other conditions for AFDC eligibility, and are indirectly able to control the number of persons who qualify for Medicaid assistance. While AFDC is limited in a majority of states to families without a father residing in the home, 24 states and two jurisdictions also extend AFDC and Medicaid coverage to families with unemployed fathers who are not receiving unemployment compensation. Seventeen states and three jurisdictions cover all children in families with income below AFDC eligibility level, regardless of the family composition or the employment status of the parents. Persons who are mandatory recipients of Supplemental Security Income (SSI), a federal program for the aged, blind, or disabled, are also automatically eligible for Medicaid, although the income limits for SSI are established by the federal government.

Optional Medicaid beneficiaries are those for whom states may receive federal matching funds but whose coverage is not required by federal legislation. This group includes medically needy families with dependent children whose incomes are above the state AFDC limit, as well as elderly persons who do not qualify for cash assistance. Many of the latter have large medical or nursing home bills.

The 30 states offering Medicaid coverage for the medically needy establish income, asset, and family-composition tests similar to those for public assistance recipients. Medically needy income levels for a family of four, as of March 1986, ranged from $13,200 in Virginia to $3804 in Kentucky and Louisiana (Health Care Financing Administration, 1988). Under the so-called spend down provision, families with incomes above these levels may also be eligible if their incomes are below this amount after deducting medical expenses incurred.

In 1987, approximately 23.3 million persons received services covered by Medicaid. This was only 400,000 more than the number who received services in 1976. However, between 1976 and 1987 the number of people living in poverty rose from 25 million to nearly 35 million. Thus, as a result of the complex set of eligibility requirements only 55 to 60 percent of the poverty population was covered by Medicaid in 1987.

Medicaid Costs

The cost of the Medicaid program has increased rapidly. Combined federal and state-local expenditures increased from $3.5 billion in 1968 to $59.3 billion in 1989 (see Table 3). Three factors explain almost all the increases in expenditures: (1) the increase in the number of Medicaid recipients covered under the AFDC program; (2) sustained medical care price inflation; and (3) the high cost of skilled nursing facilities and intermediate care facilities for the aged, poor, and disabled. Expenditures for these two items more than doubled between 1973 and 1989.

The rapid growth in the number receiving welfare payments in the late 1960s and early 1970s accounted for a large portion of the increased cost of Medicaid at this time. Since the economy was relatively prosperous during that period, most of the increase was due to the rising proportion of eligible people who applied for benefits (Palmer, 1976). Estimates indicate that the percentage of eligible people participating in AFDC increased from 60 percent to more than 90 percent.

The second major factor is the sustained inflation in medical care prices. From 1975 to 1989 medical care prices rose an average of 9 percent annually, with the prices of hospital services rising slightly faster. These higher prices were reflected in increasing Medicaid expenditures.

Annual Medicaid payments per recipient in constant 1968 "medical dollars" (expenditures divided by the medical care price index) averaged $491 in 1989 as compared to $300 in 1968. However, from 1981 1989 real per capita expenditures have remained roughly constant.

The final source of expenditure increases under Medicaid is the high cost of institutionalization for elderly, poor and disabled people who are unable to carry out normal daily activities without nursing assistance. The aged are the only sizable group for which there has been any substantial increase in expenditures in recent years. More than two thirds of Medicaid expenditures are for services to aged or disabled adults (Health Care Financing Administration, 1988).

Medicaid Recipients

The largest group of Medicaid recipients consists of dependent children under the age of 21. However, this is the group that is least costly to serve (See Table 4). Dependent children and the adults in their families constitute 70 percent of Medicaid recipients, but are responsible for only about one-fourth of Medicaid expenditures. The largest share of Medicaid payments—38 percent—is for services to the elderly, reflecting the cost of long-term nursing home services as well as the greater need for medical services within this age group. The disabled category, which includes terminally ill persons under age

Table 3. Number of Recipients, Total Payments, and Payments per Recipient Under Medicaid: Fiscal Years 1968-89

Fiscal Year	*Number of Recipients (millions)*	*Total Federal and State Payments (billions)*	*Payments per Recipient*	*Medical Care Price Index 1968-100*	*Payments per Recipient in 1968 $*
1968	11.5	$ 3.5	$ 300	100.0	$300
1969	12.1	4.4	361	106.9	338
1970	14.5	4.1	354	113.7	311
1971	18.0	6.4	356	121.0	297
1972	18.0	7.4	411	124.9	329
1973	19.6	8.6	440	129.8	339
1974	21.1	10.0	474	141.8	334
1975	22.2	12.3	554	158.9	348
1976	22.9	14.1	615	173.9	354
1977	22.9	16.3	710	192.9	368
1978	22.2	18.0	810	207.8	390
1979	21.5	20.5	953	228.0	418
1980	21.6	25.7	1,190	252.9	471
1981	22.1	30.4	1,376	280.2	491
1982	21.8	32.9	1,509	312,7	483
1983	21.5	38.7	1,800	363.2	496
1985	21.8	41.1	1,885	386.1	488
1986	22.5	44.4	1,973	415.1	475
1987	23.3	50.1	2,150	442.5	486
1988	22.9	55.1	2,406	471.4	510
1989	24.1	59.3	2,460	500.6	491

Sources: U.S. Department of Health, Education, and Welfare, Health Care Financing Administration, *Data on the Medicaid Program: Eligibility, Services, Expenditures, Fiscal Years 1966-1977* (Washington, D.C.: Institute for Medical Management, 1977), p. 34; Donald Muse and Darwin Sawyer, *The Medicare and Medicaid Data Book*, 1981 (Washington D.C.: U.S. Department of Health and Human Services, 1982), pp. 13, 20; Robert Gibson, Katherine Levit, Helen Lazenby, and Daniel Waldo, "National Health Expenditures 1983," *Health Care Financing Review 6*, No. 2 (Winter 1984): 20-21; U.S. Bureau of the Census, Statistical Abstract of the United States, 1986, 106th Edition (Washington, D.C.: U.S. Government Printing Office, 1985), p. 100; U.S. Bureau of the Census, *Statistical Abstract of the United States*, 1989, 109th Edition (Washington, D.C., U.S. Government Printing Office, 1989), pp. 95, 348 and 349; Helen Lazenby and Suzanne Letsch, "National Health Expenditures, 1989," Health Care Financing Review, Winter, 1990, Vol. 12, no. 2, p. 12; U.S. Bureau of the Census, *Statistical Abstract of the United States*, 1990, 110th Edition, (Washington, D.C., U.S. government Printing Office, 1990), p. 470.

Table 4. Medicaid Recipients and Payments by Eligibility Fiscal Year 1985

	Recipients		*Payments*[1]		
Basis of Eligibility Payment	*Number (Thousands)*	*Percent of Total*	*Dollars (Millions)*	*Percentage of Total*	*Per Recipient (Dollars)*
Age 65 or over	3,061	14.0	14,096	37.6	4,605
Blindness	80	0.4	249	0.7	3,113
Permanent and total disability	2,936	13.5	13,203	35.2	4,497
Dependent Children under age 21	9,752	44.7	4,414	11.8	453
Adults in families with dependent children	5,518	25.3	4,746	12.7	860
Other	1,214	5.5	798	2.1	657
Total	21,808[2]	100.0[2]	37,508	100.0	1,720

Notes: [1] Amounts include both state and federal share.
[2] Categories do not add up to total because of a small number of recipients who are in more than one category during the year.

Source: Health Care Financing Administration, *Medicare and Medicaid Data Book 1988*, (Health Care Financing Administration, Washington D.C., 1988), pp. 66 and 88.

65, the mentally retarded, and poor individuals with work-related disabilities, includes less than 14 percent of recipients, but accounts for about 35 percent of Medicaid payments.

As mentioned previously, most of the recent increases in Medicaid payments have gone to the aged and disabled. From 1980 to 1985 about half the growth in Medicaid payments was for disabled persons and about one third was for other persons over age 65. A significant source of growth in Medicaid payments for the disabled is the recent trend toward deinstitutionalization of the mentally retarded. The rate of growth in mentally retarded Medicaid recipients using intermediate care facilities (ICFs) has been greater than that for any other service. When the mentally retarded leave state institutions, they may become eligible for Medicaid benefits in ICFs or the community. The resulting increase in Medicaid expenditures comes from shifting costs away from state funded institutions to the federal-state Medicaid program. In addition, this change frequently results in an upgrading from the largely custodial care of state institutions to the more rehabilitative care in Medicaid-funded ICFs (Granneman & Pauly, 1982). Although there has been appreciable aging of the nation's population, it has not affected the growth of Medicaid costs. In fact, the number of recipients over age 65 actually declined from 1980 to 1985.

Distribution of Medicaid Expenditures

Medicaid expenditures are largely concentrated in a few Northern industrial states. In 1985, New York spent 20.2 percent of all Medicaid funds, and California with the second largest program, spent 11 percent. These two states together with Pennsylvania, Ohio and Illinois, accounted for 45 percent of total Medicaid expenditures (Health Care Financing Administration, 1988). The state distribution of Medicaid funds does not correspond to the prevalence of poverty or sickness. The South, with approximately 45 percent of the nation's poor, receives only 22 percent of all combined federal- state Medicaid funds.

Differences among states arise because some states cover a greater fraction of their poor population and because some have more comprehensive benefits for eligible Medicaid recipients. Average payment per Medicaid recipient in Fiscal 1985 ranged from $819 in West Virginia to $3384 in New York. The National average was $1720 (Health Care Financing Administration, 1988).

The fiscal 1983 medical benefits per family eligible for AFDC averaged $742 in South Carolina and $1698 in New York, although the national average was $1048. These differences would be of less importance if they actually reflected differences in medical care prices or state-wide differences in morbidity, but benefit patterns are unrelated to health care needs or the costs of health or medical care. For example, the average payment for physicians' services in fiscal 1983 was $491 in Alaska and $56 in Pennsylvania (Health Care Financing Administration, 1983). In 1985, 13 percent of the state of Washington's Medicaid recipients were hospitalized compared to 27 percent in South Carolina and North Dakota. In Connecticut and North Dakota, 34 percent of Medicaid recipients in 1985 received dental services under Medicaid compared to 4.2 percent in Illinois.

Medicaid data show large differences by race. The average payment on behalf of blacks in 1985 was $1199 compared to $2184 on behalf of whites.

State Discretion in Medicaid

In 1981, the Reagan administration sought to cap federal grants to states for Medicaid and to give them more discretion with regard to decisions on eligibility, benefits, and reimbursement of providers. While Congress did not go along with capping grants—choosing other means to reduce grants to the states—it did endorse granting them additional flexibility in a number of areas.

One area of flexibility concerned hospital reimbursement. Prior to the passage of the Omnibus Budget Reduction Act (OBRA), Medicaid programs had to use Medicare reimbursement principles unless they applied for a special waiver. OBRA permitted states to use any reimbursement technique as long as payments to hospitals were "reasonable and adequate." This authority has been used extensively. While some states have followed the lead of Medicare in paying on the basis of DRGs, others have implemented different types of prospective payment systems (Ginsburg, 1988).

One aspect of the flexibility provisions that may have more long-run importance is the ability of states to seek waivers from requirements to allow beneficiaries to choose their providers. It has been used in California to purchase hospital care on the basis of competitive bidding. Such bidding could not have been conducted if the program had not been able to prevent recipients from using hospitals that were not successful bidders.

The provisions allowing waiver of freedom of choice may also be important in allowing Medicaid programs greater use of alternative delivery systems. Under waiver, states have developed case management arrangements: recipients in an area must choose from among a panel of primary care physicians participating in the program and obtain all nonemergency services from that physician, or upon referral from that physician.

Provider Reimbursement

From the late 1970s through the 1980s, states have tried unsuccessfully to contain costs of the Medicaid program through the use of more stringent eligibility requirements, imposition of service cutbacks and limitations, tighter administrative controls, and postponement of increases in physician reimbursement.

Under the Omnibus Budget Reconciliation Act of 1981, federal Medicaid grants to states were reduced by 3 percent in 1982, 4 percent in 1983, and 4.5 percent in 1984; and Medicaid's rules for eligibility, benefits, and payments were altered. As a result, 750,000 beneficiaries became ineligible for Medicaid services with an estimated Medicaid savings of $3.9 billion from 1982-1985. As mentioned previously, the act also modified the long-standing freedom-of-choice policy that gave individual Medicaid recipients the freedom to obtain services from any qualified provider (Sorkin, 1986). States may now enter into arrangements to purchase laboratory services or medical devices through competitive bids, or restrict beneficiary's choice to low-cost providers.

Spending for nursing home services is the largest and most rapidly growing component of national Medicaid outlays. By 1987, nearly all states had adopted various forms of prospective reimbursement in which rates and rate increases are negotiated or determined by formulas prior to each new fiscal year.

With respect to hospital reimbursement, most states by 1987 no longer used cost-based reimbursement methods for Medicaid patients. Some states, such as New Jersey and Georgia are using experimental systems of prospective reimbursement based on diagnostic-related groupings. Most of the other states are using facility-specific budget review, rate of increase control, and other forms of prospective rate setting.

An alternative way to limit Medicaid hospital expenditures is to contract with hospitals on a competitive bid basis as California is currently doing. Arizona is requiring nearly all recipients to choose between prepaid organizations that are reimbursed on a capitation basis; all care must be provided or authorized by the health care organization, which is also at financial risk for the provision of health services.

Because state Medicaid authorities have not had to accept customary fees since 1981, the average Medicaid reimbursement for a visit to a physician has fallen to approximately 60 percent of the average charge for non-Medicaid patients. As a result, many physicians refuse to accept Medicaid patients or greatly limit their Medicaid patient load.

Nearly 60 percent of all Medicaid patients are treated by private physicians whose patient volume is comprised of at least 30 percent Medicaid patients (Council of Economic Advisors, 1986). Despite accusations that these physicians are operating "Medicaid Mills," visit length in large Medicaid practices is similar to that of non-Medicaid physicians, and prescribed ancillary services do not appear to be excessive. Medicaid doctors generally earn less than other private physicians, and the former are more likely to be older, non-Board certified, and graduates of foreign medical schools, as compared to the latter.

Between 1983 and 1987, the Health Care Financing Administration funded a multiyear evaluation of Medicaid demonstration projects in six states. The alternative delivery systems represented by the demonstrations contained a number of innovative features, most notably capitation reimbursement, case management, limitations on provider choice, and provider competition.

Primary care case-management responsibility produced significant reduction in utilization; particularly for emergency room use. The findings are particularly notable because they were detected in the first operational year of each demonstration.

Despite the reductions in utilization, however, first year program expenditures were not substantially reduced for any of the demonstration projects. This lack of cost savings in the first demonstration year is mainly the result of small reductions in inpatient use and of the basing of capitation rates on prior-year use levels (Freund, Rossiter, Fox, Meyer, Hurley, Carey, & Paul, 1989).

V. SUMMARY

The Medicare Program finances a large share of the health care costs of older people, the disabled and those with end-stage renal disease. Medicare costs have risen extremely rapidly since the inception of the program in 1965.

From 1983 to 1987, a prospective payment system based on DRG's was implemented. After full implementation there has been a slight decline in hospital admissions (unexpected) and a significant drop in hospital length of stay (expected). As a result, many medical procedures undertaken on behalf of Medicare patients are now being performed on an outpatient basis.

Most studies indicate that quality of care has not been adversely affected by the post PPS reduced length of stay. However, studies of hip fracture patients and noninsulin dependent diabetics did indicate that quality of care worsened after the DRG system was implemented.

There is no evidence that implementation of the DRG system has resulted in cost-shifting to non-Medicare hospital patients. Apparently financial incentives to shift care out of hospital have changed physician practice style for all patients.

In the early 1980s it appeared that the HI trust fund would be entirely depleted by 1990. However, due to the cost savings associated with the DRG prospective payment system, the depletion of the trust fund has been postponed until 2002-2005.

The Resource-Based Relative Value Scale (RBRVS) is an important alternative to the present practice of reimbursing physicians based on customary and reasonable fees. However, it is uncertain as to whether the former will slow the growth in physician expenditures under Medicare after it is implemented in January, 1992.

Medicaid is a combined federal-state program which provides medical assistance to about three-fifths of all low income persons. Because of state differences in eligibility criteria and access to providers, Medicaid benefits are concentrated in a small number of northern industrial states.

The rapid increase in Medicaid costs, which reflects both medical care price inflation and higher utilization, has caused both state and federal government to impose budget cutbacks and a variety of cost-containment measures. In most states, hospitals and nursing homes are presently reimbursed on a prospective cost basis. Reimbursement rates for physicians were scaled back in relative terms and many states are restricting the beneficiary's choice of provider in order to encourage patients to utilize certain low-cost providers. The relatively low reimbursement rates have reduced the willingness of some physicians to accept Medicaid patients.

From 1983 to 1987 a number of Medicaid Competition Demonstration projects were initiated. These have been quite successful at reducing utilization but have had minimal impact on program costs.

REFERENCES

Bovbjerg, R., Held, P.S., & Pauly, M.V. (1982). Pro-competitive health insurance proposals and their implications for medicare's end-stage renal disease program. *Seminars in Nephrology*, 2: 134-172.

Burwell, B., Clauser, S., Hall, M., & Simon, J. (1987). Medicaid recipients in intermediate care facilitied for the mentally retarded. *Health Care Financing Review*, 8:1.

Council of Economic Advisors. (1986). Economic Report of the President, 1985 (p. 155). Washington, DC, U.S. Government Printing Office.

Cromwell, J. & Pope, G. (1988). The impact of Medicare's prospective payment system on medical device innovation (p. 7). (mimeograph).

Dobson, A., Langenbrunner, J., Pelovitz, S., & Willis, J. (1986). The furture of policy reform: Priorities for research and demonstrations. *Health Care Financing Review*, 7: 3.

Feinglass, J. & Holloway, J. (1991). The initial impact of the medicare prospective payment system on U.S. health care: A review of the literature. *Medical Care Review*, 48 (1):96.

Fitzgerald, J.F., Fagan, L.F., Tiemey, W.M., & Dittus, R.S. (1987). Changing patterns of hip fracture care before and after implementation of the prospective payment system. *Journal of the American Medical Association*, 258:218-221.

Freund, D., Rossiter, L., Fox, P., Mayer, J., Hurley, R., Carey, T., & Paul, J. (1989). Evaluation of the medicaid competition demonstrations. *Health Care Financing Review*, 11:80, 96.

Gay, E., Kronfeld, G., Baker, S.L., & Amidon, R.L. (1989) An appraisal of Organizational response to fiscally constraining regulation: The case of hospitals. *Journal of Health and Social Behavior*, 30:41-55.

Gindburg, P. (1988). Public Insurance Programs: Medicare and Medicaid. Pp. 198-199 in H.E. Frech II (Ed.), *Health Care in America*. San Francisco, Pacific Research Institute for Public Policy.

Ginsburg, P. & Moon, M. (1984). An introduction to the medicare financing problem. *Milbank Memorial Fund Quarterly*, 62: 167.

Guterman, S., Eggers, R.W., Riley, G., Greenw, T.F., & Terrell, S.A. (1988). The first three years of medicare prospective payment: An overview. *Health Care Financing Review*, 9 (3):67-77.

Harnais, S.D., Chesney, J., & Fleming, S. (1987). The impact of the prospective payment system on hospital utilization and the quality of care: Trends and regional variation in the first two years. (mimeograph).

Health Care Financing Administration. (1983). Medicaid recipient by maintenance assistance status and by HHS region and state: Fiscal Year 1983.

Health Care Financing Administration. (1988). Medicare and Medicaid Data Book. Washington, DC, Health Care Financing Administraiton.

Hsiao, W. & Kelly, N. (1984). A reassesment. *Milbank Memorial Fund Quarterly*, 62:209.

Hsiao, W., Braun, P., & Kelly, N. (1988). Results, potential and implementation issues of the resource-based relative value scale. *Journal of the American Medical Association*, 260:2429-2438.

Hsiao, W., Yntema, D., Bruam, P., Dunn, D., & Christine, S. (1988). Measurement and analysis of intraservice work. *Journal of the American Medical Association*, 260: 2446.

Langwell, K. & Hadley, J. (1989). Evaluation of the Medicare Competition Demonstration. *Health Care Financing Review* 11 (2):77.

Meyer-Oakes, S., Oye, R.K., Leake, B., & Brook, R.H. (1988). The early effect of medicare's prospective payment system on the use of medical intensive services in three community hospitals. *Journal of the American Medical Association*, 260 (2)3146-3149.

Palmer, J. (1976). Government growth in perspective. *Challenge*, 19:43.

Roper, W. (1988). The resource-based relative value scale: A methodological and policy evaluation. *Journal of the American Medical Association* 260:2446.

Russell, L. (1989). Medicare's new hospital payment system: Is it working (p. 26). Washington, DC, The Brookings Institute.

Schramm, C.J., & Gabel, J. (1988).Prospective payment: Some retrospective observations. *New England Journal of Medicine*, 318 (25):1681-1683.

Sheffler, R.M., Gibbs, J.O., & Gurnick, D.A. (1988). The impact of medicare's prospective payment system and private sector initiatives: Blue cross experience 1980-86. Blue Cross and Blue Sheild Association in Conjunction with Research Program in Health Economics, University of California.

Sorkin, A. (1986). Health care and the changing economic environment (p. 107). Lexington, Massachusetts, D.C. Heath.

Stevens, R. & Stevens, R. (1974). Welfare medicine in America: A case study of medicaid (pp. 156-160, 282-299). New York, The Free Press.

Weinberger, M. Ault, K.A., & Vinicor, F. (1988). Prospective reimbursement and diabetes mellitus: Impact on Glycemic Control and Utilization of Health Services. *Medical Care*, 26:77-83.

PHYSICIAN PAYMENT REFORM IN THE UNITED STATES: A MAJOR STEP FORWARD

Philip R. Lee

Physician payment reform in the United States took a major step forward on January 1, 1992 when the Medicare fee schedule, enacted by Congress in November 1989, went into effect. The Medicare fee schedule was part of a comprehensive payment reform package that sought to contain the rapidly rising expenditures for physicians' services, while assuring access to cost-effective health care. There is sufficient interest among private payors (commercial and nonprofit) to indicate that the payment reforms will not be limited to Medicare.

Much of the debate among policymakers in recent years has focused on physician payment reform related to fee-for-service medicine rather than capitated group practice prepayment plans and other organized systems. This does not imply that proponents of fee-for-service payment reforms are opposed to alternative payment mechanisms. Rather, whatever the prospects for health maintenance organizations, preferred provider organizations, or other payment mechanisms, fee for service is likely to continue to play a major role in the foreseeable future, especially in the Medicare program.

Research in Human Capital and Development, Volume 7, pages 329-345.

ISBN: 1-55938-132-9

When Medicare was enacted in 1965, fee for service was the predominant method used by private third party payors to pay physicians. Fee schedules were commonly used by third parties as indemnity schedules to reimburse patients who paid physicians directly, or as service benefits to cover low-income beneficiaries (Glaser, 1989). Instead of adopting a fee schedule for Medicare in 1965, Congress chose a system of fee screens (customary, prevailing and reasonable) used by a small number of Blue Shield plans (Showstack, Blumberg, & Schwartz, 1979). The Medicare approved charge was usually the smallest of the actual charge for the service provided by the physicians, the physicians usual or customary charge (the median charge for the service by the physician in the preceding year), or the prevailing charge (the Seventy-Fifth percentile of physicians customary charges for the same service in the locality (Langwell and Nelson, 1986; U.S. Congress, House Ways and Means Committee, 1989).

Medicare pays 80 percent of the approved charge after the Part B annual deductible is met. The beneficiary is responsible for 20 percent of the approved charge. Under the CPR payment method, if the physician did not accept the Medicare approved charge as payment in full (known as accepting assignment), the patient was responsible for additional charges by the physician up to a maximum amount allowed under Medicare policy. This was referred to as extra billing (by the patient) or balance billing (by the physician).

Efforts to limit the rate of increase in expenditures for physicians services were first imposed by President Nixon in 1971, when he limited physician price increases to 2.5 percent per year. Price controls were lifted in 1974, but a new approach was implemented in 1975. Since 1975, the annual update in the prevailing charges has been limited by the Medicare Economic Index (MEI) that tied increases in Medicare prevailing charges to increases in physicians practice costs and wage rates throughout the economy. The MEI is expressed as an annual percentage increase and is a limit on the cumulative change in prevailing charges since the 1973 fee screen year (U.S. Congress, Ways and Means Committee, 1989).

Beginning in 1984, Congress took a number of additional steps to slow the rate of increase in expenditures for physicians services in the Medicare program, including a fee freeze (1984-1986), initiating the Participating Provider and Supplier Program (PAR), and limiting physician charges above what Medicare allowed on all unassigned claims (called the maximum actual allowable charge MAAC program). In addition, Congress mandated that the Health Care Financing Administration (HCFA) conduct a study of a relative value scale for physicians services and it established the Physician Payment Review Commission in 1986 to advise it on payment reform.

I. RISING EXPENDITURES FOR PHYSICIANS SERVICES

While a number of factors contributed to the actions taken by Congress to begin the process of physician payment reform, the overriding issue was the rapidly rising expenditures for physicians services. Between 1970 and 1989 Medicare spending grew at an average annual rate of 14.7 percent. This rate exceeds the growth of inflation, wages, GNP, and national health expenditures. Additionally, real per enrollee Medicare spending has risen faster than real national health spending per capita. A few facts illustrate the problem:

- Medicare expenditures for Part B (over 70% of these are for physicians services) rose from approximately $800 million in 1967 to approximately $37 billion in 1989 (Table 1);
- Part B expenditures are rising more rapidly than total Medicare expenditures, national health care expenditures, and GNP (Figure 1);
- Projections to 1994 by the Congressional Budget Office indicate a continued rapid increase in Medicare expenditures (Figure 2).

The rising expenditures for physicians' services are related to three factors: the growing number of elderly and the aging of the elderly population, the volume of services, and the price of services (Figure 3). Volume has been of growing importance in driving expenditure increases, particularly diagnostic procedures. Medicare bill summary files show the differential rates of growth for broad categories of service. Between 1980 and 1987, the proportion of Medicare physician services classified as "medical" declined from 42 percent to 34 percent. The proportion classified surgical was essentially unchanged, but diagnostic services increased from 15 percent to 21 percent (PPRC, 1988).

Two recent studies funded by the Department of Health and Human Services have increased our knowledge of the types of services that contribute disproportionately to rising expenditures. Because of limitations in the data that HCFA obtains from its carriers, the two research teams had to clean 100 percent Medicare claims files from a number of carriers. Mitchell, Wedig, and Cromwell (1989) examined Medicare spending on physicians' services from 1983 to 1986. Spending increased 29.5 percent over the period, with almost 75 percent attributable to increased services per beneficiary and changes in service mix. Spending for three types of services increased most rapidly: surgery, radiology, and specialized diagnostic tests. Surgery services per beneficiary increased 35 percent during the period, with diagnostic surgical procedures such as colonoscopy and cardiac catheterization the most rapidly increasing subcategory. Radiology procedures increased at a rate similar to surgery, but nonsurgical diagnostic tests increased 67 percent. The latter include

Table 1. Medicare Outlays, Fiscal Years 1967-1989

	Part A Hospital Insurance		*Part B Supplementary Medical Insurance*	
Fiscal Year	*Expenditures (in millions of dollars)*	*Percent increase over prior year*	*Expenditures (in millions of dollars)*	*Percent increase over prior year*
1967	$ 2,597	—	$ 799	—
1970	4,953	4.1	2,196	19.3
1975	10,612	31.6	4,170	27.0
1980	24,288	19.4	10,737	21.8
1985	48,654	15.5	22,730	11.6
1989	58,238	10.4	38,317	9.6

Source: U.S. House of Representatives, Committee on Ways and Means, 1990.

cardiac stress tests, pulmonary function tests, halter monitoring and echocardiography. In contrast to these procedures, visits were virtually unchanged.

McMenamin, West, and Marcus (1988) studied different carriers for the 1983-85 period, using somewhat different techniques. Increases in claims for outpatient surgery accounted for 40 percent of the increase in total outlays. Both increased volume of surgery and a more expensive mix of services contributed to increased claims. Substitution for inpatient surgery accounted for only 8 percent of the increase in outpatient surgery. Increased claimants was another factor. While enrollment grew 4 percent, 11 percent more beneficiaries filed claims. The authors attribute 20 percent of the growth of services to increased claimants, but some contend that increased use of electronic billing by physicians during this period may have resulted in more beneficiaries having claims.

There are a number of factors affecting the increase in the volume of billed services in the Medicare program, including the use of new technologies, expanded use of existing technologies, defensive medicine, and unbundling.

International Comparisons

In recent years, more attention has been paid to the experiences of Canada and a number of European countries in controlling the rate of increase in health care expenditures. The work of Schieber and Poullier (1991) on international comparisons of spending has been very influential in general discussions of cost containment. Many have been stunned by the difference in the proportion of gross national product spent on health services between the United States and other industrialized countries.

In 1989, 11.8 percent of GNP was devoted to health care in the United States, compared to 8.8 percent in second-ranked Sweden and 8.7 percent in third-

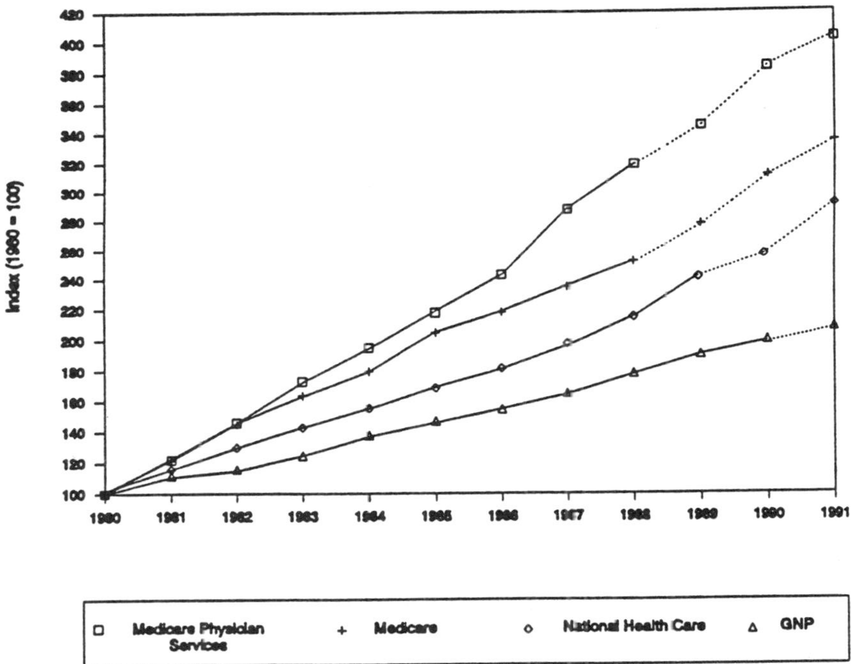

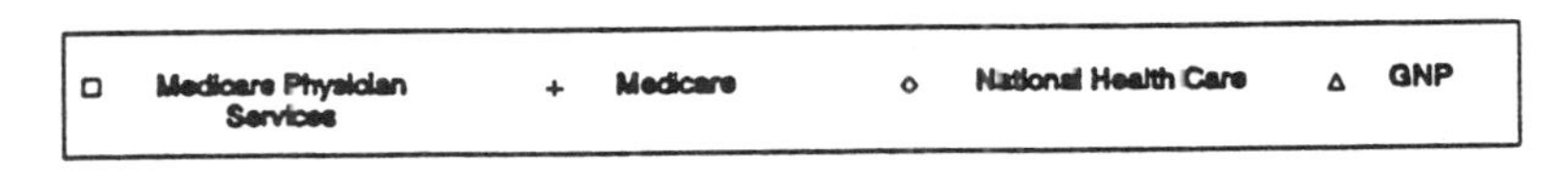

Note: .... represents projections.

Source: Health Care Financing Administration, Office of the Actuary; U.S. Department of Commerce.

Figure 1. Trends in Gross National Product and Expenditures for Medicare, Medicare Physician Services, and National Health Care 1980-1991

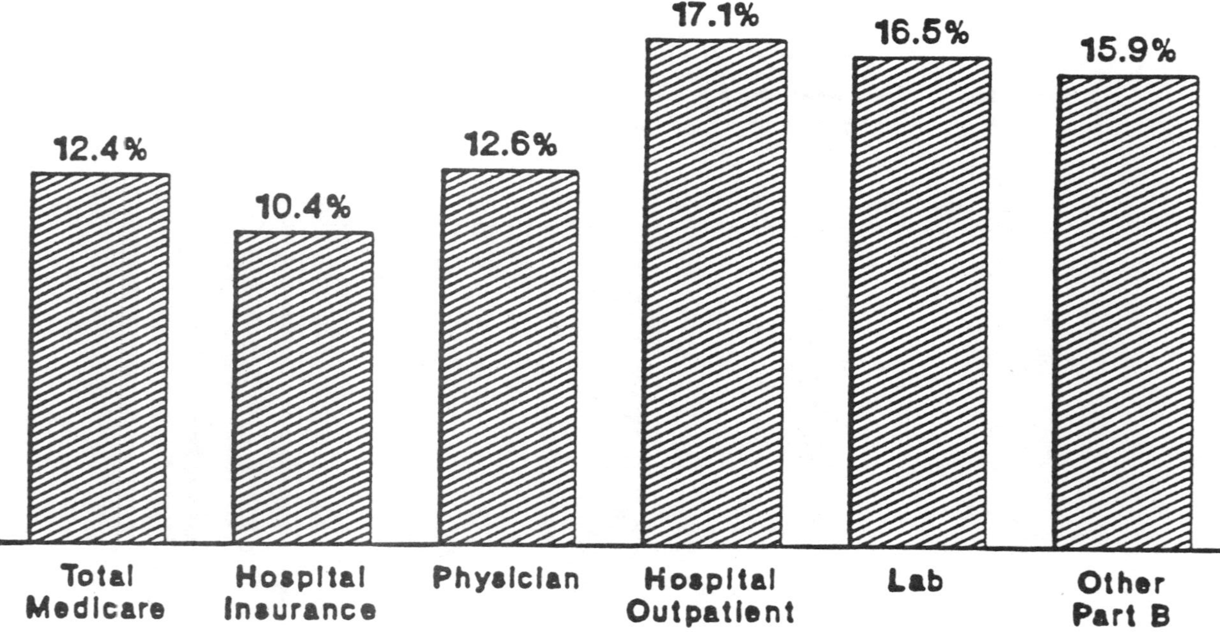

Source: Congressional Budget Office October 1988 Baseline.

Figure 2. Projected Annual Growth Rates of Medicare Outlays by Type of Service, 1988-1994

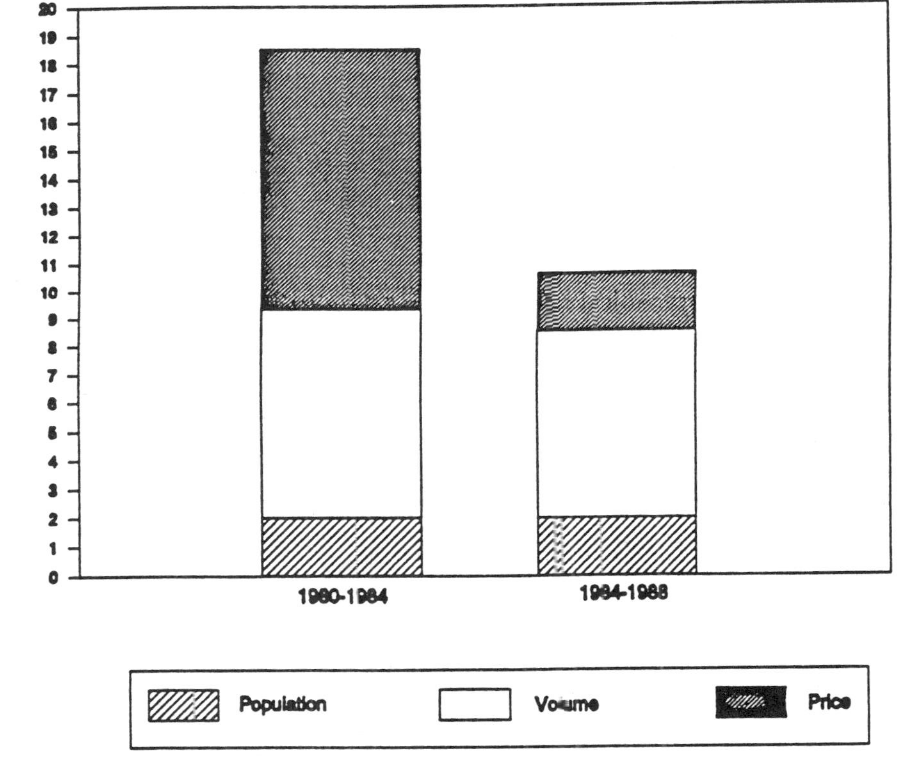

Source: PPRC, 1990.

Figure 3. Growth in Medicare Physician Expenditures by Components 1980-1988

ranked Canada and France. The lack of universal coverage in the United States makes the differences in percentage of GNP even more striking.

Per capita expenditures in the United States were 40 percent higher than Canada, the second highest country, and 71 percent higher than Switzerland, the third-ranked country.

An historical series developed by these authors shows that this gap is a recent phenomenon. Before 1980, most Western countries were experiencing increases in the proportion of resources devoted to health care, but many countries were able to stabilize the proportion, while it continued to grow in the United States. This gap has been particularly worrisome to the business community and to labor because of their implications concerning the competitiveness of the U.S. economy.

II. PHYSICIAN PAYMENT REFORM

In 1986 Congress established the Physician Payment Review Commission to recommend payment reforms because of growing concern about the rapid increase in health care costs, including expenditures for physicians services.

In considering the various options for physician payment reform in the Medicare program, the Physician Payment Review Commission carefully considered two approaches to control expenditures: limiting prices and controlling volume of services. To limit price increases and to correct the distorted incentives in the CPR method of payment, the Commission carefully examined continued use of the CPR method, with modifications; a fee schedule based on relative values; payment to physicians on a case basis (similar to the hospital prospective payment based on diagnosis-related groups); and capitation payments. To limit growth in volume, a number of alternatives were considered:

- financial incentives (e.g., expenditure target);
- organized systems of care, particularly coupled with capitation prepayment (e.g., HMOs);
- utilization and quality review;
- outcomes research and practice guidelines;
- profiling of physicians practice patterns;
- limits on physician supply; and
- limits on technology.

The Medicare Fee Schedule

After careful review of the alternatives, the Physician Payment Review Commission endorsed the concept of a fee schedule for Medicare and an expenditure target in order to control the rate of increase in expenditures for physicians services. The Commission also recommended expanded medical treatment effectiveness and outcomes research, improved utilization review and quality assurance, and continued expansion of HMOs. It did not take a position on limiting physician supply or limiting the growth of technology. In recommending these policies the Commission recognized the need to deal with both the price and volume issues.

The U.S. Congress adopted recommendations for physician payment reform in November 1989, based on the recommendations of the Physician Payment Review Commission (PPRC, 1989). The reforms, which initially will affect only Medicare payment to physicians, included:

- the establishment of a resource-based relative value fee schedule to replace the current customary, prevailing and reasonable charge payment mechanism;
- performance standard rates of increase for aggregate expenditures and volume of physicians' services; and
- limits on balance billing by physicians to protect Medicare beneficiaries from excessive charges for physician services.

In enacting these provisions for the payment of physicians in the Medicare program, the Congress initiated the most significant reform in physician payment in 25 years since the enactment of Medicare in 1965. The adoption of a fee schedule based on relative values moved to correct both geographic and interspecialty inequities in payment. The reasonable charge system of payment used by Medicare prior to 1992 had led to imbalances in relative payment levels among procedural services (e.g., surgery), imaging services, and evaluation and management services, as well as among specialists and across different geographic areas (Hsiao & Stason, 1979; Hsiao, Braun, Dunn & Becker, 1988a; Langwell & Nelson, 1986; Showstackm Blumberg, Schwartz, et al., 1979; Wilensky & Rossiter, 1986).

The resource-based payment system adopted by Congress in 1989 will alter the current economic incentives in the Medicare program and this may affect the cost, quality, and access to medical services for Medicare beneficiaries.

The Medicare fee schedule consists of a relative value scale (RVS), a geographic adjustment factor (GAF) and a conversion factor. The RVS has components for physician work (time and intensity of effort), practice expenses, and malpractice expense (PPRC, 1989). In the RVS, estimates of physician work come mostly from the resource-based relative value scale (RBRVS) study by Hsiao and his colleagues at Harvard (Becker, Dunn & Hsiao, 1988; Braun, Hsiao, & Becker, 1988; Dunn, Hsiao, & Ketcham, 1988; Hsiao, Braunn, Dunn, & Becker, 1988a; Hsiao et al., 1988b; Hsiao, Braun, Kelly & Becker, 1988c; Hsiao, Couch, & Causino, 1988d; Hsiao, Yntema, & Braun, 1988e). The project was conducted in conjunction with hundreds of physicians selected in cooperation with the American Medical Association. The studies that resulted in the physician work component of the RVS had their origins more than a decade ago in the research of Hsiao and Stason (1979) that demonstrated large inequities in payment for surgical services and nonsurgical visits. Others had also pointed out the incentives for physicians to perform procedures in the charge-based payment system (Langwell & Nelson, 1986; Showstack, Blumberg, & Schwartz, 1979; Wilensky & Rossiter, 1986).

The practice expense component of the RVS will be based on historical charges. The costs of non-physician inputs to physician services, usually referred to as practice costs, represent about 48 percent of the average physician's total revenue (Gonzalez & Emmons, 1988). The remaining 52 percent of revenue pays for the physician's inputs primarily the physician's own time and effort, or work.

Typically, practice costs include the salaries of nurses, technicians, and receptionists, and the costs of office space, equipment, medical supplies, administrative expenses, and professional liability insurance. Physicians often require different mixes of these non physician inputs in each type of practice setting and for different services.

The Commission recommended that practice costs should be incorporated into the RVS through an additive formula. Initially practice costs will be based on historical charges, but the Commission is conducting an extensive study to determine if the costs can also be allocated on a resource cost basis.

Professional liability costs are a unique and important practice cost component. They are a relatively large expense and vary dramatically by speciality and location (Posner, 1986). Premium costs increased by 17.2 percent between 1986 and 1987 according to published data from the AMA socioeconomic monitoring system (Gonzales & Emmons, 1988).

The economics of professional liability insurance are also different from other practice costs. While the markets for other non physician inputs, such as office space, are fairly competitive, the market for professional liability insurance is often a seller's market, characterized by little physician choice (Posner, 1986). Liability insurance is also a fixed cost that must be paid regardless of practice volume. The malpractice premium costs will be separated from other practice costs and will be based on historic charges.

The GAF is based on estimates of differences in input prices faced by physicians (e.g., office rents, nursing wage rates) across payment localities. The GAF used in the physician fee schedule is based on research performed by the Urban Institute and the Center for Health Economics Research (PPRC, 1989).

The conversion factor (CF), which translates these relative values into dollars, is to be calibrated so that outlays will be budget neutral. That is, the initial conversion factor must result in total payments that are the same as total payments expected under the charge-based payment method. This "budget neutrality" requirement is a key feature of the congressional mandate establishing the Medicare fee schedule.

The CF is a single national value that applies to all services paid under the fee schedule. The CF established by HCFA for 1992 is $31.01, reflecting a CF update of 1.9 percent. The process of determining the CF was very complex because it required predictions of fees for each procedure in each payment area, consistent with transition provision and prediction of the frequency with which each procedure is performed in order to establish total costs.

The fee schedule, which went into effect on January 1, 1992, represents the first stage in a transition to full implementation of the fee schedule by 1996. In the first year only about one-third of fees will be at the resource-based fee schedule, while two-thirds will still be based on historical charges. Because the fees that are increasing (evaluation and management services) are rising more rapidly than the fees that are decreasing (e.g., surgical services) an asymmetry is created in the initial year of the implementation, which results in expenditures that would exceed budget neutrality if not adjusted. A further adjustment (reduction) in the CF was made in anticipation of an increased volume and intensity of services, above current levels, in responding to the fee schedule changes. While the Commission and virtually all physician groups did not agree with the downward adjustments (Lee & Ginsburg, 1991; PPRC, 1991b), it is unlikely that Congress will overrule HCFA and mandate different rules.

Major steps toward implementing the fee schedule have taken place already. In the original legislation (the Omnibus Budget Reconciliation Act of 1989, or OBRA 89), reductions in prevailing charge screens for overvalued procedures and for radiology services were specified on the basis of preliminary versions of the RVS and the GAF, and a higher prevailing charge update was specified for office visits.

In OBRA 90, further reductions were specified for overvalued procedures and radiology, and reductions were specified for anesthesiology, pathology, and all other services (except visits and consultations) that had not been assessed as to whether they were overvalued.

Thus, when the fee schedule per se began on January 1, 1992, a portion of the change in relative payments for many services already were accomplished.

The Health Care Financing Administration (HCFA) also has taken steps toward implementation. In September 1990, HCFA published a Model Fee Schedule, which included preliminary fee schedule amounts for many services and discussed policy decisions that needed to be made. The key events to date have been the publication on June 5, 1991 of a Notice of Proposed Rulemaking (or NPRM) and the publication of the final rule on November 15, 1991. The final rules published by HCFA represent the interpretation of congressional intent by HCFA. The rules will guide carriers, providers, and beneficiaries in complying with the fee schedule implemented on January 1, 1992.

Table 2. Medicare Physician Fee Schedule Impact by Speciality (In Percent)

	1992		*1996*		*5 Year Projected Payment Increases for Physician Services*	
Specialty	*Payments per Service*	*Payments*	*Payments per Service*	*Payments*	*Average Annualized*	*Cumulative*
All physician specialties	−3	0	−6	0	12	74
Family Practice	15	16	28	30	18	125
General Practice	17	18	27	29	17	124
Cardiology	−9	−3	−17	−8	10	59
Dermatoloty	−1	0	0	2	12	77
Internal medicine	0	1	5	7	13	85
Gastroenterology	−10	−4	−18	−9	10	58
Nephrology	−6	−2	−9	−5	11	66
Neurology	−4	−2	−4	−2	11	71
Psychiatry	−2	−1	3	5	13	82
Pulmonary	−3	−1	−2	0	12	74
Urology	−6	−2	−8	−4	11	67
Radiology	−10	−4	−22	−11	9	55
Anesthesiology	−11	−4	−27	−14	8	50
Pathology	−10	−4	−20	−10	9	57
General Surgery	−8	−3	−13	−7	10	62
Neurosurgery	−10	−4	−18	−9	10	58
Ophthamology	−11	−4	−21	−11	9	55
Orthopedic Surgery	−8	−3	−11	−5	10	64
Otolarynology	2	3	3	5	13	83
Plastic Surgery	−8	−3	−13	−6	10	63
Thoracic Surgery	−14	−5	−27	−14	8	50
Clinics	−1	0	−1	1	12	75
Optometry	20	21	41	43	20	148
Chiropractic	12	13	26	28	17	122
Podiatry	6	7	14	16	15	102

Source: Health Care Financing Administration, 1991.

It has been estimated by HCFA that except for family physicians, general practitioners, and otolaryngologists, all other physicians will receive either no increase in payments in 1992 (e.g., internal medicine) or decreases in payments (all other specialties). By 1996, the effects of the fee schedule will be even more marked (Table 2). Despite the shift in relative payments, HCFA estimates that annual payments to physicians will increase by 12 percent between 1992 and 1996, resulting in five-year cumulative increases for all physicians of 74 percent, for family practitioners of 125 percent, internists 85 percent, with other increases ranging from a low of 50 percent (thoracic surgery) to a high of 83 percent (otolaryngology) (PPRC, 1991c).

In addition to the conversion factor, HCFA identified additional problems, some of which were resolved in their rules published in November, 1991. The most important problems relate to the relative value units (RVUs) that will be used in the fee schedule. The rules issued by HCFA rely primarily on the work of Professor Hsiao and his colleagues at Harvard. The Commission was quite critical of some of these values (PPRC, 1991b) and proposed an approach to correcting them in the coming year. About 1000 of the 4500 values reviewed by Hsiao were revised, but this left many unresolved problems (Lee & Ginsburg, 1991). HCFA invited comments to be submitted no later than 120 days after the publication of the final rule in the Federal Register on November 15, 1991. It is hoped that this process will permit correction of the problems before the 1993 fee schedule is announced.

The Commission has expressed particular concern that the pattern of payment for different evaluation and management services does not account for differences in the intensity of work (work per unit of encounter time) of providing different types of visits (Lee & Ginsburg, 1991).

While the Medicare fee schedule will help to correct the inequity among physicians by specialty and geographic area, it will only have a modest effect on rising costs. To slow the rate of increase in expenditures, more stringent steps were needed.

III. POLICIES TO SLOW EXPENDITURE INCREASES

Expenditure Targets: The PPRC Option

A national Medicare expenditure target for physicians' services was proposed by the Commission to slow the rate of growth of program costs by relating the update of the fee schedule conversion factor to the rate of increase in expenditures.

The Commission recommended the establishment of a national expenditure target for physicians' services under Part B to determine annual conversion factor updates under the fee schedule. The target would reflect:

- increases in inflation and practice costs using a reformulated Medicare Economic Index;
- growth and aging of the enrollee population; and
- volume of services per enrollee.

If actual expenditures during a year are equal to targeted expenditures, then the conversion factor update for the following year would be equal to the increase in practice costs. The update would be increased or decreased to reflect differences between actual and targeted expenditure increases.

Congress modified the procedure slightly and adopted the volume performance standard (VPS) as the means that will be used to determine the annual fee update for physicians.

- The VPS specifies the method by which the fee schedule conversion factor will be updated;
- fee updates will be based on increases in physicians' practice costs;
- Congress will determine the VPS and fee update in the following year; A default formula goes into effect if Congress doesn't act.

The Secretary of HHS will recommend to the Congress acceptable performance standard rates of increase for expenditures and volume of physicians' services each fiscal year. The Commission will comment on the Secretary's recommendations and make its own recommendations. Congress will then establish performance standard rates of increase. If Congress does not act after the Secretary's recommendation, the performance rates of increase will be determined through an automatic default mechanism.

The VPS for 1990 was set by Congress in OBRA 1989 at 9.1 percent. The rate of growth in expenditures between FY 1989 and FY 1990 was estimated by HCFA to be 10 percent, which exceeded the 1990 VPS by 0.9 percentage points. Payment increases annually are based on the MEI plus the reduction mandated by Congress in OBRA 1989. Congress had reduced the MEI for 1992 by 0.4 percent. This reduction, coupled with the 0.9 percent due to expenditures exceeding the VPS in 1990 will result in an MEI of 1.9 percent (3.2% in the original MEI, minus 0.4%, minus 0.9%).

The Congress established the VPS for 1991 at 3.3 percent for surgical services, 8.6 percent for non-surgical services, and 7.3 percent for all physician services. Congress has not yet established a VPS for 1992 and HCFA has proposed a VPSE of 6.5 percent for surgical services, 11.2 percent for non-surgical services, and 10 percent for all physicians services. This process will be used annually to adjust future prices in the Medicare fee schedule in response to volume changes.

IV. SUMMARY AND CONCLUSIONS

The U.S. Congress created the Physician Payment Review Commission in 1986 with a mandate to recommend policies to rationalize the payment for physicians services by the Medicare program and to slow the rate of growth of expenditures for these services. The Commission recommended a comprehensive reform package that included a Medicare fee schedule, limits on balance billing by physicians, and a volume performance standard to slow the rate of aggregate expenditure increases for physicians services.

The Medicare fee schedule adopted by Congress can serve to rationalize payments to physicians by tying them to resource costs, but further adjustments in the relative values and in the coding of services and procedures will have to take place within the next several years if this goal is to be realized.

Limits on balance billing and continuation of the PAR program will protect beneficiaries from cost shifting during the implementation of the fee schedule.

Volume performance standards should help slow the increase in Medicare expenditures, particularly if improved methods can be developed to set the annual VPS rate of increase in expenditures for physicians services.

Increased effectiveness research and practice guidelines will provide practitioners with the knowledge and means to manage available health care resources more wisely.

A slowing in the rate of increase in expenditures for physicians services can be anticipated, in part due to the fee schedule, in part due to utilization and quality review and, in part, due to volume performance standards.

Access has been excellent in the Medicare program. The payment reforms should improve access to primary care and should not adversely affect access to specialty care where prices will be reduced.

Quality should be improved because of the fee schedule, and because better information will be provided to physicians on benefits, risks, and costs of specific services.

Finally, a number of factors, beyond the policies adopted by Medicare will affect physician payment in the 1990s:

- the development of new medical technologies and procedures;
- the growth in physician supply, particularly the increased number of surgical specialists and medical subspecialists where procedures play a large role;
- the aging of the population, particularly those over age 75 years;
- the growth of managed care systems;
- developments in health care financing, particularly the likelihood that some form of universal entitlement to basic health insurance will be enacted; and

- the effectiveness of cost containment efforts in the public and private sectors, including fee schedules and expenditure targets.

Fee for service will diminish in significance, but will remain an important mode of physician payment in the 1990s. The usual, customary and reasonable (or customary, prevailing and reasonable in Medicare) system of paying physicians will be replaced by a fee schedule based on resource costs. By the mid-1990s the Medicare fee schedule will be fully implemented by Medicare and will have been adopted by the great majority of private payers. A number of state Medicaid programs will follow suit, particularly if given an incentive to do so by the Congress.

During the 1990s, HMO growth will continue. In contrast to the 1980s, group practice capitated systems and staff-model HMOs will grow more rapidly than IPAs.

Physician payment reform is but part of larger and more complex transformation of health care in the 1990s. The process has begun, but it is unlikely to be completed before the next century begins.

REFERENCES

Becker, E.R., Dunn, D., & Hsiao, W.C. (1988). "Relative Cost Differences Among Physicians' Specialty Practices." *Journal of the American Medical Association* 260: 2397-2402.

Braun, D.B., Yntema, D., & Dunn, D. (1988). "Cross-specialty Linkage of Resource-based Relative Value Scales." *Journal of the American Medical Association* 260: 2390-96.

Braun, D.B., Hsiao, W.C., & Becker, E.R. (1988). "Evaluation and Management Services in the Resource-based Relative Value Scale." *Journal of the American Medical Association* 260: 2409-17.

Dunn, D., Hsiao, W.C., & Ketcham, T.R. (1988). "A Method for Estimating the Preservice and Postservice Work of Physicians' Services." *Journal of the American Medical Association* 260: 2371-2378.

Glaser, W. (1989). "The politics of paying American physicians." *Health Affairs* 8: 129-46.

Gonzalez, M.L. & Emmons, D.W. (eds.). (1988). *Socioeconomic characteristics of medical practice, 1988*. Chicago: American Medical Association.

Hsiao, W.C., & Stason, W.B. (1979). "Toward Developing a Relative Value Scale for Medical and Surgical Services." *Health Care Financing Review*, 1, 23-38.

Hsiao, W.C., Braun, P., Dunn, D., & Becker, E.R. (1988a). "Resource-based relative values." *Journal of the American Medical Association* 260: 2347-53.

Hsiao, W.C., Braun, P., & Dunn, D. (1988b). "Results and pplicy implications of the resource-based relative-value study." *New England Journal of Medicine* 319:881-88.

Hsiao, W.C., Braun, P. Kelly, N.L., & Becker, E.R. (1988c). "Results, potential effects, and implementation issues of the resource-based relative value scale." *Journal of the American Medical Association* 260: 2429-38.

Hsiao, W.C., Couch, N.P., & Causino, N. (1988d). "Resource-based Relative Values for Invasive Procedures Performed by Eight Surgical Specialties." *Journal of the American Medical Association* 260: 2418-24.

Hsiao, W.C., Yntema, D.B., & Braun, P. (1988e). "Measurement and Analysis of Intraservice Work." *Journal of the American Medical Association* 260: 2361-70.

Langwell, K.M., & Nelson, L.M. (1986). "Physician Payment Systems: A Review of History, Alternatives, and Evidence." *Medical Care Review* 43(Spring): 5-58.

Lee, P.R. & Ginsburg, P.B. (1991). "The Trials of Medicare Physician Payment Reform." *Journal of the American Medical Association* 266: 1562-65.

McMenamin, P., West, H., & Marcus, L. (1988). *Changes in medicare part B physician charges: Final report.* Springfield, VA: Mandex Inc.

Mitchell, J.B., Wedig, G., & Cromwell, J. (1989). "The medicare physician fee freeze." *Health Affairs* 8: 21-33.

Physician Payment Review Commission. (1988). *Annual report to congress.* Washington, DC.

Physician Payment Review Commission. (1989). *Annual report to congress.* Washington, DC.

Physician Payment Review Commission. (1991a). *Annual report to congress.* Washington, DC.

Physician Payment Review Commission. (1991b). *Comments on the notice of proposed rulemaking for the medicare fee schedule* (No. 91-6). Washington, DC.

Physician Payment Review Commission. (1991c). *Survey of visits and consultations* (No. 91-1). Washington, DC.

Posner, J.R. (1986). "Trends in Medical Malpractice Insurance." *Law and Contemporary Problems* 49 (Spring): 37-56.

Schieber, G.J., & Poullier, J.P. (1991). "International Health Spending: Issues and Trends." *Health Affairs* 10 (Spring): 106-116.

Showstack, J.A., Blumberg, B.D., & Schwartz, J. (1979). "Fee-for-service Physician Payment: Analysis of Current Methods and Their Development." *Inquiry* 16 (Fall): 230-246.

U.S. Congress, House of Representatives, Committee on Ways and Means. (1990). Background materials and data on programs within the jurisdiction of the committee on ways and means. Washington, DC: Government Printing Office.

Wilensky, G.R., & Rossiter, L.F. (1986). "Alternative Units of Payment for Physician Services: An Overview of the Issues." *Medical Care Review* 43 (Spring): 133-56.

TECHNOLOGY ASSESSMENT IN TAIWAN

Gerard F. Anderson

The rapid changes in the health insurance system that are anticipated between now and the year 2000 will necessitate careful scrutiny and potential restructuring of the health care delivery system in Taiwan. Taiwan will have to examine carefully the existing supply of health care facilities and physicians, the method of setting prices for health care services, and the adequacy of the current technology assessment process before implementing national health insurance in order to be able to control costs, maintain access to essential services, and promote the provision of high quality medical care.

The first step will be a careful review of the existing supply and geographic distribution of hospitals, clinics, physicians, and other health care professionals to determine whether they are adequate to fulfill demands likely to be created by the expansion of health insurance coverage. The second step is a careful examination of the method of health care financing to determine whether appropriate incentives exist to produce the required quantity of services at equitable prices. Finally, it will be necessary to carefully examine current medical practice and scrutinize emerging technologies and procedures. All three activities are necessary in order to ensure that medical practice is appropriate, effective, and of high quality.

Research in Human Capital and Development, Volume 7, pages 347-357.

ISBN: 1-55938-132-9

I. REGULATING THE SUPPLY OF MEDICAL SERVICES

In conventional national income accounting, the level of a nation's expenditures in a particular sector is by definition a measure of the economic contribution of that sector. The recent explosion in the proportion of national income spent on computing and information processing, for example, is generally regarded as progress, rather than grounds for concern about a "computer cost explosion." Thus, the need to regulate the supply of health care services generally comes as a great surprise for individuals trained in classical economics.

Health economists on the other hand are concerned over the "value for money" in health care services. For example, the United States spends approximately 11.5 percent of the gross domestic product on health care compared to the 8.0 percent spent in most industrialized countries, yet the U.S. health status indicators are generally poorer. This type of comparison supports the widespread view that the institutions governing the organization and delivery of health care have a particular tendency to generate costs without proportional benefits.

Controlling costs without damaging quality of care or access to care is a major policy concern in most industrialized countries. An increase from the current 4.5 percent to 8.0 percent of gross domestic product in Taiwan by the year 2000 is expected as more people become eligible for health insurance benefits. An important question becomes "what will these increased expenditures be able to purchase?" Without careful monitoring, expenditures could increase without a significant improvement in health status. Based on international experience, the consensus is that unless some type of external controls are imposed on the growth of the health care sector, its financial demands will grow indefinitely. The problem is especially acute in countries with universal health insurance coverage and few regulatory controls on health care spending.

Investments in new buildings and equipment represent a significant proportion of spending by hospitals and clinics. The level and target of capital spending determine what services can be performed in which settings, and who has access to certain procedures. Of even greater importance is that capital spending will have long run implications for operating costs. Unlike most other industries where there is a capital labor tradeoff, most health economists have found that increased capital spending results in additional operating expenditures (Anderson, Erickson, & Feigenbaum, 1987). As a result, it is critical to examine the capital acquisition process if costs are to be contained and capital distributed in the most cost efficient manner.

A related issue is the geographic distribution of health care facilities. Health facilities are seldom distributed evenly within a country. Generally, there are more facilities available per capita in urban and more affluent areas and fewer services available in rural and poorer neighborhoods. This is true in countries with national health insurance programs and countries with decentralized free enterprise systems.

Taiwan currently has uneven distribution of health facilities among geographic regions and between rural and urban areas. In 1987, there were 905 hospitals and 11,294 clinics (facilities with less than 10 beds) in Taiwan (Hsaio & Lu, 1989). Taiwan has a total of 86,000 beds which is equal to 4.4 beds per 1000 population or the same proportion as the United States. Beds, however, are unevenly distributed across regions in Taiwan with the supply varying from 21.6 per 1000 population in Hwalien County and 10.6 in Chiayi City to 2.0 in Taichung County and 3.3 in Tainan City. Most of the tertiary care beds are located in Taipei. Although the government is trying to remedy the maldistribution of hospital beds through the five-year Health Plan, the economic interests of physician or owners of existing facilities is a powerful countervailing influence.

The implementation of universal health insurance in Taiwan will generate great demands on the existing health care delivery system. Hospitals, especially tertiary care facilities, will experience increased demand as insurance coverage removes financial barriers to care. It will be increasingly important to monitor the types of patients who are seen at these very sophisticated facilities to make sure that they cannot be treated at a lower cost and more effectively at a clinic or some other less sophisticated facility. Making sure that patients are seen in the most appropriate settings is going to be one of the major challenges of the next several years.

All this suggests an increased role for the Taiwan government in the health care sector. The government may want to have a direct role in regulating the supply of health care facilities. In most industrialized countries, the government controls the capital budgets of hospitals and other facilities. Through government control it is possible to constrain the growth of health care facilities and to redistribute health care services from urban areas where they tend to congregate to rural areas where they are frequently needed.

The five-year plan adopted in 1985 introduces regional planning for hospital services and requires hospitals to obtain prior approval before the construction of new beds. Examination of the U.S. experience suggest that this approach will not work unless patient care revenues and capital spending are controlled by the same regional planning body. In the United States, each local community wanted hospitals with modern physical plants, a capacity sufficient to handle all health care needs without referral outside the local community, and the most sophisticated technology available. The source of revenue for patient care for most of these facilities was national. As a result, the health planning program was unable to control capital expenditures or to encourage facilities to locate in underserved areas.

In my opinion, a successful health planning program will require that the government establish a comprehensive facility plan and maintain that plan in spite of the political pressure which will be applied. Taiwan may want to consider an approach which allows the government to build the facilities thereby giving the government even greater control than simply approving private sector applications. If the government relies on the private sector to build health care facilities there is no guarantee that facilities will be located in areas of greatest need. In fact, international experience suggests that facilities will be built in areas of existing higher concentration.

The government should also investigate a mandatory referral system which requires a patient to be seen by a primary care physician before going to a tertiary care facility. If the patient goes directly to the tertiary care facility, the insurance company can elect not to cover the person for that visit. In emergencies, of course, this requirement would be waived.

II. THE CONTROL OF HEALTH PROFESSIONALS

Many of the same problems and policy options regarding the supply of health facilities also apply to the supply of health professionals. In some ways, control of physicians may be even more difficult since Taiwan's physicians tend to occupy the top rung of the socioeconomic ladder (Hsaio & Lu, 1989). In addition to favorable social and economic status, many physicians enjoy considerable political influence. City and country medical associations are strong protectors of the physician's autonomy including opposition to government regulations to monitor the quality and appropriateness of care. The tertiary care hospitals and physicians are particularly protected since most of the political leaders receive their medical care at these institutions.

There are two aspects of the physician's practice which deserve particular attention. While both of these practices are common in Japan and South Korea as well, they deserve particular attention because of their potential impact on health care costs and medical practice. The two aspects are the ability of physicians to dispense drugs and to operate hospital beds.

In Taiwan, private physicians and hospital outpatient departments generate most of their revenues by prescribing and dispensing drugs. In 1987, the average cost of a physician visit including drugs was $10 with most of the physician's revenue derived from the dispensing of drugs. Almost half of Taiwan's health expenditures are for pharmaceuticals. Evidence has been collected which suggests that prescription patterns, particularly with respect to antibiotics, may be influenced by payment levels (Hsaio & Lu, 1989).

In addition, the practice of permitting physicians to dispense drugs has probably increased utilization of outpatient physician visits. Currently, the number of visits per capita is almost double the rate in the United States and is 50 percent greater than the rate in Japan. In order for Taiwan to control costs and to ensure that drugs are dispensed appropriately, it may be necessary to sever the link between the dispensing of drugs and physician offices.

In Taiwan, a clinic is similar to a private office of an American physician with a major difference: many clinics also operate beds for patients. These clinics provide predominantly primary care services since the physicians do not have admitting privileges in other hospitals. Because the clinic is frequently owned and operated by the physician, there is a strong economic incentive for the physician to try and fill these beds. In Korea, which has the same clinic arrangement, I conducted a study for the World Bank which found that when physicians owned and operated clinics there were several undesirable consequences (Anderson, 1989; World Bank, 1988). First, many patients were admitted unnecessarily. Second, they stayed longer than necessary and/or received too many ancillary services. Finally, some patients were prevented from transferring to a tertiary care hospital where care may have been more appropriate. In Korea, the problem of inappropriate care in clinics was exacerbated when Korea initiated National Health Insurance and more people elected to receive care in tertiary care centers leaving the clinics with unfilled beds. In Korea, the occupancy of clinics was below 50 percent in 1988 (World Bank, 1988).

Until recently, the government has done little to monitor physicians and other health professionals beyond the licensing of physicians and other health professionals. Only recently have funds been made available to develop group practice primary care clinics in rural communities. Earlier, the government increased the number of student scholarships in medical schools and required those graduates to accept lengthy assignments to practice in rural areas. In most countries, these programs have been only mildly successful. The problem is that once the obligation ends, most of the physicians leave the rural areas and migrate to the urban location. Residents in rural areas are left with the impression that their physicians are not well trained and do not want to be there, thereby further encouraging the rural citizens to seek care in urban areas where they perceive the care is much better.

III. GOVERNMENT REGULATION OF PRICE AND QUALITY OF MEDICAL SERVICES

In Taiwan, physicians and hospitals are paid fee-for-service with most of the prices set by the providers themselves. This provides strong financial incentives to perform more tests, order more drugs, and to schedule return visits. The current payment system also allows significantly higher payments to tertiary care facilities for routine services which does not discourage the tertiary care facility from providing these services. As a result, Taiwan must review its payment system before implementing universal health insurance coverage.

Taiwan has traditionally relied on competition to control prices and to ensure that hospitals and physicians provide an adequate quality of medical care. As more and more people are insured and they have to pay less and less out of their own pocket for their medical care, the policing activity of the market place deteriorates. In the United States, where 93 cents out of every dollar spent on hospital care is paid by insurance, all of the empirical evidence suggests that hospitals do not compete on the basis of price, but instead, compete on the basis of services which are available. As Taiwan implements universal coverage, this observation must be kept in mind.

Insurance companies already attempt to regulate payment rates, but without a cost accounting system, it is difficult to set hospital prices accurately. One important piece of evidence that hospital prices are being set too high is that entrepreneurs want to build and manage hospitals suggesting that they are a good financial investment. In Taiwan, physicians earn approximately six times as much as the average manufacturing worker (Hsaio & Lu, 1989). In most western European countries, the average is closer to three times (Anderson & Antebi, 1990). Unlike Korea, Japan, and most other industrialized nations, Taiwan does not have a physician fee schedule.

It is well known that payment rates can dramatically influence medical practice. I have already discussed how generation of revenues from prescription drugs can influence dispensing patterns in Taiwan. In the United States, the length of stay in the elderly dropped by almost two days when the Medicare program (which covers people over age 65) instituted a new hospital payment system which paid hospitals the same amount regardless of length of stay. The same hospital payment reform initiative has had some, but certainly less dramatic, changes on other aspects on practice patterns in hospitals (Anderson & Steinberg, 1988; Davis, Anderson, Rowland, & Steinberg, 1990).

An important step in trying to set equitable payment rates is to differentiate outputs. DRGs are a measure of hospital output and allow the government or an insurance company to compare the output of one hospital to another hospital. DRGs take into account the diagnosis, procedure, complications and/or comorbidities, age, and discharge status of the patient and then group each patient into one of 477 categories. As a result, DRGs recognize that one hospital treats relatively simple cases such as simple deliveries while another hospital treats a more complex set of surgical patients. These differences in case mix become incorporated into the hospital payment system. In the United States, approximately 40 percent of hospital revenues are paid on the basis of DRGs. In many western European countries, the governments are using or exploring the use of the diagnosis related groups (DRGs) to either set payment rates for hospitals or to set hospital budgets.

If Taiwan is going to try to control hospital expenditures and to allocate resources to hospitals efficiently and equitably, it will be necessary to institute some form of payment system which gives the government or the insurance company some ability to determine appropriate payment rates. All of the power to set prices cannot be left to the providers. Most countries are using DRGs to measure output and, therefore, to compare what is being produced at one hospital to what is being produced at another hospital. In order to introduce a payment system based on DRGs, it will be necessary to collect a minimum data set on every hospital discharge and to institute a system to allow costs or charges to be assigned to each discharge. With this minimal information, it will be possible to compare the output of hospitals and to design an equitable hospital payment system.

Reforming the physician payment system is also necessary if the system is going to be equitable and encourage the efficient provision of medical care. Both Drs Lee and Davis are more familiar with these issues and I will not discuss the issue of physician payment reform at this time.

Technology Assessment

It is difficult to determine when a particular technology or medical practice is appropriate and even more difficult to control inappropriate practices once they are identified. In most countries, including Taiwan, the physician-patient relationship is sacrosanct, and it is difficult to regulate the practice of medicine. In Taiwan the issue of where patients should receive care is likely to be an issue of primary importance given that many patients are using tertiary care facilities for common ailments that can be treated in other settings. It may also become necessary to monitor what technologies are being purchased by hospitals in order to make sure that resources are being spent wisely.

For technology assessment to be effective, it is necessary to have the appropriate supply of health facilities and health professionals and an appropriate payment system. If there are too few health facilities or health professionals, then there will be long waiting lists for care and the role of technology assessment will become a triage function which attempts to allocate resources to individuals in greatest need who will benefit the most. If there are too many health facilities or health professionals, then the responsibility of technology assessment will be to decide which services are being done unnecessarily or have only marginal benefit for the patient. In this case, the person conducting the technology assessment is frequently being opposed by the health care professional who believes that what he or she is doing is appropriate and necessary for patient care.

For technology assessment to be effective, it is also necessary to have an appropriate payment system. If the price for performing certain services is too low, then most health professionals will be reluctant to perform them. If the prices are set too high, then the temptation will be to perform more services than are medically necessary.

In the United States, there are two other barriers to implementing technology assessment recommendations or at least federal financing of technology assessment. One barrier is that pharmaceutical and health equipment manufacturers have a significant financial investment in certain products and use their influence to effect the technology assessment process.

In the United States, the government has never been able to mount an effective technology assessment program. In other countries which have more control over the health care delivery system, the technology assessment program is more effective in controlling the diffusion of new technology. Sweden and most of the Scandinavian countries are the leaders in actually using technology assessment to control the diffusion of new technology.

For the technology assessment process to be effective in Taiwan, it is also necessary to have a strong independent body which accredits health care facilities. The accrediting body must guarantee that the institutions meet certain minimal quality standards. This is necessary to ensure that the prescribed treatment will be administered properly.

I have focussed on the barriers to effective technology assessment because they appear to be more important than methodological limitations in the technology assessment process. Often, it is more difficult to implement a technology assessment finding than it is to conduct an assessment.

Within the methodology of conducting a technology assessment, the most difficult part is agreeing on the outcomes. Specifically, it is difficult to agree whether the only important outcome of an intervention is a reduction in mortality or possibly morbidity or whether patient satisfaction, activities of daily living, and the effect on family members are also relevant. It is also necessary to decide whether only medical costs are relevant or whether all costs are important including work loss, compensation for pain and suffering, and other indirect costs should be considered. Finally, it is necessary to decide from whose perspective to evaluate the outcomes. In our evaluations, we have conducted analysis from the perspective of society, the patient and the hospital. The answers obtained are very difficult depending on the perspective which is taken.

At Johns Hopkins, I helped establish a Program for Medical Technology and Practice Assessment which evaluates emerging technologies. Currently, we are examining technologies such as low osmolar contrast media, gallstone lithotripsy, and lomefloxacin. We examine the technologies primarily from a cost and quality of care perspective. In general, the new technologies are more expensive than the technologies they replace (low osmolar contrast media, for example, is 10 to 20 times more expensive than current contrast media), but may have some better actual or perceived quality. We examine the emerging technologies and make recommendations about whether hospitals or other health care providers should purchase the new technology. In making the recommendations, we present data on the cost, the expected impact on quality of life and patient satisfaction. The recommendations are presented in peer reviewed academic journals and are not binding on any institution, including the Johns Hopkins Hospital.

In the United States, technology assessment has entered a new phase of development. It is called outcomes research. Multidisciplinary teams of physicians, economists, statisticians, survey researchers, epidemiologists, and other health service researchers come together to study a particular treatment mode. In the United States nearly $50 million will be allocated each year to this type of research in 1990 and spending should double by 1992.

At Johns Hopkins, we are studying cataract surgery. More than one million cataract extractions are performed annually, making cataract surgery the most common surgical procedure performed on the elderly in the United States. Moreover, the number of cataract operations is increasing rapidly. Between 1965 and 1985, the number of cataract operations increased 500 percent while the elderly population increased by only 35 percent. Studies of geographic variations in cataract surgeries in the United States show 4 to 1 variations by region of the country. International comparisons show that the United States performs significantly more than other countries. As a result, the question becomes how many of these surgeries are appropriate.

Our study of cataract surgery has a number of specific objectives:

1. To document the variation in clinical outcomes, patient functioning, patient satisfaction and health care costs as a function of alternative strategies for management of cataracts;
2. To determine the values placed on specific clinical and functional outcomes by patients and ophthalmologists;
3. To define "appropriate" or "optimal" management strategies for different categories of cataract patients and delineate the factor(s) that determine why a particular management strategy is considered to be "optimal" for a particular category of patient; and
4. To develop a strategy for informing physicians and patients about "optimal" management strategies and a plan for evaluating the impact of intervention.

In order to meet each of these objectives, we have developed a research agenda which involves:

- An analysis of patient specific insurance claims data to determine what services patients received before and after cataract surgery in order to determine if any of them influenced the outcome.
- An analysis of claims data to determine if the specific surgical technique that was used influenced the outcome.
- A survey of patient expectations concerning improvement in their vision before the surgery and their level of satisfaction following surgery to determine how cataract surgery influenced their satisfaction.
- A survey of patient mobility pre and post surgery to determine the impact of surgery on activities of daily living.
- A survey of physicians to determine how actual practice conforms to their perceptions of efficient medical practice.
- A meta analysis of all the published literature in order to systematically analyze the multitude of existing studies.
- A decision analysis which will determine best demonstrated practice for patients with certain clinical conditions.

At the end of the project, we hope that the information, which will be widely disseminated to physicians, will influence their medical practice. In addition, the government and private insurers may use the information to establish medical practice guidelines. These guidelines would then determine what services would be paid for and under what conditions.

IV. SUMMARY AND CONCLUSIONS

Control of health care costs, efficient and effective medical care, and the provision of high quality of medical care are dependent on a number of factors. In this paper I discuss three issues; first, the need to control the supply of medical care services including hospitals and physicians; second, the need to have a payment system which rewards appropriate behavior; and third, a technology assessment program which continually evaluates emerging and existing techniques and medical practice. All three are necessary to assure that patients have access to high quality medical care at low cost.

The appropriate supply of facilities and health care professionals is necessary to ensure that there is access to essential services, but at the same time, there is not an over supply of providers who need to keep busy. Careful attention must be given, to the geographic distribution of providers as well as the total supply of providers. Based upon international experience, government control over the process is necessary to ensure an equitable distribution. A program which simply approves or disapproves applications will not be as successful in allocating resources as a system with greater government control.

Payment systems which give most of the power to set rates to the provider are unlikely to be effective in either controlling costs or promoting good medical care. It is necessary to define the output that is desired from the medical intervention and to pay accordingly. In the United States, for example, patients are classified into diagnosis related groups (DRGs) and treatment of a patient in a specific DRG is the output of the hospital.

Technology assessment is necessary to evaluate existing and emerging technologies. The major difficulty is to compare the costs, which are relatively easy to determine, and the benefits, which are much more difficult to determine. Increasingly, technology assessment requires the researcher to define the benefits of the medical intervention which can range from decreased mortality to an improvement in activities of daily living to a greater level of satisfaction with life.

REFERENCES

Anderson G. (1989). Korea: Adopting a private sector approach to achieve universal health insurance coverage. *Health Affairs.*

Anderson, G., Erickson, J., & Feigenbaum, S. (1987). Examining the relationship between capital investment and hospital operating expenditures. *The Review of Economics and Statistics.*

Anderson, G., & Antebi, S. (1990). A surplus of physicians in Israel—Any lessons for industrialized countries? *Health Policy,* (in review).

Davis, K., Anderson, G.F., Rowland, D., & Steinberg, E.P. (1990). *Health care cost containment: Lessons from the past and a policy proposal for the future.* Johns Hopkins University Press, 1990.

Foote S.B. (1987). Assessing medical technology assessment: Past, present, and future. *Milbank Memorial Fund Quarterly* 64(1): 59-80.

Hsaio, W.C., & Lu, J.R. (1989). *Taiwan's health care system and its challenge for future development.* Harvard University School of Public Health.

Steinberg, E.P., & Anderson, G. (1987). Potential "losers" under per case payment. *Annals of Internal Medicine.*

World Bank. (1988). *Korea: Health Insurance and the health sector.* Report No. 7412-KO.

LESSONS FROM THE KOREAN EXPERIENCE WITH UNIVERSAL HEALTH INSURANCE

Seung-Hum Yu

Korea as a country was completely devastated during the war from 1950 to 1953. However, in the period of two to three decades thereafter, Korea has experienced significant development both economically and socially. In the early 1960s, Korea had been typically agricultural, with 70 percent of the population living in rural areas and a per capita GNP of $100 U.S. dollars.

Korea today is one of the newest industrialized countries with 70 percent of the population living in urban areas and a per capita GNP of $5,000 dollars. A Family Planning Program and the Five Year Economic Development Plans have been successfully implemented over the past two decades.

Among the social indicators, the educational level is very high. The population of Korea is 43 million with a crude birth rate of 16 and an infant mortality rate of 12. Life expectancy is 67 for males and 74 for females (Ministry of Health and Social Affairs, 1990).

Research in Human Capital and Development, Volume 7, pages 359-368.

ISBN: 1-55938-132-9

I. HISTORICAL BACKGROUND

Laws for social security and workers' compensation were passed in 1963; however, social security legislation was unrealistic. In the early 1970s, serious social security and health care issues were first raised.

In 1977, when the fourth Five-Year Economic Development Plan began, per capita GNP was $800. Korea launched two important programs: Medical Aid for the lowest income group and the elderly, and Company Health Insurance for those firms with 500 or more employees. The former was established as a form of public assistance, the latter compulsory.

The ceiling for compulsory insurance was lowered to firms with at least 300 employees in 1979, and to those with 100 employees in 1981. In addition, health insurance for private school/university teachers and staff, the government employees, and their dependents was instituted in 1979 using the same principle under a different law.

The remainder of the nation's population that was not covered, about half of the total, were the self-employed: farmers and fishermen in rural areas as well as those employed in cottage industries. The government's plan was to be instituted in three geographical areas each in 1981 and 1982, and then expanded by 30 percent of the uninsured at a time in 1985, 1987, and 1988, respectively.

Meanwhile, beginning in 1983, insurance coverage was required for those firms employing 16 or more persons. An intolerable financial deficit, partly due to inefficient premium collection, in a pilot regional medical insurance program, had spurred heated debate on whether universal health insurance was being considered prematurely.

However, social pressure was strong enough to stir the government to action. There were three major issues concerning the uninsured. First, the uninsured paid more medical and hospital bills due to the reimbursement scheme (the insured paid less because reimbursement from insurance was set lower than existing payment levels). Second, those who were not insured urgently needed insurance because they generally did not have a regular income. Third, there was no coverage even if the uninsured wished to be voluntarily insured.

In 1986, after long debate, a final decision was made: those still uninsured in rural areas would be covered by the Universal Medical Care before January 1988 and those in urban areas before July 1989. Korea is unique in that it is the only country in the world to achieve universal medical care coverage within 12 years since its inception; every Korean is now covered for health care whenever needed.

Medical insurance coverage is summarized as follows:

Year Started	Category	Population Covered
1977	Lowest income group and the elderly	4.2 million
1977	Employees	16.5 million
1979	Government employees and teachers	4.5 million
1988	Rural residents	6.4 million
1989	Urban residents	12.6 million

II. THE KOREAN HEALTH INSURANCE SYSTEM

Social insurance originated in the Bismarck era a century ago. Under the program, insurance was compulsory for everyone and premiums/contributions were levied on the basis of individual or household income. Benefit coverage was commensurate to all insured.

Premiums for employees were shared 50/50 with employers; the government subsidized administrative expenses. For the self-employed, a premium was levied based on assets, the number of household members, and other sources of income according to a composite index formula; the government subsidized about half of the revenue because they did not have employer contributions for premium sharing.

The employees and their dependents in each firm or group of firms organized specialized insurance societies. An insurance society was a legal body akin to a cooperative, responsible for levying/collecting premiums and paying benefits.

The Korean health insurance system is operated independently on a non-profit basis. There are 154 industrial medical insurance societies. Insurance for government employees and teachers is managed by a separate corporation, an extremely large society in which four and a half million people are insured.

The self-employed belong to regional medical insurance societies, which are organized by an administrative unit such as a city or county. There are 254 regional medical insurance societies of which 117 are urban.

Reimbursement to the providers is fee-for-service, where a standard fee schedule for providers is set by the government and negotiated with the professional societies in advance, applicable uniformly nationwide. Hospital doctors are salaried as hospital employees. Practicing physicians usually have several beds in their own clinics with equipment for laboratory tests and X-rays if they wish.

Benefits are comprehensive: medical and hospital care, inpatient and outpatient drugs, basic dental care, and some herbal medical care. Excluded are cosmetic surgery, orthodontics, eyeglasses, blood, and so forth.

Beneficiaries have their choice of doctors and hospitals within their catchment areas except in the case of university hospitals (or equivalent tertiary care institutions) for ambulatory care. There are eight catchment areas: seven provincial areas and Seoul.

Co-insurance is applied; 80 percent of the total costs for inpatient care is paid by insurance. However, different copayment and deductibles apply to outpatient care to encourage the use of both primary and secondary care institutions. For clinic visits, patients pay the first $3 (U.S. currency) when the total bill is less than $15 and 30 percent coinsurance if over this amount. For hospital ambulatory visits, patients pay 40-50 percent of charges plus the examination fee.

III. IMPLEMENTATION ISSUES

First Stage (1977-1980)

The chief complaint from those insured was that they were not cared for like the uninsured were; the quality of care seemed inferior and the quantity of care insufficient. However, since the reimbursement level was lower for doctors and hospitals, the opposite was true: the insured received more care for each health dollar spent (Yu, 1983).

Providers complained about the level of reimbursement. A standard fee schedule set by the government, applicable to all doctors and hospitals, was definitely lower than their customary charges. Doctors therefore claimed that their income would be markedly decreased. But the number of patients had rapidly increased, and there was no evidence that their gross revenue had decreased appreciably (Yu, 1988b).

On the other hand, the uninsured were at a disadvantage since, due to the difference between standard costs and the fee schedule, the paid more than the insured did for similar care. Because the uninsured were generally a lower income group than the insured, the question of social justice arose.

The financial status of the program was difficult to determine because providers usually sent claims late as they were unfamiliar with the paperwork. However, the medical care utilization level and pattern changed pretty much as expected (Kim, Yu, & Kim, 1986). Hospitals, especially small ones, and the number of beds increased markedly once insurance began.

Expanding Stage (1981-1987); Pilot Regional Insurance Program

When salaried personnel (company employees, government employees, and teachers and staff) were insured, about half of the population remained uninsured: rural farmers and those self-employed. Premium collection is easy for salaried personnel since employers contribute half of the premium and the remainder is deducted from the payroll.

However, those uninsured had no regular cash income; in general, it was difficult to compute their income, deduct from their payroll, and so on. Additionally, these people typically need more insurance.

Therefore, the expansion of universal health insurance had been hotly debated. Opponents contended that once the insurance system began, the financial burden to the government would be enormous. Proponents countered that on average, people spend as much on insurance premiums as they had spent formerly on medical care.

The government tested a regional medical insurance program in three areas each in 1981 and 1982 to decide when and how to expand health insurance in rural areas and for the self-employed. Meanwhile, consolidation of all insurance schemes into a single system was proposed, as the employees' insurance had a financial surplus. There was both agreement and strong objections to this proposal.

The trial projects showed large financial deficits in all areas but one. There were two major reasons for the deficits: low premium collection and the imbalance between benefits and premiums. After several years of experience in regional medical insurance, the collection rate increased as those insured began understanding the system (Yu, 1986).

The method of collecting premiums was a problem. Premium rating was also more difficult for the newly insured because of their irregular cash income. Since a rural community is a closed society, monetary sums are relative rather than absolute.

Premiums were collected in three ways. The insured paid the insurance office directly, either insurance society staff or village chiefs collecting the premium monthly.

Geographical accessibility was also an issue. The government provided long-term loans for the construction of hospitals in remote and underprivileged areas, and it dispatched public doctors, who were exempted from active military service, to each town (population: 5,000-10,000) where there was no practicing physician.

Because transportation and communications had improved, most people could reach care facilities within half an hour except from islands and extremely remote areas. Community health practitioners (trained nurses) were dispatched to islands and remote areas with populations of less than 300 for simple care and preventive services.

As is the case in other countries, reimbursements to the providers was a continuing issue. Providers complained that the reimbursement level was too low to maintain existing facilities. If this was true, the providers would have decreased care capacities to minimize losses; however, the number of beds increased.

The government was averse to financial deficit and reviewed payment methods seriously. But due to strong resistance from the medical community, no changes were made. The primary method to control health care costs was to gradually increase the uniform fee schedule, which caused continuing conflicts with the medical profession.

Universal Health Insurance (1988-1989)

Throughout the 1980s, there was heated debate over society-managed insurance versus single system-managed insurance. If each insurance society would have been managed independently, the insured would be more cautious concerning the financial balance between premiums and benefits since each insurance society would be held responsible financially.

Under the single system on the other hand, the insured would be less sensitive to keeping a financial balance. In addition, the income of salaried personnel is easily calculated, which is not the case with rural people and the self-employed. Therefore, the former pay higher premiums than the latter.

In the end, the existing system was chosen for universal health insurance. Thus, each administrative unit has its own insurance society for regional medical insurance.

Even though the government subsidizes about half of the revenue for regional medical insurance societies, there are still financial imbalances. According to the experience from the pilot regional insurance program, stabilization is achieved in no less than two to three years since the rate of premium collection increases after three to four years.

Only two years of rural insurance and one year of urban insurance have passed. Therefore, specific issues concerning universal health insurance have not been raised yet. Several issues including the health care delivery system, reimbursement scheme, separation of prescription and drug dispensing, quality of care, claims review, and herb medicine have been discussed or debated according to the interests of professional societies or groups.

The major concern now is financial tolerability, particularly cost containment. Radical changes in the payment system to the providers will not happen in the near future.

IV. EVALUATION OF THE KOREAN HEALTH INSURANCE SYSTEM

Korea has achieved universal health insurance over the past twelve years, and this may be considered a national experiment. It is also interesting and easy to review as a case.

The goal of the system is to offer affordable, quality medical care to everyone. Every Korean can now get medical care when it is needed. A universal quality standard is met; however, there is still some discrepancy between urban and rural health care.

The efficiency of the system is still inconclusive. Whether the system will develop into a national health service like that in the United Kingdom, consolidating all insurance schemes into a single system, or in Canada, with funding through a premium or taxation, is not likely for several years since there would be insufficient rationale for such a change.

As for cost containment, the government currently sets the reimbursement scheme and controls capital investment for expensive equipment and more beds, while the insurer reviews claims. When reimbursement is insufficient, providers tend to increase the volume of their services, which is then reflected in total health expenditures. Either the government or the insurance authorities (federation of insurance societies) had proposed payment methods other than fee-for-service, but it was not adopted because of strong resistance from the providers.

Administrative costs are somewhat higher than expected. However, the substantial appropriations for public relations, health insurance education, and premium collection personnel will decrease as the system stabilizes.

The co-insurance rate seems rather high, but higher co-insurance payments are preferred over increasing premiums. Some professionals complain that the lowest income group cannot gain access to medical care because of the high copayments, but this is not apparent in reality. It is only a matter of the priorities set by each household; indeed, both urban and rural households spend more money on tobacco and recreation than on medical care in Korea.

The level of utilization is constantly increasing; consequently, total health care expenditures are also increasing. It is estimated that Korea spent about 5 percent of its GNP on health care (Kwon, 1988), which is not bad for now.

It is not known how much money or what percentage of the GNP should ideally be spent on health care. Currently, total health care expenditures in Korea are roughly equivalent to that for the consumption of tobacco. Capital investment limitations do not work very well.

To prevent unnecessary utilization, the coinsurance system is applied to inpatient care, and both coinsurance and a deductible are applied for ambulatory care. Claims concerning unnecessary treatment and overtreatment are reviewed by the insurer; less than two percent of gross claims are overturned through review.

Clients are generally happy about accessing medical care when ill without heavy financial burden. They complain about long hospitals waits, mostly at university hospitals, for ambulatory care. It is not uncommon for people to go without a referral to a university hospital for simple illnesses.

Providers are unsatisfied with the reimbursements. In the past, by limiting the number of experienced doctors, each would be well off; today however, practicing physicians are supported by a sufficient number of patients to prosper due to the increased demand (Kim, Yu, & Kim, 1986).

The ultimate goal of universal health insurance is the improvement in the health of a nation. It is presently too early to determine the success of this. Preventive care is insufficient; antenatal and delivery care are covered, but not immunization. More systematic preventive care measures are now being considered. Since the insured desire annual checkups and preventive services, many insurance societies started covering regular checkups and screening, and health education is given through leaflets or education sessions.

The main interest in each sector is different. The government is concerned with financial stability and cost containment. Providers are keen to increase the reimbursement level with minimal interference and regulation from the government. Clients are anxious to pay a lower premium and to get better care with free choices among care facilities.

Health insurance professionals are concerned with the insurance system and its management, mostly focusing on cost containment and better care. Studies have been done on these, only a limited number of which have been published in English. Studies on the quality of care, changes in utilization level and pattern, behavioral changes of clients and providers, changes in demand and supply of medical care are suggested.

V. FUTURE ISSUES IN THE KOREAN INSURANCE SYSTEM

First of all, there has been and will continue to be concern and debate over the health insurance system. National health services vs. national health insurance system, society-managed vs. unified system-managed, and alternative health care delivery system like HMO's are serious considerations. This is not just a discussion of effective and efficient aspects; there is also the matter of sociopolitical and cultural considerations.

Second, chronic and long-term care should be considered. Korea has a very limited number of chronic care facilities such as mental and tuberculosis hospitals. Care for up to six months per year is covered by insurance.

In fact, ten to fifteen percent of acute general hospital beds are occupied by long-term care patients, such as those involved in traffic accidents, worker's compensation, and other chronic care. Since the population is obviously aging and the demand for chronic care will be increasing enormously, this will have to be taken into account.

Third, cost containment should not be ignored. Advanced technology is being rapidly introduced in Korea—Computed Tomography and Magnetic Resonance Imaging. There are also the pharmaceutical companies: more than 35 joint multinational ventures are competing in Korea. It should be noted that about one third of insurance benefits are spent on drugs.

Fourth, reimbursement to the providers, the billing system, and the claims review mechanism are very complicated. The reimbursement system is expected to eventually undergo changes, albeit with difficulty.

Administrative expenses, client satisfaction, quality of care, medical care costs, and the promotion of the nation's health should all be taken into account when changes of the universal health insurance system are considered. Last but not least, the socioeconomical, political, and cultural aspects of health care should be considered deeply, not using another country as a model.

VI. LESSONS FROM THE KOREAN EXPERIENCE

First, the insurance system should be taken into account. Once a system starts, it is very difficult to change. In any country beginning an insurance system, a single system is recommended over a segmented or categorized system.

Financing through taxes is recommended when everybody is insured. Taxation is easier to implement than premium levying and collection if it is acceptable. Since it is difficult to calculate the income level of self-employed or rural people in developing countries, low income groups could be greatly burdened.

Second, the method of reimbursement should be decided before starting a system because it is important, not only to cost containment, but also to enhancing preventive services and reducing billing and reviewing efforts. Since Korea adopted the fee-for-service and third party payment methods, billing is very complicated and a standard fee schedule is applied nationwide; extra efforts in billing and reviewing claims are unavoidable.

Third, co-insurance is useful in reducing the use of unnecessary medical care by the insured and discouraging ovetreatment by the providers. Japanese insurance had full coverage until the early 1980s, when coinsurance was adopted; Korean coinsurance system was adopted from the beginning.

Fourth, Asian countries such as Taiwan are recommended not to imitate the U.S. health care system since Asian culture is quite different from Western culture, and cost containment is a serious matter. The Korean experience would be beneficial for those countries planning universal health insurance; having used trial-and-error for a decade, there have clearly been both problems and successes.

REFERENCES

Anderson, G.F. (1989). Universal health care coverage in Korea. *Health Affairs*, 852, 24-34.

Kim, I.S., Yu, S.H., & Kim, H.J. (1986). Impact of regional health insurance on the utilization of medical care by the rural population of Korea. *Yonsei Medical Journal*, 27, 138-146.

Kwon, S.W. (1988). Trends in national health expenditures. Korea Development Institute working paper No. 8809.

Moon, O.R. (1987). The national health insurance policy in Korea. The Eighth Formal Meeting of the Board, Asia-Pacific Academic Consortium for Public Health, Seoul.

Ministry of Health and Social Affairs, Republic of Korea. (1990). *Yearbook of Health and Social Statistics.*

National Federation of Medical Insurance. (1990). *1989 medical insurance statistical yearbook.*

Yu, S.H. (1983). Hospital care services between insured and non-insured patients for selected diagnosis in Korea. *Yonsei Medical Journal*, 24, 6-32.

Yu, S.H. (1986). Provision of health care protection for the rural population with special reference to the development of primary health care programs. International Social Security Association Asian Round Table Meeting on Social Security Protection for the Rural Population. Jakarta.

Yu, S.H. (1988a). Health Care Systems of Korea. In Sirageldin & Sorkin (eds.), *Health and Development*, Vol. 5. Greenwich, CT: JAI Press.

Yu, S.H. (1988b). Recent development in medical care delivery systems in the region. International Social Security Association Eighth ISSA Regional Conference for Asia and the Pacific. Seoul.

HEALTH AND THE NATIONAL ECONOMY

M. Harvey Brenner

I. INTRODUCTION

What is the importance of the national economy to the nation's health? From one viewpoint, the strongest and most pervasive findings in epidemiology—at the individual level of analysis—indicate that higher socioeconomic status is positively related to health and longevity (Antonovsky, 1967; Bunker, Gomby, & Kehrer, 1989; Kitagawa & Hauser, 1973; Report of the Research Working Group, 1980; Susser, Watson, & Hopper, 1985; Syme & Berkman, 1976; Wilkinson, 1986). Thus, one might infer that improvements in population socioeconomic status through economic growth would serve to improve health and longevity, while economic recession and decline would have the opposite effect.

However, improvements in the national economy can also give rise to errors of human adaptation that harm the national health. Many important risks to health arise out of the process of industrialization and economic growth, especially rapid growth. These health risks include the "lifestyle" diseases of "civilization" that are related to consumption of tobacco, alcohol, and fats; social isolation; and environmental contamination resulting from industrial processes. Thus, economic growth has mixed effects on the nation's health.

Research in Human Capital and Development, Volume 7, pages 369-391.

ISBN: 1-55938-132-9

Indeed, the conventional view among many in the medical community is that these health risks are the dominant factors of change in post-War mortality and that the principal sources of moderation of the health impact of these risks are health care interventions. This view interprets the central importance of socioeconomic position to health as reflecting either riskier consumption patterns or less adequate health care coverage in poorer populations.

The dominance of the conventional view has been challenged by the emerging psychobiological model of disease in which mental stresses (tension, anxiety, loss, hopelessness) and low social support increase the likelihood of illness (Engel, 1977; Henry, 1982; House et al, 1988; Karasek & Theorell, 1990; Litwak, Messeri, et al., 1989; Pearlin, 1989). This emerging model is supported by a considerable body of scientific evidence. The tendency has been to interpret the data in an individualistic perspective, focussing on subjective feelings of stress or personal coping styles and resources. Nonetheless, when the psychobiological approach has been used to understand general trends, or the role of economic change in health, it is assumed that a population's mental health status is potentially harmed by growth. This results, it is thought, from a speedier pace of social change, and a decline in family and community structures and ethnic or religious traditions (Brenner, 1990; Durkheim, 1951).

We therefore find ourselves with two formulations which appear to contradict the view that improved socioeconomic status is a fundamental and continuous source of improvement in the population's health. Yet, we can observe overarching trend declines in mortality rates in Western industrialized countries in the twentieth century (Doll, 1987; Epstein, 1990; Fries, et al., 1989; McKinlay, et al., 1989). How is this possible in the face of powerful trends of increased consumption and production risks to health, decline in family and community structure and minimal life extension attributable to health care?

Obviously, one cannot be intellectually satisfied with an outlook that harbors three unintegrated and conflicting themes. Further, as we shall see in this paper, two essential pieces of information are still missing from the story. The first is that socioeconomic status is a creature of national economic development—rather than highly individualized talent—reflecting economic growth and the distribution of national wealth. The second is that while improvement in socioeconomic status basically represents improvement in material well-being, that change has profound implications for mental status and thus for the psychobiological link to health.

The point is that respect for the individual, personal dignity and freedom, self esteem, knowledge, achievement and power—as well as the physical and nutritional necessities of life—are greatly influenced by income and wealth in societies with a market economy.

In this paper missing, but fundamental, pieces of information are introduced and examined in connection with the empirical evidence. Having identified the missing elements, the major part of this paper is then devoted to reconciling, and ultimately integrating the conflicting themes within a general systems framework. The themes, as we shall see, not only conflict in theory, but in actuality. The conflicting themes are in reality competing forces: economic growth and equality, health risks dependent on consumption and production, and health care technology. In the last analysis, the most dominant of these forces determine the trends in health and longevity.

In building the general systems framework, we therefore draw upon two strands of evolutionary theory. The first, and most traditional, regards societal development as a series of long trends involving the accumulation and diffusion of wealth and knowledge (Doll, 1987; Epstein, 1990; Fries et al, 1989). The second strand views the process of change as involving intense short-term conflict by which new technologies, ideas and institutions destroy the old; firms compete for survival in the market economy, and multiple interest groups including labor and capital, age, sex and ethnic groups conflict over the distribution of wealth and privilege (Collins, 1985; Dahrendorf, 1959, 1979).

II. THE ARGUMENT

It is the argument of this paper that stable economic growth—in conjunction with reasonable distributive equity—is in fact the *fundamental source* of improvement in health and longevity in industrialized societies, and in developing countries. Direct effects of economic growth include material benefits of wealth (e.g., nutrition, climate control, sanitation, injury control, health care access) and psychological effects of security and creativity stemming from greater control over the biological (including human) and physical environment. Indirect effects include long-term societal investments in development of the sciences and general education, by which human adaptational error can be detected and counteracted, and government expenditures that act as economic stabilizers and sources of income maintenance for vulnerable and dependent populations.

The overall process by which economic development affects health and longevity can be understood within the framework of a "basic" theory of societal evolution. Societal development, of which improved biological functioning is a principal outcome, proceeds through trial and error. The trials, or cultural experiments that produce greater human knowledge and productivity, are financed by previous investments (i.e., are based on accumulations of societal wealth). Errors of adaptation also arise out of the behavioral implications of greatly increased societal wealth or productive capacity. Such adaptational problems can become severe if the threats to health and longevity are not detected for an entire generation (e.g., smoking, alcohol and fat consumption, sedentariness, industrial carcinogens). Wealth stemming from increased productivity is in turn partly invested in knowledge development and its diffusion through education. In the long term, these tend to counteract adaptational error. The political process acts to accelerate or impede the speed at which adaptational error can be corrected.

The process of economic growth itself, a principal component of societal development, also involves major social and health costs. These arise from the problems of structural change and, especially in western industrialized societies, the business cycle (Brenner, 1976, 1979, 1984, 1991; Doll, 1987). Evolutionary changes in the economic structure are often accompanied by greater productivity and national wealth. In the short to medium-term, however, they involve large-scale migration and abandonment of earlier job skills and the destruction of work organizations, social networks and ways of life. Having developed our argument, we now seek to identify the mechanisms whereby economic growth and development are thought to lead to improved health and longevity.

III. LINKING ECONOMIC DEVELOPMENT AND HEALTH OUTCOMES

Identifying Mechanisms

What are the mechanisms whereby economic growth and development improve health and longevity in industrialized societies of the 20th century? The first, and perhaps simplest, mechanism is through the avoidance or amelioration of catastrophic, or major irretrievable losses. Such losses may involve death of family members or close associates resulting from endemic or epidemic diseases or industrial accidents. Further, the diseases would not only cause death but significant disability, which has historically been a major source of catastrophic income loss (Brenner, 1991; Cooper & Rice, 1976; Rice, 1966; Levine & Wilner, 1976).

The second mechanism has involved the avoidance of economic depressions and recessions and amelioration of their financial effects through social insurance and income support policies (Danziger & Weinberg, 1986; Palmer, Smeeding, & Torrey, 1988). The minimization of recession through long-term economic growth means that society has avoided increased mortality in virtually all chronic disease categories, as well as psychological disturbances resulting in suicide, psychiatric hospitalization, homicide and other criminal aggression.

Recession, moreover, not only affects the unemployed, and small business people and their families (Flaim & Sehgad, 1985; Horvath, 1987). It affects a far larger number of people who continue to work in firms that are financially damaged. These individuals are subject to the *fear* of loss of job, position, financial viability and career over periods of long as 10-15 years in firms that do not recover from recession. Work stress in the financially damaged firm is also at a considerably elevated level as a result of chronic instability and uncertainty, shifting employment patterns, alternating work overload and underload, and low margins for employee error resulting in strenuous efforts by management to control efficiency of production (Karasek & Theorell, 1990).

The third mechanism, avoidance and amelioration of *chronic* psychophysiologic stress, is also a byproduct of economic development (Danziger & Weinberg, 1986; Palmer, Sneeding, & Torrey, 1988). Foremost is the decline in poverty, and its consequences for damaged self-esteem and indignity that accompanies long-term growth and social policies that are focused on equity. In addition, the increase in productivity, essential to the concept of economic growth, has involved a shift from human to non-human sources of energy expenditure. This shift, in turn, has permitted children, the elderly and women to be largely exempt from demanding physical labor, and has obviously radically reduced the requirement for physically exhausting work. The advent of "human factors" engineering, in almost all aspects of production, and increasingly in services, has not only been fundamental to injury prevention but to heightened efficiency—that is, "smoothness" of man-machine interaction.

There continues to be debate about the extent to which work is overly "controlled" by management especially in a somewhat regimented, manufacturing setting. At the same time, manufacturing no longer dominates employment, and the service industries by their nature involve far less standardized activity. Considering the long-term work patterns of industrial and post-industrial society, the enormous increase in the number and types of occupations—and related ways of life—at the very least, regimentation is increasingly less of a necessity of working life. This is the fruit of continuous innovation and work opportunity that accompany economic growth. Taking this point a step further, it is escape from the slavery of dominance by human institutions (especially social class rigidities) and financial necessity that has characterized a good portion of the increased sense of human freedom of action.

In an even more general sense, however, increased control over the human and non-human environments is perhaps the fundamental factor of economic growth. These forms of control are related to increased predictability and stability that accompanies economic development. They are as much a product of knowledge development—based on investments in science and education—as they are on wealth accumulation and social policies emphasizing equity. At the individual level, the sense of increased "control" is manifested in achievement (via social mobility), mastery of work and financial processes and, finally, *creativity*—the basis of innovation that underlies growth and development. Creativity, in this sense, is related to Erikson's "generativity" (a basic requirement of human adulthood as a stage of life) and Maslow's "self-actualization" (i.e., a human need involving self-expression that comes into play after the physical, esteem and belongingness requirements are secured).

The fourth mechanism whereby economic growth increases health and longevity is through investment in health, biological and engineering sciences which result in illness prevention and amelioration (Blackburn, 1989; Monk, 1987; Moolgavkar, 1986; Nerseian, 1988; Schottenfeld, 1982; Waller, 1986). Some of the most important contributions to our understanding of disease causation and prevention in the past thirty years has come from epidemiology. Specifically, epidemiological studies have identified several of the high risk factors of chronic diseases that are prevalent in the ubiquitous human environment: consumption of tobacco, alcohol and fats; sedentarism; and toxic chemical contamination. Investments in epidemiological research have had extraordinarily high yield in actually altering the trends of mortality through stimulation of change in patterns of consumption and production. Additionally, myriad increases in technological sophistication of surgery, medicine, and clinical management have probably contributed to reductions of illness severity. We have identified the possible mechanisms whereby economic growth and development lead to improved health and longevity. We now seek systematic empirical evidence that in fact, growth and development lead to these two outcomes.

Evidence in Support of the Mechanisms

Over the past 15-20 years, research at the national level, over time, has shown that business cycle recessions and economic decline are related to increased morbidity and mortality, while economic growth has been associated with increased health and longevity (Brenner, 1980, 1984, 1987, 1991). Mental health indices, such as psychiatric hospitalization, suicide, homicide and related violence, and alcohol-related injuries, tend to increase *during* and immediately after recessions (Brenner, 1973, 1975, 1980; Catalanb & Dooley, 1982). This is also true of acute illnesses and infant mortality. (Brenner, 1973b; Frederikson & Harold, 1969). Chronic disease mortality, especially due to cardiovascular illnesses, shows a medium to long term relation to recessions that is both lagged, over at least a decade, and cumulative (Brenner, 1980, 1984, 1987, 1991; Brenner & Mooney, 1982).

The strong and consistent relations between recession and impaired population health status involve several components. Short to medium term stresses are felt by two populations: those that lose employment and/or financial standing, and those that remain employed in *firms* experiencing major financial losses, which in turn engender substantial increases in work stress. However, the most powerful recessional relations to mortality are found over the longer term. These concern, first of all, adjustment to a lower living standard (i.e., downward mobility and status inconsistency) and involve migration and the need to acquire new occupational skills and social networks. The second form of long-term recessional relations is cumulative, involving chronic stresses of intermittent economic instability in vulnerable industries, occupations and firms.

Much of the entire relation between economic change and health thus involves mental stresses. These stresses are partly direct through loss, fear, and alienation, and partly indirect through social class-related lifestyles (e.g., the consumption of alcohol, tobacco, or excess calories and sedentariness) and patterns of social support (Magnusson, 1982; Pearlin, 1989; Pearlin & Schooler, 1978).

A dynamic, quantitative model of the impact of economic change on mortality has recently been developed. In its current form this model includes:

1. long-term economic growth,
2. economic instability,
3. economic inequality,
4. adaptational error related to economic growth,
5. government sources of income stabilization and health care access, and
6. random shocks.

This model can be used to estimate the strength of each of several sources of economic change, holding constant other major sources of epidemiologic risk as well as health services and government efforts at income maintenance. The model is used in this paper to show an example of basic statistical relations for the United States during 1950-1988.

The macro, national-level evidence is largely built upon, and interpreted by, large literatures which deal with health risks to individuals. These literatures focus on low socioeconomic status, stresses of work, unemployment and social change, and biochemical risks of alcohol, tobacco, fats, and toxic chemicals (Holland et al., 1985). The existence of both individual- and national-level literatures that are consistent in their findings greatly strengthens the case for clear policy inferences and a coherent interpretation of demographic history (Kass, 1971; McKeown, 1971; McKinley, 1989).

Quantitative Historical Analysis

The research primarily discussed in this work uses quantitative historical methods. The historical perspective allows us to take account of the ecology, or environmental context, of a changing national culture, economic system, economic policies and political ideology. This contextual approach is necessary because the impact of economic events on institutions and individuals depends on changing objective political realities and culturally subjective interpretations.

This historical approach also permits us to evaluate the significance of *past* economic and social developments—especially cumulative benefits and stresses—and national investments.

In taking a developmental and dynamic perspective, this historical view also avoids the classical problem of functionalism, namely that cross- sectional or era-specific analyses describe what "is" at a moment in time rather than what is possible in the light of historical change.

At the same time, the quantitative element, with its emphasis on tests of statistical significance, allows us to assess the importance of *repeated* changes in the economy and cultural trends rather than singular events, such as a particular recession or historically specific increase in alcohol, cigarette, or fat consumption, or health expenditure.

Finally, these macro-historical approaches also help us to unravel problems that are particularly troublesome at the individual level of analysis. The classic positive relation between socioeconomic status, health and longevity has been interpreted in two opposite ways, with either socioeconomic status or health as the causal (or independent) variable. This assumes that socioeconomic status is primarily an individually generated set of attributes that can also be influenced *by* health status. Once we recognize that much of the source of individual mobility depends on national economic changes, we can ask whether health status changes *follow* changes in the national economy with little concern that the health status of the individuals subsequently affected will influence the state of the economy.

In addition, recent research in estimation of effects of unemployment (for example) on health status requires controls for other *economic* phenomena that frequently occur during recessions—when unemployment also is typically high. Business failures, financial losses and increased work stress among the employed must be specifically controlled since they frequently are responsible for stress-related health problems equal to or greater than those of unemployment. Macro-historical approaches are particularly efficient means of accomplishing this.

To examine the impact of national economic changes and policies on health, we must perform statistical tests using national level data. We cannot, for example, simply extrapolate from samples based on individual level epidemiologic studies. Even though we can derive valuable hypotheses from such studies at the micro level, we cannot use these to explain national changes and trends. In attempting to do so, we are in danger of a potential "ecological fallacy," which points to the error of assuming that we can always make inferences not only from macro to micro, but from micro to macro as well.

In the present work, a link is established between national- and individual-level studies. This link then permits inferences to national policy as well as to events in the lives of individual persons and small groups. The link between national and individual, between macro and micro is accomplished by disaggregating the national predictors of mortality according to their distribution in specific subpopulations (i.e., sex, race, region and industry groups, and varying indices of economic performance [i.e., changes in income and employment status]). At the same time overall mortality is similarly disaggregated by subpopulation and meaningful diagnoses.

IV. AN EMPIRICAL ANALYSIS

An example of recent empirical analysis of the relation between economic change and mortality can be seen in time-series linear regression equations by which we can attempt to explain United States mortality rates over the period 1944-1988.

We begin with a relatively "simple" exploratory analysis of the impact of (1) real per capita disposable income, and (2) unemployment rates on the sex- and race-adjusted mortality rate of 55-64 year olds. This type of Box-Jenkins analysis (Box & Jenkins, 1982) is initiated by finding the best forecasting model for the first (or second) differences of the 55-64 mortality rate, based on auto-regression terms and moving averages (i.e., ARIMA).

Analysis of the autocorrelation function (Berndt, 1990; Fomby, Hill, & Johnson, 1984) of the mortality rates shows that the model could be analyzed in either first or second differences. However, since a trend can still be found in first differences of the mortality rate, second differences are an appropriate choice. Tables 1-3 show the comparative differences between 1st and 2nd difference analyses of the short-term impacts of economic changes on 55-64 year mortality rates.

Table 1 shows that real per capita disposable income with a two-year (peak) lag is a statistically significant predictor of mortality rates, in addition to what could be predicted by the most sophisticated mathematical (i.e., non-causal) model.

Table 2 shows that the unemployment rate, after a two-year lag, is also a significant predictor. Table 3 further demonstrates that both the income and unemployment factors significantly enhance predictability of the mortality rate.

We now turn to a more complex analysis involving estimates of the full lag structure of the impact of economic variables on mortality. The two-year lag identified in the simple analysis represents a peak in the relation of economic changes to mortality. In fact, we usually hypothesize that the impact of economic growth and recession extend over at least a decade. The same, in terms of lag length, can be said for other derivatives of economic change that are risk factors to health—that is, the rate of consumption of tobacco, fats, alcohol and chemical production. Frequently, however, it is observed that spirits consumption and energy (i.e., fuel) consumption rates (denoting

Table 1. Box-Jenkins Multiple Regression Equation of Factors Experiencing Changes in Total Mortality Rate, Ages 55-64 United States 1944-1988

	Lag	*Coefficient*	*Standard Error*	*t-Statistic*
	First Differences			
Constant		−.282	.679E-01	−4.147
Real Disposable Income per Capital	2	−.519E-03	.200E-03	−2.592
MA	1	−.982E-01	.157	−.626
MA	2	−.212	.159	−1.337
RBAR**2 = .143				
Q(18) = 21.98				
d.f. = 41				
	Second Differences			
Real Disposable Income per Capital	2	−.458E-03	.201E-03	−2.280
MA	1	−.821	.881E-01	−9.311
RBAR**2 = .490				
Q(18) = 25.43				
d.f. = 43				

Table 2. Box-Jenkins Multiple Regression Equation of Factors Experiencing Changes in Total Mortality Rate, Ages 55-64 United States 1944-1988

	Lag	*Coefficient*	*Standard Error*	*t-Statistic*
	First Differences			
Constant		−.348	.929E-01	−3.746
Unemployment Rate	2	.277	.763E-01	3.632
AR	1	.369	.206	1.790
AR	2	.754E-01	.137	.552
MA	1	−.485	.220	−2.203
RBAR**2 = .175				
Q(18) = 24.30				
d.f. = 40				
	Second Differences			
Unemployment Rate	2	.168	.837E-01	2.00
MA	1	−.694	.130	−5.349
RBAR**2 = .490				
Q(18) = 25.43				
d.f. = 43				

Table 3. Box-Jenkins Multiple Regression Equation of Factors Experiencing Changes in Total Mortality Rate, Ages 55-64 United States 1944-1988

	Lag	*Coefficient*	*Standard Error*	*t-Statistic*
		First Differences		
Constant		−.310	.790E-01	−3.918
Real Disposable Income Per Capita	2	−.399E-03	.790E-01	−2.207
Unemployment Rate	2	.237	.780E-01	3.031
AR	1	.383	.201	1.907
MA	1	−.485	.228	−2.123
RBAR**2 = .259				
Q(18) = 25.18				
d.f. = 40				
		Second Differences		
Real Disposable Income Per Capita	2	−.447E-03	.179E-03	−2.501
Unemployment Rate	2	.880E-01	.517E-01	1.702
AR	1	−.450	.162	−2.774
AR	2	−.458	.154	−2.984
MA	1	−.675	.148	−4.548
RBAR**2 = .624				
Q(18) = 19.68				
d.f. = 40				

sedentarism) have relatively short lags (under five years) to chronic disease mortality, as would occur in the 55-64 age group.

Table 4 shows a multiple regression time-series equation, again explaining 55-64 mortality rates, in second differences. This equation allows for lag relations over 0-15 years, since the main hypothesis argues for relations over at least a decade for the majority of variables. (The Shiller procedure is used to sum the lagged relations over several years so that only one degree of freedom is expended for a single variable estimated with its full lag structure) (Shiller, 1973). In fact, a significant relation is seen for all "economic" factors (real per capita income, annual change in the real wage rate, the unemployment rate and real social welfare expenditures per capita).

The behavioral risks of consumption (cigarettes, fat, beer) and chemical production per capita, also range within 0-15 years in their relations to the 55-64 mortality rate. Spirits and total energy consumption per capita show relations over 0-6 and 0-5 years respectively.

Table 5 shows the coefficients for each year of lag in all of the ten relationships. Table 6 shows the stepwise order in which the variables were

Table 4. Multiple Time Series Regression of Relations Between Socioeconomic Environmental Factors and Total Mortality Rate, Ages 55-64 United States, 1950-1988 (Second Differences)

Order		*Cumulative Lag (Years)*	*Coefficient*	*Standard Error*	*t-Statistic*
	Economic Factors				
10	Real Per Capita Income	0-13	−.474E-02	.661E-03	−7.164
12	Real Wage Rate Annual Change	0-13	−.430E-01	.250E-01	−1.717
6	Unemployment Rate	1-14	1.492	.954E-01	15.634
2	Business Failure Rate	2-10	.186	.108E-01	17.148
8	Real Social Welfare Exp. Per Capita	0-14	−.285	.530E-01	−5.379
	Behavioral Risks				
3	Cigarette Consumption Per Capita	0-14	.423	.144E-02	29.313
7	Fat Consumption Per Capita	0-13	.752	.588E-03	12.785
5	Spirits Consumption Per Capita	0-6	9.449	.634	14.894
11	Beer Consumption Per Ckapita	4-14	.595	.161	3.691
	Production Risks				
9	Total Energy Cons. Per Capita	0-5	.382	.591E-02	6.464
4	Chemical Production Per Capita	0-12	.654	.365E-01	17.928
	Constant		.596E-01	.188E-01	3.165
	Adj. R Squared. 995				
	Durbin-Watson 1.935				
	F(12,26) = 365.342	CHOW Test: F (12,15) = .440			

entered into the model and the relative impact of each variable. Clearly, the order of entry has very minimal influence on the estimates of impact.

Table 7 presents a comparison of the coefficients indicating the impact of the predictive variables on mortality over 1950-1968 and 1969-1988. Evidently, there has been little change in those coefficients over the two periods. This lack of change is also reflected in the Chow statistical test of potential differences (Table 4).

V. POLICY IMPLICATIONS

The economy does not act on its own. It is not a given in human affairs, simply behaving as an exogenous factor that cannot be influenced. Rather, especially since the 1930s, it is the continuous product of economic policies, which represent the outcome of political struggle and changing ideologies. These

Table 5. Coefficients of Lag Structures for Relations between Economic and Social Environmental Factors and Total Mortality Rate 55-64, United States, 1950-1988

Individual Year of Lag	*Business Failure Rate*	*Cigarette Cons.*	*Chemical Production P.C.*	*Spirits Cons. P.C.*	*Unemploy-ment*	*Fat Cons. P.C.*	*Social Welfare Expend. P.C.*	*Energy Cons. P.C.*	*Real Disposal Income P.C.*	*Beer Cons. P.C.*	*Real Wages P.C.*
0		.002	.041	1.348		.411	−.026	.002	−.269E-3		−.001
1		.003	.047	1.145	.053	.461E-3	−.018	.002	−.286E-3		−.002
2	.060	.004	.085	.960	.132	.622E-3	−.009	.003	−.040E-3		−.003
3	.030	.003	.099	.766	.065	.425E-3	−.006	.010	−.367E-3		−.003
4	.014	.001	.105	.527	051	.234E-3	−.008	.006	−.439E-3	.049	−.004
5	.011	.004	.075	.314	.036	.216E-3	−.018		−.473E-3	.044	−.004
6	.015	.004	.106	.100	.028	.535E-3	−.018		−.473E-3	.044	−.004
7	.019	.003	.056		.038	.667E-3	−.021		−.311E-3	.032	−.004
8	.019	.003	.047		.092	.796E-3	−.020		−.342E-3	.045	−.002
9	.020	.003	.057		.034	.623E-3	−.018		−.405E-3	.052	−.004
10	.025	.004	.035		.141	.585E-3	−.018		−.405E-3	.052	−.004
11		.001	.048		.038	.723E-3	−.020		−.428E-3	.045	−.004
12		.000	.036		.010	.475E-3	−.021		−.081E-3	.021	−.004
13		.000			.033		−.022		−.227E-3	.022	−.002
14		.002			.069		−.018			.020	
SUM.	.213	.038	.836	5.160	.820	7.065E-3	−.253	.025	−4.209E-3	.437	−.046

Table 6. Multiple Time Series Regression of Relations Between Socioeconomic Environmental Factors and Total Mortality Rate, Ages 55-64 United States, 1950-1988 (Second Differences)

			Coefficients for Each Stage of Stepwise Model Development (T-Statistics in Parentheses)										
Order	*Name*	*Cumulative Lag (Years)*	*Stage 1*	*Stage 2*	*Stage 3*	*Stage 4*	*Stage 5*	*Stage 6*	*Stage 7*	*Stage 8*	*Stage 9*	*Stage 10*	*Stage 11*
1	Constant	0	−.563E-01	.110	−.538E-01	−.424E-01	−.442E-01	.147E-01	.216E-01	.297E-01	.511E-01	.586E-01	.596E-01
			(−.390)	(−.887)	(−.765)	(−.659)	(−.838)	(.380)	(.647)	(.957)	(2.283)	(3.013)	(3.165)
2	Business Failure Rate	2-10	.275	.282	.297	.314	.228	.220	.209	.208	.195	.189	.186
			(4.206)	(5.297)	(10.104)	(11.458)	(7.469)	(10.181)	(11.017)	(11.871)	(15.402)	(17.044)	(17.148)
3	Cigarette Consumption Per Capita	0-14		.376E-01	.412E-01	.424E-01	.406E-01	.452E-01	.440E-01	.438E-01	.441E-01	.419E-01	.423E-01
				(4.438)	(8.791)	(9.868)	(11.458)	(17.237)	(19.145)	(20.581)	(29.169)	(28.482)	(29.313)
4	Chemical Production Per Capita	0-12			.867	.855	.811	.741	.716	.685	.655	.616	.654
					(9.142)	(9.868)	(11.2930	(14.249)	(15.725)	(15.548)	(20.638)	(20.659)	(17.928)
5	Spirits Consumption Per Capita	0-6				5.317	5.733	7.427	7.784	8.043	8.279	9.018	9.449
						(2.835)	(3.722)	(6.600)	(7.960)	(8.829)	(12.768)	(14.970)	(14.894)
6	Unemployment Rate	1-14					.824	1.032	1.184	1.203	1.302	1.400	1.492
							(4.197)	(7.210)	(9.875)	(14.738)	(17.111)	(15.634)	
7	Fat Consumption Per Capita	0-13						.706E-02	.685E-02	.704E-02	.747E-02	.766E-02	.752E-02
								(5.848)	(6.548)	(7.251)	(10.762)	(12.736)	(12.785)
8	Real Social Welfare Exp. Per Capita	0-14							−.310	−.237	−.261	−.288	−.285
									(−.444)	(−2.683)	(−4.150)	(−5.255)	(−5.379)
9	Total Energy Cons. Per Capita	0-5								.194E-01	.332E-01	.414E-01	.382E-01
										(2.488)	(5.464)	(7.138)	(6.464)
10	Real Per Capita Income	0-13									−.421E-02	−.481E-02	−.474E-02
											(−5.521)	(−7.050)	(−7.164)
11	Beer Consumption Per Capita	4-14										.541	.595
												(3.309)	(3.691)
12	Real Wage Rate Annual Change	0-13											−.430E-01
													(−1.717)
	Adjusted R Square		.305	.538	.860	.883	.922	.961	.971	.975	.987	.991	.991
	Durbin-Watson		2.699	2.746	.2984	2.677	2.239	1.780	2.051	2.202	1.763	1.924	1.935

Table 7. Multiple Time Series Regression of Relations Between Socioeconomic Environmental Factors and Total Mortality Rate, Ages 55-64, United States (Second Differences) Comparison of 1950-1988, 1950-1968, and 1969-1988

Order		*Cumulative Lag (Years)*	*Coefficient 1950-1988*	*Coefficient 1950-1968*	*Coefficient 1969-1988*
	Economic Factors				
10	Real Per Capita Income	0-13	−.474E-02	−.378E-02	−.468E-02
12	Real Wage Rate Annual Change	0-13	−.430E-01	−.840E-01	−.612E-01
6	Unemployment Rate	1-14	1.492	1.622	1.458
2	Business Failure Rate	2-10	.186	.198	.180
8	Real Social Welfare Exp. Per Capita	0-14	−.285	−.215	−.236
	Behavioral Risks				
3	Cigarette Consumption Per Capita	0-14	.423	.439	402
7	Fat Consumption Per Capita	0-13	.752E-02	.796E-02	.657E-02
5	Spirits Consumption Per Capita	0-6	9.449	10.476	10.244
11	Beer Consumption Per Capita	4-14	.595	.787	.445
	Production Risks				
9	Total Energy Cons. Per Capita	0-5	.382E-01	.461E-01	.355E-01
4	Chemical Production Per Capita	0-12	.654	.655	.681
	Constant		.596E-01	.631E-01	.636E-01
	Adj. R Squared .994				
	Durbin-Watson 1.935				
	F(23,26) = 365.342	CHOW Test: F (12,15) = .440			

policies include the macroeconomic (fiscal and monetary industrial), income distribution (taxation, welfare, social security, unemployment insurance), international trade, and investment in overall scientific development.

Policies that directly counteract the adaptational error arising from the economic growth process include industrial regulation (especially of chemical production) and occupational safety and health. National investments in general education and in the health sciences and their application (particularly through mass communication) are among the most powerful indirect policies that offset adaptational error.

Health care *delivery* policy is another important area of overall health policy. It may, however, act more through income redistribution than through direct improvement of health by medicine or surgery. In the major diseases of the western industrialized world—chronic physical disorders and mental health problems—health care plays a significant but not major role in comparison with the principal groups of risk factors associated with the economy: income, employment, education, consumption, and production.

Nevertheless, in the United States among many other countries, health care delivery policy has come to be regarded as the only health policy. The political arrangement that ties health policy entirely to delivery and financing of health care is tragically flawed. It deflects the public's attention away from the causes of illness and from the primary policies which normally affect health and longevity.

Reasons for the absence of an overall health policy coordinated with economic policies are several: the extensive specialization of government functions, which also parallels academic diversification; an ideological frame of reference that emphasizes individualism and "freedom of will" for citizens in their economic and social affairs; the absence of social responsibility for policies affecting large proportions of the population, the legitimacy of profound economic inequalities; and a basic mistrust of government as antilibertarian.

The intensely individualistic ideology in the United States makes it all but impossible for policy makers or citizens—and often specialists—to understand the sources of the society's health at the national level. It prohibits the development of integrated societal policies to deal directly with these issues, and serves to make physicians and laypersons alike feel that health risks are either uncontrollable or dependent on individual behavioral proclivities.

Reasonable well-being for the population can be obtained with (for example) relatively conservative macroeconomic policy and liberal social (especially "welfare" and social security) policies. There is a danger, however, that the welfare statist approach may, if the government sector becomes too large, serve to reduce national investments required for industrial development. A plausible middle ground can be reached in both types of policies where measures of social well-being are explicitly taken as criteria.

Along the same lines, it is possible to so over-regulate or over-tax industry that the resulting economic (including employment) losses inflict greater harm on the population's health. Here again, one must confront ideological perspectives with empirical data on probable health implications.

VI. CONCLUSIONS: HEALTH AND ECONOMIC CHANGE

Longevity Patterns and Their Interpretation

In Western societies—especially the United States—age-specific trends in mortality have been falling for well over a century. And they continue to fall.

In addition, in virtually all countries, socioeconomic status is the central factor which determines differentials in mortality and morbidity—historically and contemporaneously. Moreover, research over the past two decades has shown that, within countries over time, mortality tends to decline in relation to long-term economic growth and it tends to increase following business cycle downturns.

These facts would seem to indicate that sustained economic growth is, and has been, the backbone of increase in health and longevity in modern industrialized societies. Similarly, the occurrence of economic decline, and enlargement of socioeconomic differentials, are a major source of harm to the health of national populations.

This description of trends and population distribution of health and longevity is consistent with the classical formulations of social development and modernization theory that have been basic to the social sciences since the mid-eighteenth century. This perspective includes the writings of many of the major economic, political and sociological thinkers of the last two centuries. They express the view that there are basic interrelations among developments in the economy, science and political equality and that these are the bedrocks of societal progress. Our further addition would be that these bases of progress are also the foundation of human biological adaptation, and thus the long-run increase in health and longevity.

Tradeoffs Between Economic Growth and Health

Despite evidence both over time and among populations of the central importance of economic position to health, two views have developed among scientists since the 1950s which assume health progress to be in basic conflict with the output of continued economic growth.

The first of these views arises out of the findings of modern epidemiology. Epidemiological research has shown that in industrialized societies where chronic disease is the principal source of ill health and mortality, consumption of fats, alcohol and tobacco, chemical production, sedentariness, and social isolation are among the most important risks. And these health risks are historically associated with economic growth and prosperity. Indeed, the most *optimistic* scenario in this view is that the major epidemiologic risks move through time like long-term epidemics, derived from economic growth, which subside for a time only to be reignited by a newly created risk factor.

The second view assumes that investments in health care technology, stemming from economic growth, have significant short-term effects on survival but almost no important impact on chronic disease processes and the level of morbidity (i.e., illness). In this perspective the slight gain in life expectancy is offset by more than concomitant gains in degenerative illness rates which increase with the aging process. The net perverse effect is that health care investments increase morbidity rates and thus the cost of health care as well as the dependency of the older population on the finances and emotional sustenance of the young.

An Integrated Approach

Which of these views is closest to the truth: increased health and life span based on social development consequent upon economic growth; unlimited epidemic illnesses stimulated by economic growth, or the increased degeneracy of aging fostered by economic development?

It is apparent that because there are some important factual data to support each view, there must be some truth to each. And the question of whether we envision economic growth as the source or enemy of health and longevity must take into account the data which appear to support those opposing views. We therefore require an integrated perspective which must finally indicate that economic growth has both profoundly beneficial and damaging effects on health and life. The key problem is to specify the conditions under which economic growth is the central benefactor or villain.

However, in order to fully describe the integrated, multifactor perspective through which we can observe the mixed effects of economic growth, additional elements of the story must be identified. First of all, it will be necessary to understand how it is that economic growth benefits health in an era in which chronic disease and psychic disorders are preeminent. In order to do so we shall have to introduce literatures which involve psychophysiology and social functioning, and which bear on the question of quality of life. Second, it will be important to consider in depth the issue of "epidemic" eruptions and decline in health risk factors and their connections to the process of economic growth.

The principal elements of the integrated view can be identified at this point. Fundamentally, economic growth is the basis of improved population health and longevity. Economic growth is the source of enhanced nutrition, sanitation, climate control, fertility control and reduced physical requirements of work. It also provides the material grounding for political developments which maximize equality in the distribution of the national wealth. It is the basis of investment in the creation of knowledge which is, in turn, a prime source of human adaptation, predictability, and person-environment fit. Economic growth also provides the resource base for satisfaction of variable human wants through the increased ability to demand goods and services, taking into account the shifting values of society and individuals. It is the basis of achievement, stability, and mastery of the environment. It therefore lays the foundation for human freedom and dignity and confidence in the future.

Related critical benefits of sustained economic growth involve the prevention of economic recession—perhaps the major source of stress in Western societies. In the short-term, recession involves economic failure and in the longer term for those populations which undergo late recovery, or do not recover, it signifies permanent downward social mobility and relative deprivation (i.e., economic inequality).

Economic growth, however, is achieved at considerable human cost. Six main costs of economic growth can be identified: necessary and irretrievable loss stemming from obsolescence and a changed social structure, family dynamics and culture; the threat of such losses, resulting from processes of innovation—and the societal conflict that results from such threats; loss of control in the workplace, where machines schedule, monitor or otherwise heavily influence human activity; "adaptative error," which stems from increased consumption and production, based on greater availability of disposable income and investment capital without concomitant increases in human knowledge of health risks, and resulting in large-scale damage to population health (e.g., alcohol, tobacco, fats, chemicals); accidents arising out of the need to adjust to new innovations, to increased demand for higher production or to the design of complex industrial systems with minimal slack for human error; and long-term damage to the natural environment.

These health risks associated with economic growth can come dangerously close to offsetting many of its benefits. In fact, if unchecked, some of the costs of economic growth can be so high as to threaten, or even override, the entire trend of biological advantage inherent in economic development.

Reversing the damage caused by some of the outcomes of growth requires important shifts in societal policy which, interestingly, are usually financed or facilitated by *further* economic growth. Thus, wealth production can be instrumental in correcting the problems of growth, but only if major changes in social policy are pursued. These policies depend on long-term investments, short-term expenditures, or a psychological environment of economic prosperity that influences the political process.

Amelioration of the damaging effects of both recession and worker obsolescence is accomplished through the financing of direct income supports (unemployment, poverty, disability) and retraining and migration to new worksites. Considerable and continuous financing is also required in order to ease industrial innovations into the workplace via lengthier and slower training, extra personnel, and redesign of machine-worker interactive equipment as well as the design of industrial systems with greater slack for error. Similarly, the degree of regimentation in work systems, and intolerance for error, can be greatly mitigated through the use of greater industrial democracy—but this also depends on the existence of well-financed industries—that is, that are not desperately fighting recession, or structural change for their survival.

These secondary benefits of economic growth extend not only to prevention and amelioration of economic loss and work stress. They relate, as well, to the prevention and moderation of epidemic patterns of adaptational error. Adaptational errors depend for their severity (i.e., health damage) on the lack of scientific knowledge and on the absence of substitute products and alternative behavioral patterns which are not health risks. Minimization of such health damage depends on the financing of science and regulatory policy and on the economic feasibility of product adjustments and substitutions. Finally, environmental destruction and contamination are, in the long-term, correctable by alternative technologies which require considerable societal investments for both research and development and the replacement of older technologies.

A final word should be said about the economic growth-related ability to finance the health care industry, even though there is little evidence as yet that it contributes in a major way to the health and longevity of national populations. Suppose, in fact, that policymakers only minimally utilize additional capital made available by economic growth to finance the research and new technological developments that reduce the health risks arising out of that growth. In that case, we shall find that growth itself may produce more harm than benefit. If so, mortality trends may well cease to decline and morbidity rates may increase over the longer term. In this way, the radically pessimistic scenario of health care technology investment might well come to fruition. Namely, heroic medicine increasingly saves the lives of this morbid population, only to leave them in a state of continued, or even elevated, illness and a financial and emotional drain on society.

Recapitulation

To recapitulate, evidence from data across countries shows economic position to be the most powerful discriminator of health and longevity among individuals. This finding is supported at national levels with data showing that, other factors controlled, economic development is the prime factor in mortality decline. And these data are in turn supported by analyses which indicate that departures from economic growth through recession or alteration in the economic structure that increase inequality, involve considerable risks to illness and mortality.

While these findings conform to theories of modernization and human progress in adaptation, important modifications in this theme are needed. There is evidence that economic growth itself poses major health risks involving losses due to obsolescence of skills and traditions, damage to community structure, social conflicts over threats of such losses, loss of control due to mechanization, errors of adaptation involving risk-laden consumption and production (especially chemical), accidents related to adaption to innovation and overly complex systems, and environmental degradation.

At the same time, under specific policy conditions, benefits of economic growth act to minimize recession, ameliorate the harshest effects of economic loss and obsolescence, and machine dominance of work and regimentation. Investments stemming from economic growth involving science, education, and new products provide the capacity for either preventing or greatly curtailing the severity and duration of epidemic movements of chronic or infectious disease or violence. Investments in health care technology have shown significant yet relatively small health/longevity impact, but health care research and development also depend on financing which results from the production of national wealth.

It is therefore clear that given continued economic growth, that is reasonably equitable in its distribution, and a major commitment to investment in science and the political diminution of the costs of economic growth—especially errors of adaptation—it becomes possible to envision the continuance of the biological adaptation process. This requires that national *health* policy focus primarily on the aggressive pursuit of factors which promote economic growth and social equity. And it requires major national investments in epidemiological science and the technologies and products that minimize health risks. Such aggressive pursuit has not been characteristic of policy history in the United States.

The general public, much of the medical profession, and a great many economists assume that it is fundamentally health *care* that historically and contemporaneously benefits health, although this assumption pays no attention to the predominant relation of economic position to health and barely acknowledges the importance of consumption and production factors. The health care industry in the United States absorbs more than a tenth of national wealth, while the overwhelming economic policy, consumption and production issues receive minimal attention from the standpoint of the nation's health.

Indeed, to the extent that health care expenditures remain the principal vehicle of health policy, and illness prevention receives minimal resources, the peculiar scenario of demographic pessimism is realized. In that situation, medical technologies enable the diseased and disabled—especially elderly—population to survive a bit longer. This further increases the level of population morbidity and dependency as well as health care and general welfare costs to society.

REFERENCES

Antonovsky, A. (1967). "Social class, life expectancy, and overall mortality." *Milbank Memorial Fund Quarterly*, 45, 31 73.

Berndt, E. (1990). *The practice of econometrics*. Reading MA: Addison-Wesley.

Blackburn, H. (1989). Trends and determinants of CHD mortality: Changes in risk factors and their effects. *International Journal of Epidemiology*, 18, (supplement 1), S210-S215.

Box, G., & Jenkins, G. (1982). *Time series analysis: Forecasting and control*. San Francisco: Holden Day.

Brenner, M.H. (1973a). *MentaliIllness and the economy*. Cambridge: Harvard University Press.

Brenner, M.H. (1973b). Fetal, infant, and maternal Mortality during periods of economic instability. *International Journal of Health Services* 3:145-159.

Brenner, M.H. (1975). Trends in alcohol consumption and associated illnesses: Some effects of economic changes. *American Journal of Public Health*, 65, 12, 1279-1292.

Brenner, M.H. (1976). Estimating the social costs of national economic policy: Implications for mental and physical health and criminal aggression. U.S. Congress, Joint Economic Committee. Washington DC: Government Printing Office.

Brenner, M.H. (1979). Mortality and the national economy: A review and the experience of England and Wales, 1936-1976. *The Lancet* (September 15): 568-573.

Brenner MH. (1980). Impact of social and industrial changes on psychopathology: A view of stress from the standpoint of macro societal trends. In L. Levi (ed.). *Society, stress and disease: Working life* (Volume 4, pp. 249-260). Oxford University Press.

Brenner, M.H. (1984). Estimating the effects of economic change on national health and social well-being. U.S. Congress, Joint Economic Committee. Washington DC: Government Printing Office.

Brenner, M.H. (1987). Economic change, alcohol consumption, and heart disease mortality in nine industrialized countries. *Social Science and Medicine* 25:119-13.

Brenner, M.H. (1990). Recession and mortality: The experience of major industrialized countries. In R. Veenhoven (ed.), *International economic crisis*. Netherlands: Reidel.

Brenner, M.H. (1991). Health, productivity, and the economic environment: Dynamic role of socioeconomic status. In G. Green & F. Baker (eds), *Work, Health, and Productivity*. Oxford University Press, New York.

Brenner, M.H. & Mooney, A. (1982). Economic change and sex-specific cardiovascular mortality in Britain 1955-1976. *Social Science and Medicine* 16:431-442.

Bunker, J., Gomby, D., & Kehrer, B. (1989). Pathways to health: The role of social factors. Menlo Park CA: Kaiser Family Foundation.

Catalano, R. & Dooley, C. (1982). Economic predictors of depressed mood and stressful life events. *Journal of Health and Social Behavior* 18:292-307.

Collins, R. (1985). *Three sociological traditions*. New York: Oxford University Press.

Cooper, B.S. & Rice, D.P. (1976). The economic cost of illness revisited. *Social Security Bulletin* 39:21-36.

Dahrendorf, R. (1979). *Life chances*. Chicago: University of Chicago Press.

Dahrendorf, R. (1959). *Class and class conflict in industrial society*. Stanford University Press.

Danziger, S.H. & Weinberg, D.H. (eds.). (1986). *Fighting poverty: What works and what doesn't*. Cambridge: Harvard University Press.

Doll, R. (1987). Major epidemics of the 20th century: From coronary thrombosis to AIDS. *Journal of the Royal Statistical Society* 150:4:373-395.

Durkheim, E. (1951). *Suicide*. Glencoe, IL: Fress Press.

Engel, G. (1977). The need for a new medical model: A challenge for biomedicine. *Science* 196, 129-136.

Epstein, S. (1990). Losing the war against cancer: Who's to blame and what to do about it. *International Journal of Health Services* 20:1:53-71.

Fomby, T., Hill, R., & Johnson, N. (1984). *Advanced econometrics*. New York: Springer-Verlag.

Frederikson, H. (1969). Feedback in economic and demographic transition. *Science*, 837-847.

Fries, J. et al. (1989). Health promotion and the compression of morbidity. *Lancet*, (March 4):481-483.

Henry, J. (1982). The relation of social to biological processes in disease. *Social Science and Medicine* 16:369-380.

House, J. et al. (1988). Social relationships and health. *Science*, 241, 540-545.

Karasek, R., & Theorell, T. (1990). Health work: Stress, productivity, and the reconstruction of working life. New York: Basic Books.

Karasek, R., & Theorell, T. (1990). The environment, the worker, and illness: Psychological and physiological linkages. Pages 83-116 in *Health Work*. New York: Basic Books.

Kass, E. (1971). Infectious diseases and social change. *Journal of Infectious Diseases* 123:110-114.

Kitagawa, E., & Hauser, P. (1973). Differential mortality in the United States: A study in socioeconomic epidemiology. Cambridge: Harvard University Press.

Levine, D.S., & Wilner, S.C. (1976). The cost of mental illness-1974. *Statistical Note 125*. Washington DC: U.S. National Institute of Mental Health.

Litwak, M. et al. (1989). Organizational theory, social supports, and mortality rates: A theoretical convergence. *American Sociological Review*, Volume 54 (February):49-66.

Magnusson, D. (1982). Situational determinants of stress: An interactionist perspective. In L. Goldberger & S. Breznitz (eds), pp. 36-48 in *Handbook of Stress: Theoretical and Clinical Aspects*. New York: Free Press.

McKeown, T. (1971). A sociological approach to the history of medicine. In G. McLachain & T. McKeown (eds). *Medical History and Medical Care*. New York: Oxford University Press.

McKinlay, J. et al. (1989). A review of the evidence concerning the impact of medical measures on recent mortality and morbidity in the United States. *International Journal of Health Services* 19(2):181-208.

Monk, M. (1987). The epidemiology of suicide. *Epidemiologic Review*, 51-69.

Moolgavkar, S.H. (1986). Carcinogenesis modeling: From molecular biology to epidemiology. *Annual Review of Public Health*, 151-170

Nerseian, W.S. (1988). Infant mortality in socially vulnerable populations. *Annual Review of Public Health*, 361-378.

Palmer, J., Smeedling, T., & Torrey, B.B. (eds). (1988). *The vulnerable*. Washington DC: The Urban Institute Press.

Pearlin, L. (1989). The sociological study of stress. *Journal of Health and Social Behavior*, 30 (September):241-256.

Pearlin, L., & Schooler, C. (1978). The structure of coping. *Journal of Health and Social Behavior*, 19 (March):2-21.

Report of the Research Working Group. (1980). *Inequalities in health: The Black report*. London: Department of Health and Human Services.

Rice, D.P. (1966). *Estimating the cost of illness*. Washington, DC: Government Printing.

Schiller, R.J. (1973). A distributed lag estimator derived from smoothness priors. *Econometrica* 41:775-788.

Shottenfeld, D., Fraumeni, J.F., Jr. (1982). Cancer epidemiology and prevention. WB Saunders, Philadelphia (The Bible).

Susser, M., Watson, W., & Hopper, K. (1985). *Sociology in medicine, third edition*. New York: Oxford University Press.

Syme, S.L. & Berkman, L.F. (1976). Social class, susceptibility, and sickness. *American Journal of Epidemiology* 104:1-8.

Waller, J.A. (1986). Prevention of premature death and disability due to injury. In Last, J.M. (Maxcy-Rosenau) (eds.), *Public Health and Prevention*. 12th Edition. Appleton Century Croft, Norwalk, CN. Pp. 1543-1576.

Wilkinson, R.G. (ed.). (1986). Class and health—Research and longitudinal data. London: Tavistock.

J A I P R E S S

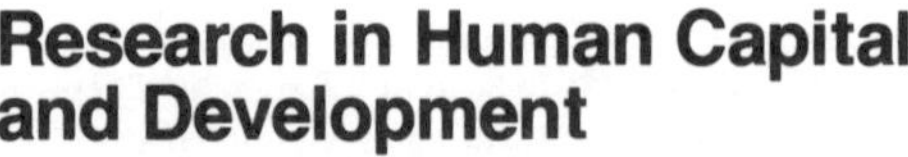

Research in Human Capital and Development

Edited by **Alan Sorkin,** *Department of Ecomonics, University of Maryland*

REVIEW: "The idea of developing RHCD into a forum for important empirical and theoretical research is a brillant one and will definitely be fruitful in the years to come... Without a doubt the book is an extremely valuable contribution to research on human capital theory."

— *The Paristan Development Review*

Volume 1, 1979, 258 pp. $73.25
ISBN 0-89232-019-2

CONTENTS: Introduction, *Ismail Sirageldin.* **PART I: HEALTH AND FERTILITY. Relevance of Human Capital Theory to Fertility Research: Comparative Findings for Bangladesh and Pakistan,** *Ali Khan.* **Health and Economic Development: A Theoretical and Empirical Review,** *Robin Barlow.* **Health, Nutrition, and Mortality in Bangladesh,** *W. Henry Mosley.* **Discussion,** *Ismail Sirageldin.* **PART II: EDUCATION AND MANPOWER. College Quality and Earnings,** *James N. Morgan and Greg J. Duncan.* **Some Theoretical Issues in Manpower and Educational Training,** *Mohiuddin Alamgir.* **Barriers to Educational Development in Underdeveloped Countries: With Special Relevance to Venezuela,** *Kristin Tornes.* **Manpower Planning and the Choice of Technology,** *S.C. Kelley.* **The Growth of Professional Occupations in U.S. Manufacturing: 1900-1973,** *Carmel Ullman Chiswick.* **Summary and Discussion,** *Alan Sorkin.* **PART III: DISTRIBUTION AND EQUITY. Equity Social Striving, and Rural Fertility,** *Ismail Sirageldin and John Kantner.* **Index.**

Volume 2, Equity, Human Capital and Development
1981, 224 pp. $73.25
ISBN 0-89232-098-2

Edited by **Ali Khan** and **Ismail Sirageldin,**
The Johns Hopkins University

CONTENTS: Introduction and Summary, *Ali Khan and Ismail Sirageldin.* **PART I: MEASURES AND PARADOXES. Measures of Poverty and their Policy Implications,** *Koichi Hamada and Noriyuki Takayama.* **Paradoxes of Work and Consumption in Late 20th Century America,** *Nathan Keyfitz.* **PART II: THEORETICAL ISSUES. A Model of Economic Growth with Investment in Human Capital,** *Ronald Findlay and Carlos A.*

Rodriguez. **The Influence of Nonhuman Wealth on the Accumulation of Human Capital,** *John Graham.* **The Changing Role of Breastfeeding in Economic Development: A Theoretical Exposition,** *William P. Butz.* **PART III: CASE STUDIES. The Effects of Income Maintenance on School Performance and Educational Attainment in the U.S.A.,** *Charles D. Mallar and Rebecca A. Maynard.* **An Analysis of Education, Employment and Income Distribution Using an Economic Demographic Model of the Philippines,** *G.B. Rodgers.* **The Welfare Implications of Relative Price Distortions and Inflation: An Analysis of the Recent Argentine Experience,** *Ke-Young Chu and Andrew Feltenstein.* **Index.**

Supplement 1, Manpower Planning in the Oil Countries
1981, 276 pp. $73.25
ISBN 0-89232-129-0

Edited by **Naiem A. Sherbiny,** *The World Bank*

CONTENTS: Series Editor's Introduction, *Ismail Sirageldin.* **Editors Introduction,** *Naiem A. Sherbiny.* **PART I: OVERVIEW AND METHODOLOGY. The Issues,** *Jan Tinbergen.* **Structural Changes in Output and Employment in the Arab Countries,** *Maurice Girgis.* **The Modeling and Methodology of Manpower Planning in the Arab Countries,** *M. Ismail Sirageldin.* **Vocational and Technical Education and Development Needs in the Arab World,** *Atif Kubursi.* **PART II: CASE STUDIES. An Econometric/Input-Output Approach for Projecting Sectoral Manpower Requirements: The Case of Kuwait,** *M. Shokri Marzouk.* **A Macroeconomic Simulation Model of High Level Manpower Requirements in Iraq,** *George T. Abed and Atif Kubursi.* **Sectoral Employment Projections with Minimum Data Base: The Case of Saudi Arabia,** *Naiem A. Sherbiny.* **PART III: POLICY ISSUES. Labor Adaption in the Oil Exporting Countries,** *M. Ismail Sirageldin.* **Labor and Capital Flows in the Arab World: A Policy Perspective,** *Naiem A. Sherbiny.* **Index.**

Volume 3, Health and Development
1983, 364 pp. $73.25
ISBN 0-89232-166-0

Edited by **David Salkever** and **Ismail Sirageldin,**
The Johns Hopkins University
and **Alan Sorkin,** *University of Maryland.*

CONTENTS: PART I: CONCEPTS AND MEASURES. A Conceptual Model of Health, *Hector Correa.* **A Conceptual Framework for the Planning of Medicine in Developing Countries,** *Peter Newman.* **Health and Development: A Discussion of Some Issues,** *Oscar Gish.* **PART II: HEALTH IN HUMAN CAPITAL FORMATION. Adolescent Health, Family Background, and Preventive Medical Care,** *Linda Edwards and Michael Grossman.* **An Economic Analysis of the Diet, Growth and Health of Young Children in the United States,** *Dov Chernichovsky and Douglas Coate.* **The Demand for Prenatal Care and the Production of Healthy Infants,** *Eugene M. Lewit.* **Life Environments and Adult Health: A Policy Perspective,** *Anthony E. Boardman and Robert Inman.* **Summary and Discussion, Part II,** *David Salkever.* **PART III: HEALTH IN DEVELOPMENT. Correlates of Life Expectancy in Less Developed Countries,** *Robert N. Grosse and Barbara H. Perry.* **The Power of Health,** *Wilfred Malenbaum.* **Health Planning in the Sudan,** *Ronald J. Vogel and Nancy T. Greenspan.* **Health Expenditure in a Racially Segregated Society—A Case Study in South Africa,** *M.D. McGrath.* **Analytical Review of the World Health Organization's Health Manpower Development Program 1948-1978,** *W.A. Reinke and T. Fulop.* **Summary and Discussion, Part III,** *Alan Sorkin.*

Volume 4, Migration, Human Capital and Development
1986, 285 pp. $73.25
ISBN 0-89232-416-3

Edited by **Oded Stark,** *Havard University and Bar-Ilan University*

CONTENTS: Introduction, *Oded Stark.* **Human Capital and the Labor Market Adjustment of Immigrants: Testing Alternative Hypotnheses,** *Barry R. Chiswick.* **International Trade Theory and International Migration,** *Wilfred J. Ethier.* **What's In a Name?. Country-of-Origin Influences on the Earnings of Immigrants in the United States,** *Guillermina Jaso and Mark R. Rosenzweig.* **Emigration, Employment and Accumulation: The Miners of Southern Africa,** *Robert E.B. Lucas.* **Urban External Economies and Optimal Migration,** *Vibhooti Shukla and Oded Stark.* **Differential Migration, Networks, Information and Risk,** *J. Edward Taylor.*

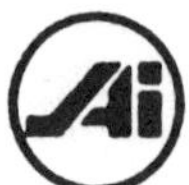

Volume 5, Public Health and Development
1988, 293 pp. $73.25
ISBN 0-89232-508-9

Edited by **Ismail Sirageldin,** *The Johns Hopkins University* and **Alan Sorkin,** *University of Maryland*